OTOLARYNGOLOGY RESEARCH ADVANCES

# DEAFNESS, HEARING LOSS AND THE AUDITORY SYSTEM

# OTOLARYNGOLOGY RESEARCH ADVANCES

**Handbook of Pulmonary Diseases: Etiology, Diagnosis and Treatment**
*Krisztián Fodor and Antal Tóth (Editors)*
2009. ISBN: 978-1-60741-898-6

**Snoring: Causes, Diagnosis and Treatment**
*Eugene Lefebvre and Renaud Moreau (Editors)*
2010. ISBN: 978-1-60876-215-6

**Snoring: Causes, Diagnosis and Treatment**
*Eugene Lefebvre and Renaud Moreau (Editors)*
2010. ISBN: 978-1-61668-854-7 (Online Book)

**Handbook of Pharyngeal Diseases: Etiology, Diagnosis and Treatment**
*Aaron P. Nazario and Julien K. Vermeulen (Editors)*
2010. ISBN: 978-1-60876-430-3

**Deafness, Hearing Loss and the Auditory System**
*Derick Fiedler and Rowland Krause (Editors)*
2010. ISBN: 978-1-60741-259-5

**Laryngeal Diseases: Symptoms, Diagnosis and Treatments**
*Oldrich Nemecek and Viktor Mares (Editors)*
2010. ISBN: 978-1-60876-107-4

OTOLARYNGOLOGY RESEARCH ADVANCES SERIES

# DEAFNESS, HEARING LOSS AND THE AUDITORY SYSTEM

**DERICK FIEDLER**

AND

**ROWLAND KRAUSE**

EDITORS

Nova Science Publishers, Inc.
*New York*

**LIBRARY OF CONGRESS CATALOGING-IN-PUBLICATION DATA**

Deafness, hearing loss, and the auditory system / editors, Derick Fiedler and Rowland Krause.
   p. ; cm.
 Includes bibliographical references and index.
 ISBN 978-1-60741-259-5 (hardcover)
 1. Hearing disorders. 2. Deafness. I. Fiedler, Derick. II. Krause, Rowland.
 [DNLM: 1. Hearing Loss--etiology. 2. Hearing Loss--pathology. 3. Hearing Loss--therapy. WV 270 D2773 2009]
 RF290.D427 2009
 617.8--dc22
                    2009041960

*Published by Nova Science Publishers, Inc.*  ✦ *New York*

# CONTENTS

# PREFACE

Noise-induced hearing loss is one of the most common occupational diseases. Approximately 30 million workers in the USA alone are exposed to hazardous noise at work. There is no effective treatment for permanent hearing loss resulting from excessive noise exposure. Furthermore, the condition can be easily prevented using preventative measures such as personal hearing protection devices or hearing protectors. This book summarizes the evidence for the effectiveness and safety of different types of hearing protective devises among workers exposed to noise in the workplace. Furthermore, sensori-neural hearing loss is a frequent complication of radiotherapy of head and neck tumours, when the auditory pathways have been included in the radiation field. This book focuses on reviewing three aspects of radiation-induced SNHL which have significant impact on modern-day medicine. Otoacoustic emissions (OAEs) are a promising technique for the early detection of mild hearing loss. The authors of this book re-evaluate recently published OAE data and its role in hearing loss evaluation. Other chapters provide new insights into our understanding of the influence of chronic sublethal hypoxia on functional integrity of the auditory system, interventions in hearing impairment due to perinatal asphyxia and the effects of clinical studies using rTMS in tinnitus patients

Chapter 1 - The ventral complex of the lateral lemniscus (VCLL) is a group of neurons thought to play an important role in coding the temporal aspects of sound. This review chapter will examine the current literature available describing the anatomy, physiology, cellular morphology and spatial organisation of the VCLL and its constituent neurons. Studies included in this chapter are distinguished by species and include both *in vivo* and *in vitro* data. Intracellular and extracellular responses to noise and tone bursts from VCLL neurons, as well as 3-dimensional reconstructions of the VCLL illustrating the functional distribution of various auditory response properties are highlighted. An examination of the ongoing and controversial search for a tonotopic distribution within the VCLL is presented along with arguments on both sides. Finally, a powerful, fast inhibitory circuit within the VCLL is described that may co-ordinate the timing of higher brain centre responses. This and other possible functional roles are proposed in an attempt to uncover the significance of these enigmatic nuclei in mammalian auditory processing.

Chapter 2 - Excessive noise exposure can lead to metabolic and/or mechanical effects resulting in alterations of the structural elements of the organ of Corti. Besides occupational noise exposure, there are several sources of leisure noise exposure attributing to noise-induced hearing loss (NIHL). These leisure noise exposures include exposure to loud music or even participation in non-musical activities. The major sources of the former activities are attendance at discotheques, nightclubs and live concerts, and usage of personal music players. Recently, it was estimated that the prevalence of leisure noise in the UK has tripled since the early 1980s. Therefore, an increase in prevalence of NIHL in adolescents and young adults is assumed, especially in the mainstream media. Epidemiologic literature is, however, more equivocal. The lack of hearing deterioration is most likely explained by the fact that leisure noise exposure is insufficient to cause important hearing loss. Nevertheless, the effects of leisure noise exposure on the auditory system of young people is a cause for concern. The purpose of this chapter is to review the sources of leisure noise in relation to their contribution in life-time noise exposure of individuals and to present epidemiologic data regarding NIHL in young people caused by leisure noise. Differences in attitude of young people regarding leisure noise exposure and usage of hearing protection are discussed, as well as the importance of prevention and sensitization campaigns. Moreover, short- and long-term effects of several leisure noise sources are reviewed. Shortcomings in the current literature are stressed, and proposals for additional research regarding the usefulness of several audiological tests to detect minimal cochlear damage after exposure to loud leisure noise are pointed out.

Chapter 3 - Sensori-neural hearing loss is a frequent complication of radiotherapy of head and neck tumours, when the auditory pathways have been included in the radiation field. This chapter focuses on the review of three aspects of radiation-induced SNHL that have a significant impact on modern day medicine: 1) effect of radiation on retro-cochlear nervous pathways, 2) cellular and molecular processes involved in radiation-induced ototoxicity, 3) combined ototoxic effects of radiation and cisplatin. A model of radiation-induced damage of the sensor-neural auditory system has been proposed, which is based on the concept of dose-dependent, reactive oxygen species related cochlear cell apoptosis without significant damage to the retro-cochlear pathway. This model supports the feasibility of cochlear implantation, should one be clinically indicated in such patients. It can explain clinical observations such as radiation-induced sensori-neural hearing loss being dose-dependent and affects the high frequencies more than the lower frequencies. It also opens up the possibility of preventive strategies targeted at different stages of the apoptotic process. The use of anti-oxidants which target upstream pathways, appear promising. In particular, it may have a major role in chemo-radiation where combined ototoxic effects lead to significant sensori-neural hearing loss.

Chapter 4 - As early as 1931, immune dysfunction was hypothesized as the impairment of the inner ear's function. Since then, a variety of antigens have been described and implicated in immune-mediated hearing loss. Among these are collagen, heat shock protein-70, myelin protein P0, glycolipids, β-tubulin protein, calcium binding protein S-100β, Raf-1 protein and more recently β-actin, cochlin, β-tectorin and choline transporter-like protein 2. Of these target autoantigens, cochlin and β-tectorin seem to be specifically expressed in the inner ear. The validity of these proteins as autoantigens and their utility as clinical marker - or more importantly as predictors of hearing loss - is yet to be determined. Central to their utility is their ability to distinguish between individuals with or without immune-mediated hearing loss. Identifying one or more proteins as autoantigens predictive of hearing loss, would provide an opportunity to diagnose, treat and possibly monitor immune-mediated inner ear hearing loss.

Chapter 5 - Acute severe or lethal hypoxia is well known to damage the immature auditory system. However, limited information is available about whether chronic sublethal hypoxia also damages this system. Previous studies in animal experiments showed that chronic sublethal hypoxia adversely affects the immature cerebral cortex. Recent studies have revealed that chronic sublethal hypoxia damage functional integrity of the immature auditory system in both human infants and animal models of chronic sublethal hypoxia. In human infants, a typical clinical problem that is associated with chronic sublethal hypoxia is bronchopulmonary dysplasia (BPD), a major perinatal problem that often leads to neurodevelopmental deficits. In recent years, the influence of this problem on the immature brain has attracted considerable attention. The understanding of the influence of chronic sublethal hypoxia associated with BPD on the immature auditory system remains very limited. Brainstem auditory function has recently been studied in very preterm infants who suffered chronic sublethal hypoxia due to BPD. In the maximum length sequence brainstem auditory responses the components that reflect central auditory function were significantly abnormal, while the components that reflect peripheral neural function of the auditory system did not show any major abnormalities. The results suggest that chronic sublethal hypoxia damage neural conduction, reflecting impaired myelination and synaptic dysfunction, in the immature central auditory system, with no major effect on neural function of the peripheral auditory system. Newborn rats reared in chronic sublethal hypoxia showed a significant reduction in myelination in major white tracts and a patchy distribution of the residual myelination in the auditory brainstem. There was also a reduction in myelin basic protein expression. It appears that chronic sublethal hypoxia inhibits myelination and the expression of myelin basic protein in the auditory brainstem. These recent novel findings provide new insights into our understanding of the influence of chronic sublethal hypoxia on functional integrity of the very immature auditory system.

Chapter 6 - The pathophysiology of tinnitus remains incompletely understood and treatment is elusive. Recent neurophysiological and neuroimaging data suggest that some forms of tinnitus are associated with synchronized hyperactivity in the auditory cortex. Therefore targeted modulation of tinnitus-related cortical hyperactivity has been considered as a new promising treatment strategy. Repetitive transcranial magnetic stimulation (rTMS) is a non-invasive method for modifying neural activity in the stimulated area and at a distance along functional anatomical connections. This chapter will summarize the effects of clinical studies using rTMS in tinnitus patients.

This technique can be applied in two different ways in diagnosing and treating tinnitus patients. One approach uses single sessions of high-frequency rTMS applied to the temporal cortex. This method has shown success in suppressing tinnitus transiently during the time of stimulation and has been suggested as a predictor for treatment outcome of direct electrical epidural stimulation with implanted electrodes. Low-frequency rTMS is an efficient method to selectively reduce the abnormally increased activity in cortical areas. Several small controlled studies demonstrated beneficial effects in tinnitus patients after repeated sessions of low-frequency rTMS. In some patients, treatment effects outlasted the stimulation period by twelve months and more. However, available studies are characterized by the high inter-individual variability of treatment effects and only moderate effect sizes. Basic research should focus on a better understanding of the neurobiological effects of this technique. Clinical studies with larger sample sizes can provide more information on the impact of patient-related (e.g. hearing loss, age, tinnitus-duration) and stimulation-related (e.g. frequency, target control) factors on treatment outcome.

Chapter 7 - The ear is a complex organ system that contains a diversity of cell and tissue types and as such the elucidation of the various biological factors that can contribute to deafness can be quite challenging. The starting point for any such investigation is generally a comprehensive search of the biomedical literature to see what factors have already been determined to play a role and in what ways. The overwhelming volume of biomedical literature available, however, can often make uncovering such information difficult as standard keyword based search techniques often fail to narrow down search results into readily manageable quantities. This study will demonstrate the use of the informatics technique of text mining via regular expression based pattern matching as a means of uncovering the various genetic causes of deafness described in the biomedical literature. Several genetic causes of deafness can be linked to genes encoding proteins of the myosin family. As such, a text mining technique is illustrated that will match the expression of myosin variants to various parts of the ear in an effort to better elucidate the roles of myosins in the normal and aberrant function of the ear.

Chapter 8 - Multicellular organisms have separate compartments of different compositions. In the cochlea of the inner ear separation between endolymph and perilimph, two compartments with very different sodium and potassium ion concentrations, is necessary for normal hearing. This compartmentalization is achieved by tight junctions (TJs), which form the major selective barrier of the paracellular pathway between epithelial cells. TJ strands contain at least five types of membrane-spanning proteins. To date, mutations in five different TJ membrane integral proteins have been associated with hearing loss. Mutations in claudin 14 and in tricellulin are associated with hereditary hearing loss in humans. Claudin 9-, claudin 11- and claudin 14-mutant mice are deaf. In zebrafish, a mutation of the *cldnj* gene leads to abnormal auditory and vestibular functions. There are different etiologies for hearing loss associated with each of these proteins, including hair cell loss, reduced endocochlear potentials, and abnormal embryonic development of the inner ear. Nevertheless, in all cases the underlying cause is dysfunction of the paracellular barrier. These findings elucidate the crucial role played by TJs in the auditory apparatus, and enhance our understanding of the hearing process. This knowledge will be further enhanced by identification of hearing-related phenotypes associated with additional TJ proteins and generation of additional animal models in years to come.

Chapter 9 - *Introduction:* Noise-induced hearing loss is one of the most common occupational diseases. Approximately 30 million workers in the USA alone are exposed to hazardous noise at work (WHO 2002). There is no effective treatment for permanent hearing loss resulting from excessive noise exposure. The condition can be easily prevented using preventative measures such as personal hearing protection devices or hearing protector (i.e., earplugs, earmuffs).

*Objective:* To summarize the evidence for the effectiveness and safety of different types of hearing protective devices among workers exposed to noise in the workplace.

*Methods:* A systematic review of the literature was conducted. The authors searched the Cochrane Central Register of Controlled Trials (CENTRAL); Pubmed; EMBASE; LILACS and; Current Controlled Trials for ongoing trials. The date of the last search was 16th February 2009. Studies were included if they had a randomized or quasi-randomized design, if they were among noise exposed (> 80 dB(A)) workers and, if there was at least two hearing protectors to be compared. The reviewer selected relevant trials, assessed methodological quality and extracted data.

*Results:* Two studies were included with a total of 46 participants. It was not possible to combine the included studies in a meta-analysis. Both included studies evaluated earplugs as hearing protectors. The representations of meta-analysis with only one study showed that participants that worn HL SmartFit had fewer number of difficulties per number of conversations compared to E-A-R Push-Ins earplugs. In addition, participants reported higher rate of satisfaction wearing HL SmartFit when compared to E-A-R Push-Ins or Sonomax SonoCustoms.

*Conclusion:* The evidence found in this review showed that the HL SmartFit earplug is more effective compared to E-A-R Push-Ins foam earplug and Sonomax SonoCustoms regarding the number of difficulties per number of conversations and satisfaction. Future trials should have standardized outcomes measures such as attenuation, speech intelligibility and audibility (hear communication) in the noise environment, worker acceptance of HPDs and the likelihood that workers will wear them consistently, hearing loss thresholds by audiometric test, costs and others.

Chapter 10 - Perinatal asphyxia is an important risk for acquired hearing impairment in infants and children. Selection and implementation of a proper plan to intervene in hearing impairment requires accurate information about all frequencies important for speech and language development. Thus, it is crucial to obtain detailed information about cochlear function in infants with hearing impairment. Distortion product otoacoustic emissions (DPOAEs) have been widely used to examine cochlear function in infants. Recent studies found that infants after perinatal asphyxia showed a decrease in DPOAE pass rates at most frequencies in the first few days after birth. The decrease occurred mainly between 1 and 5 kHz, particularly 1 and 2 kHz. Overall DPOAE pass rate was also decreased. These results suggest that perinatal asphyxia damages the neonatal cochlea, which occurs mainly at the frequencies 1-5 kHz, particular at 1 and 2 kHz. At 1 month the decreased DPOAE pass rates did show any improvement. It seems that the impairment detected in the first few days after birth is unlikely to improve in later neonatal period. Follow-up studies revealed that at 6 months after birth DPOAE pass rates were increased slightly at most frequencies, but were decreased slightly at some other frequencies. At 12 months infants after perinatal asphyxia still demonstrated a decrease in DPOAE pass rates at most frequencies, particularly 1 and 2 kHz. Similarly, overall DPOAE pass rates were also decreased. The same was true for the comparison of the pass rates at 12 months with those at 6 months. These longitudinal prospective studies of DPOAEs indicate that hypoxia-ischemia that is associated with perinatal asphyxia adversely affects cochlear function. The major affected frequencies are 1 and 2 kHz. At 1 year, cochlear function remains relatively poor. Therefore, cochlear function, mainly at 1 and 2 kHz, is impaired after perinatal asphyxia, which is persistent during the postnatal development, with only slightly improvement. These findings provide useful information for selecting and implementing early interventions in hearing impairment due to perinatal asphyxia.

Chapter 11 - Otoacoustic Emissions (OAEs) are a promising technique for the early detection of mild hearing loss. The correlation between OAE levels and the audiometric threshold level has been well-established for transient-evoked OAEs (TEOAEs), Distortion products (DPOAEs) and stimulus-frequency OAEs (SFOAEs). Spontaneous OAEs are also correlated with minima of the audiometric threshold microstructure. The use of TEOAEs in neonatal hearing screening tests is widely accepted. The diagnostic potential of OAEs has not been fully exploited yet, partly due to intrinsic limitations (OAE responses cannot be measured at all in the profoundly hearing-impaired subjects) that permit their application only to subjects with mild or medium hearing loss levels (HL < 40-50 dB), partly because the OAE generation mechanisms are quite complex and not yet fully understood. The constant improvement of innovative acquisition and analysis techniques and the better understanding of cochlear mechanics are improving the effectiveness of OAE techniques in at least three main diagnostic fields:

(a)  objective evaluation of the hearing threshold level

(b)  objective evaluation of the frequency resolution of hearing (cochlear tuning)

(c)  monitoring small modifications of the hearing functionality in subjects with normal-hearing or mild hearing loss.

As regards the first two applications, at the present stage, the OAE techniques can surely be considered as an important objective complement to the correspondent psychoacoustical techniques, i.e. Tonal Audiometry (TA) and the measure of the Critical Bandwidth (CB). OAE measurements can also complement the information coming from other objective techniques, such as the Auditory Brainstem Response (ABR). The third use of OAEs is very promising to monitor the hearing function of subjects exposed to noise, particularly in the case of professional exposure. Some recent studies suggest indeed that OAEs could be more sensitive than TA for this specific diagnostic task.

In this study the authors report a re-analysis of recently published OAE data of a population of subjects with long-term exposure to industrial noise and of another group of subjects exposed to intense noise in a discotheque, before and after exposure. The results show the potential of OAE-based tests in all the three above-mentioned tasks:

(a)  dichotomous OAE-based tests can be effective for detecting hearing loss down to sub-clinical levels (10 dB HL);

(b)  cochlear tuning can be objectively estimated from the OAE latency;

(c)  OAE levels are sensitive indicators of noise exposure in subjects with normal hearing or mild hearing loss.

Chapter 12 - The audiovestibular system can be affected by an immunological etiology; the presence of immune mediated sensorineural hearing loss (IMSNHL) as part of or in combination with other autoimmune diseases is well documented in the literature. Hearing loss can be caused by autoimmune disorders localized to the inner ear or secondary to systemic immune diseases (Cogan's syndrome, juvenile chronic arthritis, ulcerative colitis, Wegener's granulomatosis, scleroderma, pulseless disease, and SLE). A systemic autoimmune disorder can be present in fewer than one-third of cases

The clinical presentation of immune inner-ear disease is extremely variable and depends on the type of immune reaction and on the site of injury within the inner ear. IMSNHL typically presents with an idiopathic, progressive unilateral and successive bilateral rapidly progressive sensorineural hearing loss; the course of the hearing loss occurs over weeks to months and is most common in middle-aged women; it may be accompanied by tinnitus and vertigo and is almost always unilateral.

IMSNHL is still a diagnostic and therapeutic dilemma, and predicting recovery from it is very difficult. Different factors may influence a prognosis: e.g., severity of hearing loss, duration of symptoms before treatment, presence of vertigo, type of audiogram, and age of patients. The therapeutic approaches normally used for this pathological condition include the systemic and local administration of cortisone, vasoactive agents, anticoagulants, vitamin complexes, a cytotoxic agent and plasmapheresis. These drugs can be effective in reversing such hearing loss, although at the cost of occasionally severe side effects.

Currently, evaluating the importance of an autoimmune phenomenon in the genesis of inner-ear disease is difficult because the clinical and biological criteria of autoimmune deafness have not yet been well defined. A positive response to treatment is a criterion for the diagnosis of immune inner-ear disease.

This chapter aims to assess the effect of sodium enoxaparin on the recovery of hearing in patients affected by ISSNHL. Sodium enoxaparin was administered subcutaneously at a dose of 4,000 IU once a day for 10 days.

Sodium enoxaparin is a particular kind of heparin with a low molecular weight (LMWH) and is endowed with a high antithrombotic activity.

The literature does not report any therapeutic protocols for autoimmune IMSNHL treatment with sodium enoxaparin or other kinds of unfractionated heparin. Our decision to use enoxaparin was based both on the pathogenesis of this condition and on evaluation of the other classes of drugs currently used.

Chapter 13 - The authors studied the molecular basis of NSHL in the Volga-Ural region. The Volga–Ural region of Russia is of particular interest, because its ethnic populations mostly belong to the Turkic, Finno-Ugric, and Slavonic linguistic groups and have complex ethnogenesis and combine the Caucasian and Mongoloid components in various proportions. A total number of 100 patients of Tatars, Russian or mixed ethnicity and 768 population samples were analyzed by PCR-SSCP followed by direct sequencing of the *GJB2* gene. The *GJB6* gene deletion and the common non-syndromic deafness-causing mitochondrial mutations were also tested when appropriate. The 35delG mutation was predominant among patients from Volga-Ural region. Mutation 312del14 in *GJB2* gene is the second most frequent cause of non-syndromic hearing impairment in the Volgo-Ural region.

The authors' data testify to the founder effect and suggest an eastward distribution of 35delG, since its frequency in Finno-Ugric populations gradually decreases from Estonia to Komi. The question whether the Volga-Ural region could be one of the founder sources for the 235delC and 167delT mutations, widespread in Asia and Israel community, is open. Also, the 312del14 mutation in *GJB2* is the second most frequent cause of non-syndromic hearing impairment in the Volga-Ural region.

Chapter 14 - A case is presented of a 70-year-old man with a profound sensorineural hearing loss in the right ear since childhood and who developed sudden severe hearing loss in the left ear at age 63. Eventually, after he received cochlear implants in both ears, he started to present behavioural auditory processing skills associated with binaural hearing, such as improved ability understanding speech in the presence of background noise, and sound localization. Responsiveness and outcomes were measured using cortical auditory evoked potentials, speech perception in noise, sound localization performance , and a self-rating questionnaire. The results suggest that even after more than 50 years of unilateral deafness it is possible to develop binaural interaction and sound localization.

Chapter 15 - Ototoxicity is defined as the tendency of certain therapeutic agents to cause functional impairment and cellular degeneration of the inner ear and of the eighth cranial nerve. Cisplatin (cis-diamminedichloroplatinum II; CDDP) is the first generation platinum-containing antitumoral drug known to be effective against a variety of solid tumors. Ototoxicity has been observed in up to 36% of patients receiving cisplatin. Risk factors for cisplatin ototoxicity include renal insufficiency, co-administration with aminoglycosides and/or radiation therapy, and increased cumulative doses. Monitoring for ototoxicity should be individualized: an audiogram (high frequencies and ultrahigh frequencies) should be obtained at the onset of therapy, before each successive dose, and with the onset of symptoms. Second generation platinum derived drugs have been developed in order to minimize the toxic effect on the inner ear.

Only 1% of intracellular platinum (Pt) is bound to nuclear DNA with the great majority of the drug available to interact with other cellular targets. The quantification of Pt inside the inner ear by quadrupole inductively coupled plasma mass spectrometry (ICP-MS) has shown the presence of Pt-biomolecules in nuclear, cytosolic and mitochondrial fractions. The Pt-biomolecules binding could play a role in ototoxicity since the complexes were different depending on the drug and represents a future outlook in the management of cisplatin ototoxiciy.

Although classically the most prominent change seen in the cochlea after cisplatin administration consists of loss of outer hair cells (OHCs), new directions in the research allowed us to provide a main role to the supporting cells (Deiter's cells) since they appeared more sensitive than outer hair cells.

*In vitro* and *in vivo* experiments have shown that apoptotic cell death is the primary mechanism of cisplatin antitumoral action. A novel investigation has shown that cisplatin induces apoptosis in hair cells, supporting cells, spiral ganglion cells, stria vascularis cells and spiral ligament fibrocytes by the activation of caspases, evoking an intrinsic pathway of pro-apoptotic signalling. This innovative idea has facilitated the development of several strategies to prevent oxidative stress-induced apoptosis of inner ear cells that have been exposed to cisplatin. However, the loss of the population of some type of inner ear cells could be irreversible, and then it would be necessary to replace these cells. The conversion of inner ear stem cells to sensory neurons and the search of a possible common pathway of inner ear damage need to be explored and they will lead the future trends in inner ear research.

Chapter 16 - Modeling of the perceptual masking properties of the Human Auditory System is investigated. An artificial neural network is trained to model the perceptual masking map of the human auditory system. Successful application of the model to data hiding is demonstrated.

Chapter 17 – Automatic speech recognition (ASR) broadly encompasses the recognition of human speech by a machine or by some artificial intelligence. The recognition process should be robust, that is, it should accurately recognise the spoken word in the presence of speaker variabilities, word perplexities, and speech corrupted by noise which are introduced during transmission and in the communication channels itself. Research in the past several decades has produced speech processing techniques like the short-time Fourier transform (STFT), the linear prediction (LP) and autoregressive (AR) methods, and the mel-frequency cepstral coefficients (MFCC), which have contributed significantly to robust speech recognition. The ability of the human auditory system to recognize speech in adverse and noisy conditions has motivated speech researchers to include features of human perception in speech recognition systems. Particularly in the early 1980s, several computational models of the auditory periphery based on physiological measurements of the response on individual fibres of the auditory nerve were proposed. These "cochlear models" only provided marginal improvements at higher computational costs when applied to speech recognition. As a result, a decline in the interest in auditory models was observed until computing resources were able to meet the intensive computational requirements of such models. In recent years, there has been a resurgence in perceptual speech processing after research provided evidence that it may lead to improved recognition performances.

This chapter describes several psychoacoustic properties of the peripheral auditory system applied to a speech recognition front-end. Dynamic behaviour of the auditory nerves are incorporated in speech parametrization utilizing temporal processing, so that time domain information as appropriate time constants are incorporated in speech parameterization. A simplified method of synaptic adaptation as determined by psychoacoustic observations in an auditory nerve is described. It utilizes a high pass infinite impulse response (IIR) temporal filter to enhance the signal onsets and the subsequent dynamic and the steady-state characteristics. Speech features are extracted in the temporal mode utilizing a zero-crossing algorithm. The two-tone suppression as observed in the non-linear response of the basilar membrane is described in a zero-crossing auditory front-end using a temporal companding strategy. This may introduce asymmetric gain control without degrading the spectral contrast. The word recognitions are evaluated by continuous density hidden Markov models and are shown to provide improvements over conventional parameterizations in clean and noise conditions. Some of these perceptual algorithms may also benefit people with sensorineural hearing loss and may be implemented in hearing aids and cochlear implants for the hearing impaired through VLSI implementations.

Commentary - It remains to be seen if the use of acupuncture in the treatment of ear disorders can be supported by solid well-designed research. Although it is unrealistic to expect it to work in established hearing defects due to cochlear hair-cell loss, it will be interesting to find out if it is of value in treating potentially reversible conditions such as early sudden hearing loss and Meniere's disease.

In: Deafness, Hearing Loss and the Auditory System
Editors: D. Fiedler and R. Krause, pp.1-79

ISBN: 978-1-60741-259-5
©2010 Nova Science Publishers, Inc.

*Chapter 1*

# THE VENTRAL COMPLEX OF THE LATERAL LEMNISCUS: A REVIEW

*David A.X. Nayagam[1]\*, Janine C. Clarey[1] and Antonio G. Paolini[2]*
[1]The Bionic Ear Institute, 384-388 Albert St., East Melbourne, Victoria, Australia
[2]School of Psychological Science, La Trobe University, Australia

## ABSTRACT

The ventral complex of the lateral lemniscus (VCLL) is a group of neurons thought to play an important role in coding the temporal aspects of sound. This review chapter will examine the current literature available describing the anatomy, physiology, cellular morphology and spatial organisation of the VCLL and its constituent neurons. Studies included in this chapter are distinguished by species and include both *in vivo* and *in vitro* data. Intracellular and extracellular responses to noise and tone bursts from VCLL neurons, as well as 3-dimensional reconstructions of the VCLL illustrating the functional distribution of various auditory response properties are highlighted. An examination of the ongoing and controversial search for a tonotopic distribution within the VCLL is presented along with arguments on both sides. Finally, a powerful, fast inhibitory circuit within the VCLL is described that may co-ordinate the timing of higher brain centre responses. This and other possible functional roles are proposed in an attempt to uncover the significance of these enigmatic nuclei in mammalian auditory processing.

## LIST OF ABBREVIATIONS

| | |
|---|---|
| 2-DG | 2-Deoxyglucose |
| AM | Amplitude Modulation |
| AMPA | α-amino-3-hydroxy-5-methyl-4-isoxazolepropionic acid |
| AP | Action Potential |
| AVCN | Anteroventral Cochlear Nucleus |
| BDA | Biotinylated Dextran Amine |
| CF | Characteristic Frequency |

---

\* Corresponding Author

| CN | Cochlear Nucleus |
|---|---|
| CNIC | Central Nucleus of the Inferior Colliculus |
| CV | Co-efficient of Variance |
| DAB | 3,3'-diaminobenzidine |
| dB | Decibel |
| DCN | Dorsal Cochlear Nucleus |
| DNLL | Dorsal Nucleus of the Lateral Lemniscus |
| DPO | Dorsal Periolivary Nucleus |
| EPSP | Excitatory Post-Synaptic Potential |
| FM | Frequency Modulation |
| FSL | First Spike Latency |
| GABA | γ-aminobutyric acid |
| HRP | Horseradish Peroxidase |
| IC | Inferior Colliculus |
| ILD | Interaural Level Disparity |
| INLL | Intermediate Nucleus of the Lateral Lemniscus |
| IPSP | Inhibitory Post-synaptic Potential |
| ISI(H) | Interspike Interval (Histogram) |
| ITD | Interaural Temporal Disparity |
| LNTB | Lateral Nucleus of the Trapezoid Body |
| LSO | Lateral Superior Olive |
| LVPO | Lateroventral Periolivary Nucleus |
| MGN | Medial Geniculate Nucleus |
| MNTB | Medial Nucleus of the Trapezoid Body |
| MSO | Medial Superior Olive |
| NBQX | 2,3-dihydroxy-6-nitro-7-sulfamoyl-benzo[f]quinoxaline-2,3-dione |
| NLL | Nuclei of the Lateral Lemniscus |
| OCA | Octopus Cell Area |
| PST(H) | Post-stimulus Time (Histogram) |
| PVCN | Posteroventral Cochlear Nucleus |
| RMP | Resting Membrane Potential |
| RPO | Rostral Periolivary Nucleus |
| SOC | Superior Olivary Complex |
| SD | Standard Deviation |
| SPL | Sound Pressure Level |
| TC | Tuning Curve |
| VCL | Ventral Complex of the Lateral Lemniscus |
| VCN | Ventral Cochlear Nucleus |
| VNLL | Ventral Nucleus of the Lateral Lemniscus |
| VNLLa | Ventral Nucleus of the Lateral Lemniscus (anterior region) |
| VNLLc | Ventral Nucleus of the Lateral Lemniscus (columnar region, in echolocating species) |
| VNLLd | Ventral Nucleus of the Lateral Lemniscus (dorsal region) |
| VNLLm | Ventral Nucleus of the Lateral Lemniscus (multipolar region, in echolocating species) |
| VNLLv | Ventral Nucleus of the Lateral Lemniscus (ventral region) |
| VNTB | Ventral Nucleus of the Trapezoid Body |

# INTRODUCTION

The ventral complex of the lateral lemniscus (VCLL) is a group of neurons that is embedded within the lateral lemniscal tract. Connecting the brainstem with the midbrain, this pathway is a major component of the mammalian auditory system. Despite the large number of studies of this region, the function of this group of cells and their role in auditory processing is unknown.

The aim of this chapter is to collate what is known about the VCLL, as there has not been a review of this body of literature for over half a decade. The current chapter will examine the results of anatomical and electrophysiological studies, both *in vivo* and *in vitro*, from a wide range of species. Ultimately, this compendium of our current understanding of the structure and function of the VCLL will provide a basis for future studies to pose more insightful questions and perform pertinent experiments to uncover the significance of this part of the auditory brain.

# GENERAL OVERVIEW OF THE ASCENDING AUDITORY PATHWAY

The cochlea's efferent fibres form the auditory nerve (the cochlear division of the vestibulocochlear nerve or cranial nerve VIII) and synapse on the most rostral aspect of the medulla (ponto-medullary junction) on neurons of the dorsal and ventral cochlear nuclei (DCN and VCN, respectively) (Berne et al., 1998). These nuclei are the source of axons that form the basis of the entire ascending central auditory system. They provide a wide range of modes of neural integration. The different types of cells in the cochlear nuclei (CN) form the basis of at least four parallel systems in the auditory brainstem (Young, 1998).

The axons from the cochlear nuclei course out along three primary pathways: the dorsal acoustic stria, the intermediate acoustic stria and the trapezoid body. The trapezoid body contains fibres bound for both of the superior olivary complexes (SOC; on each side of the brain stem). These binaural SOC nuclei are concerned with sound localisation based on interaural temporal and level disparities (ITD and ILD, respectively). The medial superior olive (MSO) discriminates auditory signals on the basis of phase differences, the lateral superior olive (LSO) on the basis of intensity differences (Kandel et al., 1991). Axons stemming from these superior olivary nuclei connect with the crossed and uncrossed axons travelling up bilaterally from the cochlear nucleus, via the dorsal and intermediate stria, to form the lateral lemnisci, which terminate in the inferior colliculi (IC). Figure 1 shows a stylised overview of the ascending auditory pathway of mammals.

The lateral lemnisci are important neuronal fibre tracts in the ascending auditory pathway. Each lateral lemniscus streams dorsally in humans (rostrally in four legged animals) through the nuclei of the lateral lemniscus (NLL). At this stage, some fibres synapse and there is an extensive crossing between the two sides via the commissure of Probst.

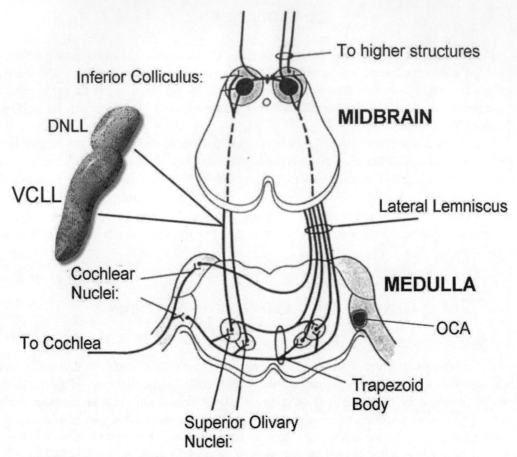

Figure 1. General overview of the ascending auditory pathway.
The central auditory pathways extend from the cochlear nucleus (CN) to the primary auditory cortex. The lateral lemniscus is one of these three main pathways. Formed from crossed and uncrossed axons from the CN and superior olivary complex (SOC), it courses dorsally (rostrally in four-legged animals) to the inferior colliculus (IC) passing through the nuclei of the lateral lemniscus (NLL) along the way, where some fibres terminate. The dorsal nucleus of the lateral lemniscus (DNLL) as well as the ventral complex of the lateral lemniscus (VCLL) are illustrated (not to scale). Also illustrated is the octopus cell area (OCA; not to scale) of the CN, which contains cells that project to the VCLL.

Ultimately, the lateral lemniscal fibres all synapse in the IC. Here the neurons are arranged tonotopically and are predominantly binaural. These IC cells mainly project to the ipsilateral medial geniculate nucleus (MGN) of the thalamus, via the brachium of the inferior colliculus. The MGN gives rise to the auditory radiation, which ends in the ipsilateral auditory cortex, found within the transverse temporal gyrus of the temporal lobe in humans (Kandel et al., 1991).

It seems clear that, at least from above the level of the CN, there are extensive bilateral interactions in the ascending pathway, in contrast to some other sensory systems. Decussation of pathways occurs at many stages throughout the ascending auditory system. The second order neurons of the CN, project bilaterally to higher areas (Nolte and Angevine, 1995) making it possible for sound localisation and other binaural processes to be performed within the brainstem itself.

As well as ascending projections and commissural connections, there is also a significant amount of feedback in the auditory system. Primarily, projections from the auditory cortex descend to the MGN and IC. There are also projections from the IC to the SOC, CN and NLL. Furthermore, many of the auditory nuclei including the lemniscal nuclei contain intrinsic projections. These will be discussed in more detail later.

The present review concentrates on the rat auditory system as a model for the human brainstem. The general organisation of the rat auditory system is essentially equivalent to that of other terrestrial mammals, including humans. Here, specific differences between the NLL of the rat and other mammalian species have been identified and will be discussed below. The species under investigation will be routinely identified where appropriate for ease of comprehension.

## ANATOMY OF THE NUCLEI OF THE LATERAL LEMNISCUS

The NLL are anatomically and functionally distinct cell groups situated in the pons between the lower brainstem and the auditory midbrain intercalated with fibres of the lateral lemniscus. The lemniscal nuclei have been extensively studied in echolocating bats (Zook and Casseday, 1982a, b; Covey and Casseday, 1986; Metzner and Radtke-Schuller, 1987; Zook and Casseday, 1987; Ross et al., 1988; Covey and Casseday, 1991; Covey, 1993a; Huffman and Covey, 1995; Vater et al., 1997) and in these animals are thought to play a vital role in echolocation. The current review will concentrate on findings from non-echolocating species, which lack the specialisations necessary for echolocation. In non-echolocating species, there is contention as to the parcellation of the NLL. Studies on cat (Adams, 1979; Glendenning et al., 1981; Malmierca et al., 1998), rat (Caicedo and Herbert, 1993; Merchán and Berbel, 1996), rabbit (Batra and Fitzpatrick, 1999), opossum (Willard and Martin, 1983) and guinea pig (Schofield and Cant, 1997) have identified different nuclei within the NLL; however, the delineations are not uniform across species. Some studies have identified two (rat: Merchán and Berbel, 1996; opossum: Willard and Martin, 1983; cat: Adams, 1979; Whitley and Henkel, 1984; Adams, 1997), whilst others have identified three nuclei (guinea pig: Schofield and Cant, 1997; cat: Glendenning et al., 1981): the dorsal, ventral and intermediate nuclei of the lateral lemniscus (DNLL, VNLL and INLL respectively). Whilst the DNLL is widely considered a separate structure both anatomically and physiologically (cat: Aitkin et al., 1970a; Glendenning et al., 1981), the distinction between the INLL and the VNLL is not so well established. Furthermore, different studies have divided the VNLL into one (rat: Merchán and Berbel, 1996; guinea pig: Malmierca et al., 1996; gerbil: Nordeen, 1983), two (cat: Roth et al., 1978; bat: Zook and Casseday, 1982b; Covey and Casseday, 1986), or sometimes three (rabbit: Batra and Fitzpatrick, 1997; guinea pig: Schofield and Cant, 1997; cat: Adams, 1979) subdivisions. A consensus is yet to be reached on whether the INLL should be classified as part of the VNLL or as a separate entity and whether the VNLL is a single nucleus or is made up of subdivisions. The differences across species no doubt play a large role in this debate; analogies may not be as straightforward as a one-to-one correlation between species. Therefore, for the purposes of this chapter the term, ventral complex of the lateral lemniscus (VCLL; after Merchán et al., 1997), has been adopted to encompass both the VNLL including its various subdivisions, as well as the INLL (see below). This nomenclature

(VCLL) is equivalent to the term "ventral *nuclei* of the lateral lemniscus" popularised by Oertel and Wickesberg (2002) who also felt it best to represent the various ventral clusters of the NLL as a single nuclei with subdivisions. However, the term ventral complex of the lateral lemniscus (VCLL) avoids ambiguity when using the abbreviation "VNLL" to describe only the ventral *nucleus* of the lateral lemniscus (without including the intermediate nucleus of the lateral lemniscus) Figure 2 shows the parcellation of the rabbit VCLL as well as the inputs, outputs and cell types within the various parts of the structure. These topics will be discussed below.

## VCLL Parcellation

Many researchers have conducted studies over the years, using different species, to gain a better understanding of the spatial organisation of this particular part of the auditory system, from the early classical anatomy studies (Held, 1893; van Gehuchten, 1906; Cajal, 1909) to the abundance of contemporary studies in morphology and functional projections (rat: Bajo et al., 1993; Caicedo and Herbert, 1993; Merchán et al., 1994; Merchán and Berbel, 1996; Kelly et al., 1998a; Kelly et al., 1998b; Zhao and Wu, 2001; Nayagam et al. 2006; Kelly et al. 2009; rabbit: Batra and Fitzpatrick, 1997; opossum: Willard and Martin, 1983; mouse: Willard and Ryugo, 1983; mole: Kudo et al., 1990; guinea pig: Schofield and Cant, 1997; ferret: Moore, 1988; cat: Adams, 1979; Glendenning et al., 1981; Whitley and Henkel, 1984; Spangler et al., 1985; Smith et al., 1993; Adams, 1997; Saint Marie et al., 1997; bat: Schweizer, 1981; Zook and Casseday, 1982a, b; Covey and Casseday, 1986; Vater and Feng, 1990; Huffman and Covey, 1995). Based predominantly on cytoarchitecture and projection patterns, different studies have parcellated the VCLL to different degrees. The differences between studies are due in part to the different species used and in part to the criteria for classification used. The arguments involved in the delineation of the internal subdivisions of the VCLL are in many regards closely linked with the arguments for and against the classification of the INLL as a separate nucleus. A difficult aspect of distilling these findings is the different nomenclature used by different authors, which may refer to equivalent regions. The present review, has adopted the terminology proposed by Schofield and Cant (1997) in guinea pig and subsequently adopted by Oertel and Wickesberg (2002) in their review chapter, who discussed ventral, dorsal and anterior divisions of the VNLL (VNLLv, VNLLd, VNLLa respectively) and a separate INLL. The major findings across non-echolocating species are correlated, where possible, to these divisions of the VCLL. Table 1 summarises key literature from non-echolocating species with regard to the various putative parcellations of the VCLL. Note that whilst some authors omit the 'N' in their abbreviations, e.g. ILL, VLL etc. it has been re-inserted throughout this chapter for continuity.

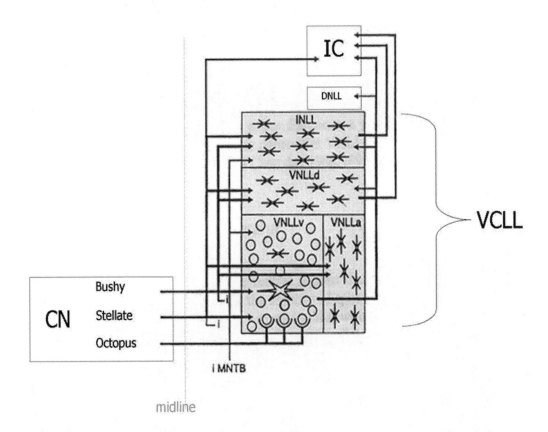

- Modified from Oertel and Wickesberg (2002): with kind permission from Springer Science and Business Media.

Figure 2. Diagrammatic representation of the parcellation of the ventral complex of the lateral lemniscus. Schematic shows the various putative sub-divisions of the ventral nucleus of the lateral lemniscus (VNLL), including the ventral, dorsal, and anterior regions (VNLLv, VNLLd, VNLLa respectively). Also shown is the INLL, which lies dorsally to the VNLL in some species. Collectively these structures are termed the VCLL. The different regions are characterised by the presence of different neuron types or distributions in certain species. The parcellation and morphological distribution presented in this figure is derived from a study in guinea pig (Schofield and Cant, 1997). The VNLLv contains predominantly spherical bushy cells (circles), which are innervated by specialised calyx-like synapses (arcs) from octopus cells in the contralateral posteroventral cochlear nucleus (PVCN). Multipolar cells (stars) and giant cells (large stars) have also been identified in the VNLLv of some species. The VNLLd and VNLLa are distinct from the VNLLv due to the characteristic lack of spherical bushy cells. Both these regions contain mainly multipolar cells. VNLLa and VNLLd are separated from one another based on the directionality of the dendrites, in the VNLLa the dendrites are aligned with the lemniscal fibres, whereas in the VNLLd they lie perpendicular to the ascending fibres. The major excitatory input to the VCLL stems from the various cells of the contralateral cochlear nucleus. The VCLL also receives minor inputs from the ipsilateral CN and the ipsilateral medial nucleus of the trapezoid body (MNTD). The major VCLL projection is to the ipsilateral IC but there are also minor projections to the ipsilateral DNLL, and from the INLL to the medial geniculate nucleus (MGN) on both sides. Major projections are denoted with heavy lines and minor projections are denoted with light lines.

## Table 1. Summary of major papers investigating VCLL parcellation.

| Author(s)/Year | Species | Parcellation | Techniques | Notes |
|---|---|---|---|---|
| Caicedo and Herbert (1993) | Rat | INLL exists | Nissl stain (Thionin) | Didn't examine VNLL |
| Merchán and Berbel (1996) | Rat | VNLL | Nissl stain (Cresyl Violet), Retrograde tracing (BDA, HRP/Biocytin) from IC | Continuous helicoidal laminae throughout the ventro-dorsal extent of the structure |
| Kelly et al. (1998a) | Rat | VNLL, INLL | Nissl stain (Cresyl Violet) | Uses terms VNLL and INLL but no evidence for separate nuclei |
| Kelly et al. (1998b) | Rat | VNLL, INLL | Retrograde tracing (Fluorogold) from IC | |
| Malmierca et al. (1996) | Guinea Pig | VNLL | Nissl Stain (Cresyl Violet) | Used Caicedo and Herbert's (1993) study as a basis |
| Schofield and Cant (1997) | Guinea Pig | VNLLa VNLLd VNLLv INLL | Nissl stain (Cresyl Violet), Antero/Retrograde tracing to/from VCN | Divisions based on differences in cell types and their packing density.. |
| Batra and Fitzpatrick (1997) | Rabbit | VNLLd, VNLLm, VNLLl | Extracellular electrophysiology + Nissl stain (Thionin) | VNLLd = INLL VNLLm = VNLLa VNLLl = VNLLv |
| Willard and Martin (1983) | Opossum | VNLL | Nissl / Golgi / Fibre and HRP stain | |
| Glendenning et al. (1981) | Cat | INLL, VNLL | Antero/retrograde tracing (autoradiographic and degeneration) to/from VCN, Nissl staining and 2-DG | INLL had similarities and differences with both VNLL and DNLL. Lateral tegmentum may correspond with VNLLa |
| Whitley and Henkel (1984) | Cat | VNLL with 3 zones | Autoradiographic tracing from IC | Based on projections, some variations along dorso-ventral axis identified following Adams (1979). Dorsal zone = INLL |
| Adams (1979) | Cat, Human | VNLL with 3 zones (cat) or 2 zones (human) | Nissl / Protargol stain, retrograde tracing (HRP) from IC | Dorsal, middle and ventral zones identified based on cytological differences in cell type. Dorsal zone = INLL and is absent in humans |
| Malmierca et al. (1998) | Cat | VCLL | Retrograde tracing (BDA) from IC | Arbitrarily defined dorsal, middle and ventral regions. Dorsal region = INLL and had different clustering pattern |
| Nayagam et al. (2006) | Rat | VCLL, (VNLL + INLL) | 3D reconstructions of intracellular electrophysiological recording sites; Nissl stain (Thionin) | Dorsal region contains cells with different response properties, providing evidence for INLL |
| Kelly et al. (2009) | Rat | VNLL, INLL | Single and double labelled retrograde tracing (Flurogold, Fluoro Ruby, Fast Blue) from IC, DNLL, INLL and VNLL; Nissl stain (Cresyl Violet) | Distinct projections to each subdivision of the VCLL and IC suggesting anatomical and functional seperation f the INLL |

Species, divisions of VCLL described, and techniques used to gather evidence are shown. Note that whilst some authors omit the 'N' in their abbreviations, e.g. ILL, VLL etc., it has been re-inserted throughout this review for continuity. Abbreviations: 2-DG, 2-Deoxyglucose; BDA, biotinylated dextran amine; HRP, horseradish peroxidase.

## Ventral VNLL

The ventral part of the VNLL (VNLLv) is characterised primarily by a population of compact and distinctive cells similar in shape and afferent synapses to the spherical bushy cells of the CN (sometimes described in the literature as 'globular' cells, Schofield and Cant, 1997). These cells appear dark with Nissl stain and are distributed in alternating dense and loosely packed bands (Schofield and Cant, 1997). They have also been described as oval shaped and resembling the principal cells of the medial nucleus of the trapezoid body (MNTB) because of their appearance and also because they are covered in endbulbs (otherwise known as calyces) (Adams, 1979).

The VNLLv has been identified in several species including humans (Adams, 1997), cats (Adams, 1979, 1997), rabbits (Batra and Fitzpatrick, 1999 - termed VNLLl), guinea pigs (Schofield and Cant, 1997), mice (Willard and Ryugo, 1983) and moles (Kudo et al., 1990). It is represented to varying degrees in different species, and is prominent in humans (38% of VNLL) compared with cats (4%, Adams, 1997). In guinea pigs, the VNLLv is the largest and most complex subdivision of the VNLL and its borders have been delineated from the adjacent structures based on cytoarchitecture and inputs from the CN (Schofield and Cant, 1997). In this and most non-echolocating species, the VNLLv is not a homogeneous cell group, containing giant neurons, multipolar cells (cat: Henkel, 1983), elongated cells (cat: Adams, 1979), as well as the characteristic bushy cells (guinea pig: Schofield and Cant, 1997). This is not to say that segregation between cell types does not exist within the VNLLv. In guinea pigs, the globular cells are preferentially located rostrally, whereas the giant cells are most numerous in the posterior and medial portion of the subnucleus (Schofield and Cant, 1997). Similarly in cats, giant cells of the VNLLv are more common posteriorly and medially (Henkel, 1983) but globular cells are found ventrally (Adams, 1979). In mice (as well as some echolocating bats) the segregation is almost complete with globular cells isolated to a single, almost homogeneous subdivision of the VNLLv (mouse: Willard and Ryugo, 1983; bat: Zook and Casseday, 1985; Covey and Casseday, 1986; Vater and Feng, 1990).

In many species, the borders of the VNLLv are not distinct and there is considerable overlap with neighbouring regions (Adams, 1979). However, in echolocating bats, the VNLLv is thought to correspond with a distinct and highly segregated group of bushy cells known as the columnar region (see below). In rats, opossums and some cat studies, the VNLLv has not been specifically identified (rat: Merchán and Berbel, 1996; Nayagam et al., 2006; opossum: Willard and Martin, 1983; cat: Glendenning et al., 1981). However, these studies have concurred that small, round, darkly staining bushy cells, akin to those that characterise the VNLLv are present within the VNLL. Glendenning et al's study (cat: 1981) found small darkly staining cells preferentially distributed ventrally, in agreement with previous cat studies (Adams, 1979). However, in rats these cells have been identified interspersed throughout the VNLL (M.S. Malmierca, personal communication in: Oertel and Wickesberg, 2002).

The VNLLv receives a variety of thick and thin axonal inputs (see below). Bushy, T stellate and octopus cells in the contralateral CN are the main sources of these inputs (various species: Cant and Benson, 2003; guinea pig: Schofield and Cant, 1997; cat: Glendenning et al., 1981; Adams, 1997). The thick axon projection from the octopus cell area (OCA) of the contralateral PCVN is considered to have important functional ramifications. Studies have identified large secure calyx-like terminal endings on bushy cells in the VNLLv that receive input from the OCA (guinea pig: Schofield and Cant, 1997; cat: Adams, 1997). In guinea pigs the thick axons from the OCA only innervated cells in the VNLLv (Schofield and Cant, 1997), whilst thin axons arising from multipolar and spherical bushy cells terminate throughout the VCLL (Schofield and Cant, 1997). A minor projection from the ipsilateral VCN, as well as the ipsilateral MNTB, also targets cells of the VNLLv. The importance of the VNLLv, and more specifically the bushy (globular) cells that characterise this region and their connection with octopus cells of the contralateral posteroventral cochlear nucleus (PVCN) will be discussed below.

### Anterior VNLL

The anterior division of the VNLL (VNLLa) in guinea pigs contains only multipolar cells with dendrites orientated parallel with lemniscal fibres (Schofield and Cant, 1997). This region appears to be an interstitial nucleus, in that it is a cluster of cells located within the fibres of the lemniscal tract. In guinea pig, it has been classified as a separate part of the VNLL based on its ascending projection to the contralateral IC (Schofield and Cant, 1997). The VNLLa has been identified in guinea pig (Schofield and Cant, 1997) and rabbit (termed VNLLm, Batra and Fitzpatrick, 1997), although not in the same relative anatomical position. In the rabbit a lightly staining interstitial cluster of multipolar cells termed 'VNLLm' was defined on physiological grounds in a similar location to VNLLd in guinea pig (see below), however, the cell densities of these two regions do not correlate. Hence, Batra and Fitzpatrick (2002b) surmised that the region termed VNLLa in guinea pigs correlated with their VNLLm in rabbit, as the cells in these two regions appeared to have similar responses. The VNLLa has not been identified *per se* in the cat (Aitkin et al., 1970a; Guinan et al., 1972b; Adams, 1979; Guinan et al., 1972a). A cluster of cells medial and adjacent to the VNLL classified by Glendenning et al. (1981) as the lateral tegmentum may correspond with Schofield and Cant's (1997) VNLLa, however, this has yet to be shown conclusively. It is unlikely that the paralemniscal zone defined in cats (Henkel and Edwards, 1978; Henkel, 1981; May et al., 1990), a region involved in acoustically driven motor responses, corresponds with the VNLLa in guinea pigs or VNLLm in rabbits (Batra and Fitzpatrick, 2002b) as it lies outside the boundaries of the VNLL.

Schofield and Cant (guinea pig; 1997) suggested that the reason the VNLLa is undefined in most studies, including rat, could be that it has been overlooked due to its light staining and the scattered distribution of cells amongst the lemniscal fibres. It may be that the cells are incorporated into or relocated to a different area of the VNLL, an idea supported by Batra and Fitzpatrick (rabbit; 2002b). Schofield and Cant (1997) also acknowledge the possibility that in other species the VNLLa simply does not exist.

### Dorsal VNLL

There is some confusion in the literature and thus it is important to make the distinction between the dorsal division of the VNLL (VNLLd) and the INLL. In some studies the region defined as VNLLd (cat: Adams, 1979; Whitley and Henkel, 1984; rabbit: Batra and Fitzpatrick, 1999) correlates with the region that has come to be known in other studies as INLL (Glendenning et al., 1981). In the present review, VNLLd refers to the dorsal region of the VNLL as well as cell areas surrounding the VNLLv, which are distinguished from VNLLv by their lack of spherical bushy cells. The INLL is considered separately and will be discussed below.

The VNLLd in guinea pigs is populated primarily with multipolar cells, elongated to give the appearance of horizontal striations (orthogonal to the direction of lemniscal fibres) and arranged into loose vertical columns. These arrangements are not as distinct as in the adjacent INLL; this difference allows these two regions to be set apart. The guinea pig VNLLd also contains a small number of giant cells that have an elongated soma and stain more darkly than the multipolar cells, however not as many as in the neighbouring reticular formation, which allows the border between these regions to be distinguished (Schofield and Cant, 1997).

In rat and some cat studies the VNLLd has not been specifically identified, however differences in the fibro-dendritic structure and cell types of the VNLL along its dorsoventral axis have been reported (various species: Merchán et al., 1997; rat: Merchán and Berbel, 1996; cat: Malmierca et al., 1998). Rat-specific differences will be discussed further below.

## Arguments for and Against the INLL Subdivision

All studies have agreed that there are *at least* two nuclei of the lateral lemniscus (DNLL, VNLL). However, not all studies have concurred with the three-subdivision nomenclature (DNLL, INLL, and VNLL) with some researchers finding the INLL was a dorsal part of the VNLL (rat: Merchán and Berbel, 1996; cat: Adams, 1979; Whitley and Henkel, 1984; Adams, 1997). The early classical studies recognised the two subdivisions (DNLL and VNLL) on the basis of delimiting fibre bands and cytoarchitecture (Held, 1893; van Gehuchten, 1906). However, later studies, especially on the bat (Zook and Casseday, 1979; Covey and Casseday, 1991), began to distinguish the INLL as a separate nucleus (rat: Kelly et al., 1998b; guinea pig: Schofield and Cant, 1997; cat: van Noort, 1969; Brunso-Bechtold and Thompson, 1978; Roth et al., 1978; Glendenning et al., 1981; Saint Marie et al., 1997). The pivotal argument in favour of three nuclei came from a comprehensive study by Glendenning et al. (1981) in the cat. This study was in part addressing the work of Zook and Casseday (1979), who reported a heavy projection from the lateral nucleus of the trapezoid body (LNTB) of the bat to the region equivalent to the INLL in the cat. Addressing this discovery, Glendenning et al. (1981) performed a series of tracing studies, both retrograde and anterograde, in an attempt to elucidate the ascending projections to the various nuclei of the lateral lemniscus. They concluded that the region known as the INLL shared similarities as well as differences with the VNLL and DNLL. Like the VNLL it received a major projection from the contralateral VCN, a projection not received by the DNLL. However, it also received a large projection from the SOC, a projection pattern similar to the DNLL but unlike the VNLL. In at least two respects it was also found to be different to both the VNLL and DNLL: it received a large projection from the MNTB and a small projection from the LNTB. On these 'connectivity' grounds, Glendenning et al. (1981) argued in favour of defining the INLL as a separate nucleus within the lateral lemniscus of the cat. Glendenning et al.'s (1981) findings were supported by other researchers and across other species (rat: Moore and Moore, 1987; Caicedo and Herbert, 1993; cat: Spangler et al., 1985). Some researchers were able to distinguish the INLL from the VNLL based on cellular cytoarchitecture. Schofield and Cant (1997) reported that the most dorsal region of the VNLL could be distinguished from the dorsally bordering INLL by the orientation or arrangement of the constituent neurons (see above). A recent study (Kelly et al., 2009) provides strong support to the arguments for parcellating of the NLL into 3 separate divisions (DNLL, INLL, and VNLL) based on the distinct projections patterns revealed by tract-tracing experiments in a large sample of rats.

The opposing view is one that suggests that the INLL is not a separate nucleus, but a dorsal division of the VNLL. Merchán and Berbel (rat; 1996) are the foremost advocates of the non-existence of the INLL as a separate nucleus and, furthermore, that the VNLL is a single nucleus, with no subdivisions (see above). Their argument on the basis of connectivity and cytoarchitecture is that there is no fundamental distinction between INLL and VNLL in the rat. A subsequent study in the rat by Kelly et al. (1998b) supported this view. An alternate approach by some researchers is to distinguish between monaural and binaural nuclei. In bats, Covey and Casseday (1991) used the terms "monaural nuclei" or "monaural complex" to describe the INLL, and the two monaural subdivisions of the VNLL that are present in the bat. Nonetheless, they still acknowledge the INLL as a separate nucleus. Malmierca et al. (cat; 1998) used the term VCLL to include the ventral and intermediate nuclei and the gamut of subdivisions identified by other researchers in a variety of species using various criteria (rat: Caicedo and Herbert, 1993; guinea pig: Malmierca et al., 1996; Schofield and Cant, 1997; cat: van Noort, 1969; Adams, 1979; Glendenning et al., 1981; bat: Covey and Casseday, 1991). However, Malmierca et al. (1998) outlined four fundamental features of the dorsal VCLL region (that corresponds with the INLL of other studies): 1) Different clustering pattern of fibrodendritic laminae (cat: Malmierca et al., 1998); 2) Different extent of labelling in the projection to the IC (cat: Whitley and Henkel, 1984); 3) Contains cells that are apparently excitatory rather than inhibitory (rat: Riquelme et al., 1998; Riquelme et al., 2001; cat: Saint Marie et al., 1997; bat: Winer et al., 1995; Vater et al., 1997); and 4) Receives glycinergic input from the MNTB (cat: Glendenning et al., 1981; Spangler et al., 1985).

An intracellular and extracellular electrophysiological approach to identifying dorsoventral differences within the rat VCLL based on neural responses was performed by Nayagam et al. (2006). This study revealed that the dorsal part of the VCLL contained a population of cells that responded differently to acoustic stimulation compared to cells in the remainder of the structure. These differences (discussed in more detail below) provided physiological evidence for considering the dorsal part of the VCLL as a separate structure.

Despite some fundamental similarities, anatomical differences do exist between species. Bats and cats especially seem to differ significantly from rats, mice and guinea pigs (see below). In humans there doesn't appear to be a dorsal division of the VCLL that corresponds with the INLL of other species, which receives input from the MNTB. This is understandable given the dearth of cells in humans in the region where the MNTB would be (Adams, 1997). The INLL certainly is the most controversial of the nuclei of the lateral lemniscus, if indeed it is a separate nucleus at all. One thing is certain, the region known as the INLL is different in some ways to the rest of the VCLL, be that a difference on cytoarchitectonic (cat: Stotler, 1953; van Noort, 1969), hodological (cat: Brunso-Bechtold and Thompson, 1978; Roth et al., 1978; Adams, 1979; bat: Zook and Casseday, 1979) or on electrophysiological grounds.

## VCLL Parcellation in Echolocating Species

In studies performed on echolocating bats, it has become widely accepted that the monaural NLL are significantly hypertrophied and unusually ordered in structure (Zook and Casseday, 1982b; Zook and DiCaprio, 1988). The VCLL in these echolocating animals seems to contain three distinct nuclei, with morphologically distinct cell populations; the INLL, the VNLL columnar region (VNLLc) and the VNLL multipolar region (VNLLm)[1] (Covey and Casseday, 1986, 1991; Huffman and Covey, 1995; Vater et al., 1997). The bat INLL is a large region, possibly larger than DNLL and VNLL combined, but lacking in any distinct form or shape (Zook and Casseday, 1979).

The three regions are separated based on their constituent neuronal types. The INLL contains mainly elongate neurons with several long dendrites that extend from either side of the soma orthogonally to the ascending fibres of the lateral lemniscus, but parallel to the fibres that enter the nucleus (Covey and Casseday, 1991). The VNLLc is made up of densely packed neurons, distributed in columns (hence the name) between bundles of lateral lemniscal fibres. Almost all  neurons in the VNLLc are of the same type and are very similar to spherical bushy cells of the anteroventral cochlear nucleus (AVCN). They are round or oval shaped, with one main dendrite that branches profusely from the soma. Some of the branches appear to extend parallel to the ascending fibres of the lateral lemniscus (Zook and Casseday, 1982a; Covey and Casseday, 1986, 1991). The VNLLm on the other hand contains mainly multipolar type cells (hence the name). These neurons' somas and dendrites do not appear to have any consistent orientation with respect to the fibres of the lateral lemniscus. The cells are larger than those in the VNLLc and have several sparsely branching thick dendrites with no apparent directional preference (Covey and Casseday, 1986, 1991).

In non-echolocating mammals such as the cat, guinea pig, mouse and rat, the same principal cell types are found in the VCLL as in the bat's VCLL (rat: Nayagam et al., 2006; mouse: Willard and Ryugo, 1983; guinea pig: Schofield and Cant, 1997; cat: Adams, 1979). However, as previously discussed, the different neuron types are not as clearly segregated as they are in the echolocating bat (Covey and Casseday, 1991). These characteristic differences in the neurons of each subdivision, coupled with enhanced segregation of cell types, allows the VCLL of the echolocating bat to be parcellated without the controversy of its non-echolocating counterpart.

In the bat, there is a projection from the MNTB to the INLL as well as the VNLLc (Covey, 1993b). This is different to the cat where the projection from the MNTB to the INLL is what sets it apart from the VNLL (Glendenning et al., 1981).

## VCLL Anatomy and Parcellation in the Rat

Different rat atlases have published plates showing the stereotaxic size, shape and position of the VNLL and INLL. These plates are not consistent with each other over different editions of the atlases (Paxinos and Watson, 1998; Swanson, 1998; Paxinos and Watson, 2005). However, in general the VCLL extends dorsoventrally ~2.5 mm, lateromedially ~1.2 mm and rostrocaudally ~1.2 mm at its largest extents. It is centred ~2.6 mm lateral of the midline, ~7 mm ventral of the cortical surface and ~8.2 mm caudal to Bregma.

The borders of the VCLL in the rat have been studied by Merchán and Berbel (1996) and Caicedo and Herbert (1993), as well as defined in various rat brain atlases (Paxinos and

---

[1] The multipolar region of echolocating species VNLL (VNLLm) should not be confused with the VNLLm defined by Batra and Fitzpatrick (1997) in the rabbit, which refers to the middle zone of the VNLL.

Watson, 1998; Swanson, 1998; Paxinos and Watson, 2005). Different rat atlases have published plates showing the stereotaxic size, shape and position of the VNLL and INLL. These plates are not consistent with each other over different editions of the atlases (Paxinos and Watson, 1998; Swanson, 1998; Paxinos and Watson, 2005). However, in general the VCLL extends dorsoventrally ~2.5 mm, lateromedially ~1.2 mm and rostrocaudally ~1.2 mm at its largest extents. It is centred ~2.6 mm lateral of the midline, ~7 mm ventral of the cortical surface and ~8.2 mm caudal to Bregma.

Merchán and Berbel (1996) reported on the anatomic location, cytoarchitecture and morphology of the rat VCLL and described the dorsal border of the VCLL as sharp and easily defined. They claim that the horizontal cell group, a narrow band of tightly packed flat neurons, forms the border between the VNLL and the DNLL. This supported the work of Bajo et al. (1993), as well as Caicedo and Herbert (1993). However, it is contrary to studies in the cat which reported that although the VNLL is separated from the INLL by fibres, the border is not well defined and regions of overlap occur (Glendenning et al., 1981). Laterodorsally the border with the nucleus sagulum is clear, as the latter contains smaller and more densely packed neurons. Similarly, the lateroventral border is distinct within the lateral limb of the lemniscus. The lemniscal fibres, which surround the VCLL, define the rostral and caudal limits of the nucleus. In the medial and ventral zones, the borders are more blurred due to the absence of clear anatomical landmarks. On the ventral aspect, the proximity to the ventral nucleus of the trapezoid body (VNTB) makes the border more difficult to establish. However, the different orientations of the fibre fascicles that traverse the two nuclei allow the border to be distinguished. The VCLL is crossed ventrodorsally by lemniscal fibres, where the fibres of the trapezoid body cross the VNTB lateromedially. Thus, neurons in the VCLL are oriented vertically, as opposed to neurons in the VNTB which are oriented horizontally. Although more ambiguous than the other borders, the medial border may also be defined as cells of the neighbouring reticular formation are smaller and more loosely arranged than in the VCLL (Merchán and Berbel, 1996).

The most prominent anatomical study of the rat VCLL favoured a classification scheme that treated the VCLL as a single nucleus containing a homogeneous cellular morphology based on cytology (Merchán and Berbel, 1996). However, the authors of this study acknowledge similarities to earlier findings in cats (Adams, 1979) and bats (Covey and Casseday, 1991) which proposed three divisions of the VCLL. Although they admit to observing cytoarchitectural differences between the dorsal, middle and ventral zones of the rat VNLL, they are careful to avoid the word 'division'. Differences, they claim, may be explained by assuming the fibro-dendritic laminae within the VCLL forms a helicoidal shape. The different patterns of the helicoid's coils may underpin the disparities in the VCLL's appearance. The wide dorsal zone seems to show coils that are more open; the middle zone's coils are horizontal and closely bunched giving the neurons a denser appearance; and the ventral zone has coils that are more open and obliquely oriented. Merchán and Berbel (1996) proposed that perhaps these coiling differences match the subdivisions proposed in bats and cats. They emphasise that their 3D reconstructions revealed a homogeneous pattern within the VCLL and therefore argue against parcellating the nucleus into sub-nuclei.

A comprehensive physiological study which examined the VCLL based on a large sample of neural response properties to dichotically presented acoustic stimuli was performed by Nayagam et al. (2006). They constructed a 3-dimensional model of the rat VCLL from Nissl stained sections and reconstructed the location of their electrophysiological recording sites within this model. By examining the distribution of cells with common neural response properties the authors were able to propose a parcellation for the VCLL. They found the dorsal part of the VCLL, the region corresponding with the INLL in other species, contained a different functional population of cells than the ventral portion of the nuclei. This description of dorso-ventral distinctions within the rat VCLL is in line with descriptions from other species (rabbit: Batra and Fitzpatrick, 1997; guinea pig: Schofield and Cant, 1997; cat and human: Adams 1979), the rat atlases and a subsequent tracing study (Kelly et al., 2009), but contrasts with descriptions from some anatomical tracing studies of the rat VCLL (Merchán and Berbel, 1996).

Morphological and tracing studies have not agreed on structural sub-divisions within the rat VCLL. However, the most recent data from electrophysiological and tract-tracing studies (Nayagam et al., 2006; Kelly et al., 2009) suggest that the INLL is a separate subdivision of the VCLL. It is important to consider the various putative parcellations in other species when studying functional responses from the rat VCLL. A lot of the debate is a matter of semantics: how exactly does one define a 'nucleus'? Various definitions (be they based on cytoarchitecture, projection patterns, response types or something else) may well lead to different interpretations.

## Cytoarchitecture and Morphology of VCLL Neurons

There are several types of neurons found in the INLL as well as the VNLL and its various subdivisions. The VCLL contains cells that resemble bushy and stellate cells of the CN (rat: Zhao and Wu, 2001; guinea pig: Schofield and Cant, 1997; cat: Adams, 1979; Glendenning et al., 1981). There is little information on VCLL neuronal morphology in non-echolocating species that includes the structure of the dendrites. A comprehensive study (Zhao and Wu, 2001), performed on rats, identified four main classes of cell: stellate (I, II, and elongate) and bushy. They separated morphological classes based on the number, length and orientation of dendrites, size and shape of soma, and extent of dendritic branching.

### Cytoarchitecture and Morphology of INLL Neurons

In the cat, the INLL seems to contain predominantly multipolar cells and, to a lesser extent, horizontal cells that have finely dispersed Nissl substance and often lack a cap of Nissl substance around their nuclei. These cells resemble the multipolar cells found in the DNLL (Adams, 1979). Adams (1979) refers to the INLL as a dorsal division of the VNLL (VNLLd). In contrast, the cells of the bat INLL were very different to those of the DNLL and VNLL. Most of the INLL cells in bat are elongate or globular, and their dendrites are oriented orthogonally to the ascending lateral lemniscal fibres (Covey and Casseday, 1986). There is also a scattering of multipolar cells in this division, albeit less densely packed than in the ventral divisions. The multipolar cells here lack the columnar arrangement observed in the ventral divisions (Covey and Casseday, 1986). The Covey and Casseday (1986) study on bats also distinguished a transitional zone anteriorly, which contained medium sized globular, multipolar, and elongate cells that had a columnar organisation.

## Cytoarchitecture and Morphology of VNLL Neurons

In the echolocating bat, the multipolar (VNLLm) and the columnar (VNLLc) regions of the VNLL and their cell types are distinctive and well defined. The columnar region in particular has very distinct cytoarchitectural features; it is populated almost exclusively with small darkly staining cells (~10μm in diameter), with round or oval somas, little cytoplasm and eccentric nuclei. These cells are described as reminiscent of spherical bushy cells in the AVCN[2] in their oval to round shape and their single thick dendrite which extends some distance from the soma before branching profusely (Covey and Casseday, 1991). At least some of these dendritic branches extend parallel to the ascending fibres of the lateral lemniscus. As mentioned previously, the cells in this area are tightly packed and arranged in columns parallel to the fibres of the lateral lemniscus (Zook and Casseday, 1979; Covey and Casseday, 1986). Ventral to the columnar region is the multipolar region, or VNLLm. Most of the cells in this area have many large dendrites radiating from an irregularly shaped soma. There is also a sparse distribution of globular and elongate cells in this area. Although the cells in this multipolar region do have some preponderance to be distributed in columns, it certainly lacks the distinctive columnar organisation found in the adjacent (dorsal) VNLLc (Covey and Casseday, 1986). Furthermore, the somas and processes of cells in the VNLLm have no consistent orientation relative to the lateral lemniscal tract (Covey and Casseday, 1991). The columnar region in the moustache bat is in a different location; in this species it is the most ventral of the lateral lemniscal structures (Zook and Casseday, 1982b).

In non-echolocating species, the cell types are not so well defined. The cat VNLL contains medium and large multipolar cells in the dorsal VNLL and globular cells in the ventral zone of the VNLL (Adams, 1979, 1981). Much of the cytoarchitecture revealed in cats and guinea pigs has already been discussed. The predominant cell types discovered in these species were globular cells, giant cells, multipolar cells and vertical cells. In several species, the globular cells are segregated from other cell types (at least partially); in cats they are concentrated in the ventral region of the VNLL (Adams, 1979) and in guinea pigs their population is more numerous in the rostral zone of the ventral VNLL (VNLLv rostral) (Schofield and Cant, 1997). The segregation peaks in mice (and some bats), where they are almost completely isolated from other cell types (mouse: Willard and Ryugo, 1983; bat: Zook and Casseday, 1985; Covey and Casseday, 1986; Vater and Feng, 1990). The neuron types described by Schofield and Cant (guinea pig; 1997) correlate to some degree with the more recent study by Zhao and Wu (2001) in rat. Humans have an increased proportion of globular cells in the VNLL, although these data come from one study only (Adams, 1997).

## Cytoarchitecture and Morphology of VCLL Neurons in the Rat

One of the most cited anatomical studies in the rat VCLL found, using a combination of Nissl stained sections and injections of the tracer biotinylated dextran amine (BDA), that the VCLL seems to contain only flat stellate neurons (Merchán and Berbel, 1996). They found neurons and fibres were oriented in parallel and form anisotropic fibrodendritic laminae in the VCLL. However, in light of studies that found multiple neuronal types in the VCLL of other species (opossum: Willard and Martin, 1983; cat: Adams, 1979; bat: Zook and Casseday, 1982b), the existence of other morphological classes of neurons in the rat VCLL would seem

---

[2] This differs with the same authors' claim in their 1986 study that the cells of the VNLLc are almost exclusively "small darkly staining round to oval *multipolar* cells." Covey and Casseday, 1986, p. 2927. [italics added]

likely. Merchán and Berbel (1996) acknowledged these previous studies, particularly the Covey and Casseday (1991) bat study, and claimed that findings of elongate neurons in the INLL, round and oval neurons in the VNLLc, and multipolar neurons in the bat VNLLm may not be incompatible with the results in the rat. 3D reconstructions of the rat VCLL reveal a helicoidal lamina formed by the cells, dendrites and fibres. Merchán and Berbel (1996) argued that differences in the pattern of coiling of this lamina underlies differences in neuronal shape and appearance of each division, and may explain why other studies have identified different cell classes when it is possible that there may be only one type of cell orientated in different ways.

A more recent rat study by Zhao and Wu (2001) filled individual cells with Neurobiotin to allow direct observation of their dendritic structures (Figure 3). In this study, the authors were able to distinguish four types of neurons in two categories – bushy and stellate. The stellate neurons were of three types: stellate I, stellate II and elongate. The cell bodies of the bushy cells were round or oval, with short to medium length dendrites that bifurcated profusely into many fine endings (Zhao and Wu, 2001). These cells were found mainly in the ventral area of the VNLL. The stellate cells had fewer dendritic branches than the bushy cells. The dendritic arbors of stellate I cells had no directional preference. Elongate cells had a similar number of dendrites to stellate I, however, their cell bodies were elongated and possessed dendritic trees that ran along the longitudinal axis of the cell body. The stellate II cells had longer but fewer dendrites than the other two types. The various cell types were distributed throughout the VNLL with distributions similar to other mammals such as guinea pigs and cats.

Different types of neurons were preferentially located in different regions of the rat VNLL (Zhao and Wu, 2001). Bushy and stellate I cells from this study were localised mostly in the ventral area of the VNLL, whereas stellate II and elongate cells were localised mostly in the dorsal area. Similarly, cat and guinea pig oval and globular cells (guinea pig: Schofield and Cant, 1997; cat: Adams, 1979), which Zhao and Wu (2001) correlate with their own stellate II cells, were located mainly in the dorsal and middle zones. Zhao and Wu (2001) state that the dendritic morphology of neurons is an important feature for distinguishing neuronal types. Acknowledging the work of Merchán and Berbel (1996), they conceded that because all the cells found in the VNLL had three to seven primary dendrites, they could all be seen as multipolar cells of the same neuronal type. However, they go on to point out that upon closer examination of the dendritic morphologies, they were able to identify differences between cell types, and thus consider the VNLL to be a heterogeneous neuronal group.

The dendritic pattern of the VCLL neurons may give a clue as to their functional role: large dendrites that extend over a range of lemniscal fibres may integrate inputs from a range of frequencies, whereas small dendritic fields may be more narrowly tuned. The dendritic trees of bushy cells in the rat VCLL are smaller and more compact with a greater degree of bifurcation but a more restricted coverage than the dendritic trees of stellate cells which radiated away from the cell body and covered a relatively wide area (Zhao and Wu, 2001). Stellate II neurons (with their longer dendrites) receive input from a wider range of fibres than stellate I neurons. Elongate neurons (with their dendrites orientated in parallel with the fibres) may be involved in integrating information from a narrow band of frequencies, however, due to a small pool of results, this is merely conjecture and requires further study. All four neuron types identified by Zhao and Wu (2001) had axonal collaterals that terminated near the cell's dendritic area in a feedback mechanism.

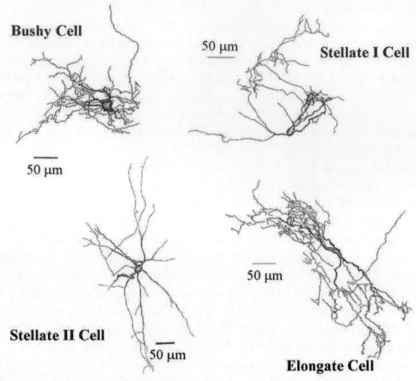

- Modified from Zhao and Wu (2001): with kind permission from John Wiley and Sons, Inc.

Figure 3. Morphology of Neurobiotin labelled neurons of the VCLL.
Camera lucida drawings of four Neurobiotin-labelled cells of the rat VCLL. The cells shown are typical examples of the four morphological types described by Zhao and Wu (2001). In all cases dorsal is at the top of the page.

In comparison with other species, it was found that the dendritic morphologies of bushy cells in the rat VNLL resembled the equivalent short compact dendritic morphologies of cells in the bat VNLLc, and cat and mouse CN (mouse: Wu and Oertel, 1984; cat: Osen, 1969; Brawer et al., 1974; bat: Covey and Casseday, 1991). The only difference being that the bushy cells in the rat VNLL appear to possess three to six primary dendrites, as opposed to one or two thick primary dendrites in the VNLLc and CN (Zhao and Wu, 2001). Parallels were also found between the dendritic features of the stellate II neurons (characterised by a small number of long dendritic branches) and multipolar neurons found in the medial section of the mouse VNLL (Willard and Ryugo, 1983) and the bat VNLLm (Covey and Casseday, 1991).

Nayagam et al (2006) filled several cells in the VCLL with Neurobiotin in the course of gathering their electrophysiological recordings *in vivo*. These cells were reconstructed digitally and their position was located within a 3D model of the VCLL. The morphologies of the cells correlated with those described previously by Zhao and Wu (2001), supporting the description of the VCLL as containing heterogeneous cell types.

## TOPOGRAPHY AND TONOTOPICITY WITHIN THE VCLL

Tonotopy refers to the spatial arrangement of frequency specific regions where sound is received, perceived or transmitted. Here, it refers to topologically neighbouring neurons in the brain that represent similarly adjacent tonal frequencies. Tonotopicity is well established as the basic principle of organisation within the mammal auditory system, from the cochlea to the cortex (for review see: Irvine, 1992). Studies have shown that the CN (various species: Masterton and Imig, 1984; cat: Bourk et al., 1981; rat: Saldaña, 1993), the LSO and MSO (cat: Elverland, 1978; Casseday and Covey, 1983; Henkel and Spangler, 1983), the DNLL (rat: Merchán et al., 1994; Kelly et al., 1995), and the central nucleus of the inferior colliculus (CNIC) (rat: Clopton and Winfield, 1973; Ryan et al., 1988; Kelly et al., 1991; Saldaña and Merchán, 1992; guinea pig: Malmierca et al., 1995; cat: Rose et al., 1963; Merzenich and Reid, 1974; Semple and Aitkin, 1979) contain neurons and fibres that are spatially oriented in isofrequency planes.

Uncovering the tonotopic arrangement, if one exists, of a given nucleus is an important step towards understanding the function of that nucleus. For example, it has become well established that in the CNIC single neurons are tuned to sound frequencies and are organised along isofrequency contours that preserve the tonotopic gradient established in the cochlea. High frequencies are represented by neurons located ventromedially and low frequencies by dorsolaterally located neurons within the CNIC (rat: Clopton and Winfield, 1973; Flammino and Clopton, 1975; Kelly et al., 1991; Kelly et al., 1998a; rabbit: Syka et al., 1981). These studies in the IC have been confirmed with both c-fos and 2-deoxyglucose (2-DG) mapping (rat: Coleman et al., 1982; Huang and Fex, 1986; Friauf, 1992). The reason that the tonotopicity of the IC has been singled out by way of example, is because there is a significant projection from the VCLL to the ipsilateral IC (rat: Beyerl, 1978; Ito et al., 1996; Merchán and Berbel, 1996). Hence, the nuclei that are the source (CN) and target (IC) of the VCLL are tonotopically organised; does it follow that, assuming a point-to-point connection, the VCLL too will be tonotopically arranged? As it turns out, this is not necessarily true.

The issue of a tonotopic arrangement in the VCLL is a highly contentious one (for review see Glendenning and Hutson, 1998). As yet, no clear layout has been agreed upon in the VCLL of rats and other mammals. Some researcher's data favour a progressive dorsal to ventral, high to low frequency, quasi-linear model (rat: Friauf, 1992; cat: Aitkin et al., 1970a), whilst others' findings suggest a more haphazard distribution, often involving multiple frequency gradients within the nuclei (bat: Covey and Casseday, 1995; Covey and Casseday, 1986; Metzner and Radtke-Schuller, 1987; Covey and Casseday, 1991). More recently, some studies have suggested a concentric lamina model with a helicoid (rat: Merchán and Berbel, 1996) or mosaic (cat: Malmierca et al., 1998) arrangement; and still others maintain that there is no tonotopicity evident in the VCLL based on various lines of evidence (cat: Adams, 1979; Glendenning et al., 1990; Glendenning and Hutson, 1998; Guinan et al., 1972a). The best way to establish a tonotopic arrangement within a given nucleus is by way of reconstructing electrophysiological recording sites. Tracing studies can only demonstrate topography of inputs and outputs. In many cases, topography of an area's connections correlates with or implies tonotopicity, as pathways through the auditory system tend to conserve the point-to-point connections of the original cochleotopicity. In the case of the VCLL, there are conflicting results and the electrophysiological data has so far not validated the findings of anatomical tracing studies that have shown a tonotopic arrangement.

## Tonotopic Organisation in the VCLL

One of the prime difficulties in describing the organisation of the VCLL is that electrophysiological studies in different mammals have yielded a diverse and complex set of results that are not easily generalised. Aitkin et al. (1970a) proposed a weak dorsal to ventral, high to low frequency representation in the cat VCLL based on a subset of their electrophysiological penetrations. However, a later electrophysiological study by Guinan et al. (cat: 1972b; 1972a) failed to confirm this finding, and found no evidence for any tonotopic trends. Similarly, 2-DG methods showed no evidence for a tonotopic map in the VCLL of the cat (Glendenning and Hutson, 1998). A medial to lateral, high to low frequency spread was found within the INLL of the horseshoe bat by Metzner and Radtke-Schuller (1987), however, no single tonotopic gradient could be discerned in the VNLL. Covey and Casseday (1991) reported multiple tonotopic maps with the VNLLc, VNLLm and INLL of the echolocating bat based on a series of electrophysiological recordings. There has only been a limited amount of electrophysiological work performed in the rat that has addressed the issue of tonotopicity (Kelly et al., 1998a; Zhang and Kelly, 2006a; Nayagam et al. 2006).

An early study by Aitkin et al. (1970a) which investigated the tonotopic organisation and discharge characteristics of cells in the cat VCLL and DNLL to monaural stimulation, mapped out the characteristic frequencies (frequency at which the cell responds with the lowest threshold; CF) obtained from a small sample of extracellular recordings. They concurred with earlier cytoarchitectonic studies (see above) which considered the DNLL and VCLL as separate midbrain structures in the cat. They found that in each of these regions neuron CFs were roughly distributed with low frequencies to high respectively dorsal to ventral (Aitkin et al., 1970a; Aitkin et al., 1970b). In the DNLL, the distribution of neurons with low and high CFs suggested that the tonotopic organisation is not strictly low to high, dorsal to ventral, but rather a concentric onion-like distribution of low to high, from inside to outside (Saint Marie et al., 1999). The VCLL progression was even less clear and this may have been caused by a non-optimal orientation of the electrode penetration with respect to the gradient of tonotopicity (Aitkin et al., 1970a). This study became accepted as the benchmark for many years despite contrary evidence from Guinan (1972b; 1972a) who did not find a tonotopic gradient within the cat VCLL using similar electrophysiological recordings. Adams (1979) also did not find evidence for tonotopicity in cat VCLL using tracing techniques. More recently, challenges to Aitkin et al.'s (1970a) proposal have surfaced.

Covey and Casseday (1986) originally performed a detailed anatomical tracing study combined with electrophysiology of the tracer injection sites to attempt to elucidate tonotopicity within the VCLL of echolocating bats (see below). In a subsequent study, Covey and Casseday (1991) attempted to find separate tonotopic representations in each cytoarchitectural and connectional subdivision using standard electrophysiological techniques. They found that the individual monaural nuclei of the bat lateral lemniscus (INLL, VNLLc and VNLLm) each have a complete tonotopic representation. Furthermore, their results suggest a concentric 'onion like' organisation within the INLL and the VNLLm, with high frequencies represented more centrally and low frequencies more peripherally. The

VNLLc was found to contain more broadly tuned units that, where possible to identify a CF, were arranged with low frequencies represented dorsally and high frequencies ventrally, similar to the original Aitkin (cat; 1970a) findings.

How do these findings in the bat relate to the dispute over the frequency representation within the cat VCLL (Aitkin et al., 1970a; Adams, 1979; Guinan et al., 1972a) and whether or not it is tonotopically organised? Assuming the connections in the cat and the bat are similar, which some studies have suggested is likely (cat: Warr, 1966; van Noort, 1969; Warr, 1969; Roth et al., 1978; Glendenning et al., 1981), Covey and Casseday (bat; 1986) the cat VCLL would be expected to have multiple rather than single tonotopic representations. Covey and Casseday (bat; 1991) point out that although other studies on cat found either a single dorsal to ventral tonotopic representation (Aitkin et al., 1970a) or no tonotopicity (Guinan et al., 1972b; Guinan et al., 1972a), it is possible that multiple tonotopic organisations were missed because of the small sample sizes. They suggest that there is a homology between connections in the echolocating bat and other mammals, with the exception of a small binaural area in the ventral nucleus of the cat.

In the rat, Kelly et al. (1998a) made electrophysiological recordings from single neurons of the DNLL, but in the process recorded from cells of the INLL and other surrounding structures as well. They reported that reconstructions of electrode penetrations along several angles oblique to the dorsoventral axis did not reveal any patterns of tonotopicity within the DNLL or the INLL, both from individual animals and across the sample. However, the authors do concede a number of limiting factors that may impede their ability to detect tonotopic organisation. These factors are: a relatively high margin of error in localising extracellular recordings due to the small size of the nucleus, difficulty in sampling enough neurons to cover the full range of frequencies in a single electrode penetration, and non-linear maps are difficult to detect with straight electrodes (Kelly et al., 1998a). Furthermore, as this study used extracellular recordings, despite efforts to ensure that recordings were of neurons and not fibres of passage, a possibility of contamination exists. A more recent and more detailed extracellular electrophysiological study of the rat VCLL has also reported a lack of apparent tonotopicity along the dorsoventral axis (Zhang and Kelly, 2006a), however they did not examine possible 3D tonotopic distributions along the rostrocaudal or lateromedial axes.

Nayagam et al. (2006) recently used a combination of intracellular electrophysiology and 3D computer-assisted reconstructions of VCLL recording sites to create a more accurate map of the VCLL than previously attempted. This technique reduces the constraints previously faced by the extracellular electrophysiological studies without 3D reconstructions and allows a greater degree of insight into potential tonotopicity. The data from their study did not reveal any clear evidence of tonotopicity, even when rotated and examined from all directions (Figure 4). They did not report any frequency organisation within single tracks or when reconstructed across many animals. However, this technique would not be able to show a helical or complex mosaic tonotopic distribution if the position of the helix/mosaic was different, with respect to the VCLL, from one animal to another.

The overall picture from electrophysiological studies is that there is no obvious tonotopicity within the VCLL. Certainly in non-echolocating species, with the exception of the indistinct single gradient proposed by Aitkin (cat; 1970a), no evidence for tonotopicity has been demonstrated. However, the possibility of tonotopicity cannot be completely ruled out. This lack of obvious tonotopicity is unusual amongst brainstem nuclei and some have described the VCLL as unique based on this characteristic (cat: Glendenning and Hutson,

1998). Table 2 summarises results of studies investigating potential tonotopicity in the VCLL of non-echolocating species using electrophysiological techniques.

**Table 2. Tonotopic organisation in the VCLL determined by electrophysiological studies in non-echolocating mammalian species.**

| Author(s)/Year | Species | Tonotopicity | Techniques |
|---|---|---|---|
| Aitkin et al. (1970a) | Cat | Dorsal – Ventral; Low – High frequency | Extracellular recordings *in vivo* |
| Guinan et al. (1972b; 1972a) | Cat | No evidence found | Extracellular recordings *in vivo* |
| Kelly et al. (1998a) | Rat | No evidence found | Extracellular recordings *in vivo* |
| Zhang and Kelly (2006a) | Rat | No evidence found | Extracellular recordings *in vivo* |
| Nayagam et al. (2006) | Rat | No-evidence found | Intracellular recordings *in vivo* with 3D reconstructions |

## Topographic Organisation of the VCLL with Respect to Inputs and Outputs

Anatomical tracing studies, using restricted injections of retrograde tracer into the IC, as well as injections of anterograde tracer into the VCLL itself, have attempted to describe the topography of the VCLL with respect to the established tonotopicity of the target IC nuclei. The major projection from the VNLL to the IC is inhibitory, and it is not necessarily the case that projection neurons in the VNLL have the same CF as their IC target (various species: Oertel and Wickesberg, 2002). This is an important point to bear in mind when reviewing results from anatomical tracing studies. Tracing studies can highlight the organisation of neurons' connections as well as visualise the organisation of the underlying fibrodendritic laminae of a given nucleus. The arrangement of the extracellular matrix and the fibrodendritic laminae of the VCLL is uncertain. Different visualisation techniques have yielded different results across species. Many descriptions of the VCLL topography have been proposed, including horizontal bands of spindle neurons (rat: Moore and Moore, 1987; cat: Roth et al., 1978; Adams, 1979; Brunso-Bechtold et al., 1981), fibres in a ladder rung pattern known as cross-bridges (cat: Glendenning et al., 1981; Spangler et al., 1985) and multiple laminae representations in bats (Covey and Casseday, 1991). Table 3 summarises the results of studies investigating potential topographic organisations of the VCLL in non-echolocating species using tracing and activation techniques.

Merchán and Berbel (1996) interpret the various aforementioned descriptions of topography (horizontal bands, cross-bridges, and multiple laminae) in the VCLL as consistent with a helicoidal organisation. Their rat study lends support to the spiral organisation first proposed by Willard and Martin (1983) in the North American opossum. Willard and Martin (1983) also considered the VCLL a single nucleus and described the dendritic arrangement within the VCLL as a tightly woven helical spiral that encircles columns of lemniscal fibres.

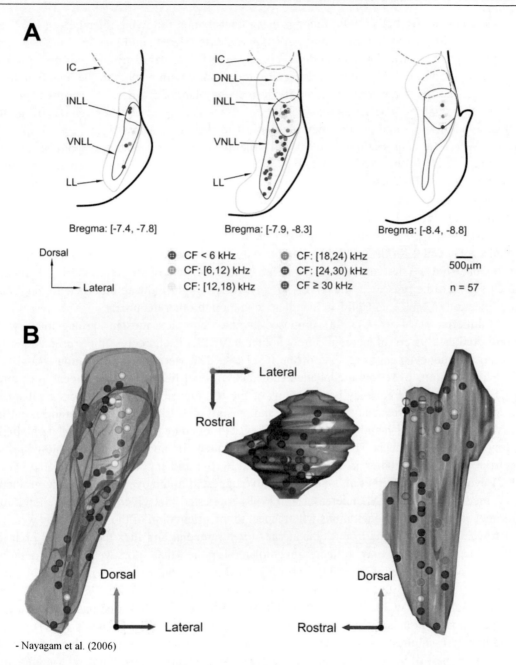

Figure 4. Spatial distribution of intracellular unit's CF within the VCLL.
**A:** Standard coronal sections of the rat's VCLL collapsed from 3 rostrocaudal ranges (given in Bregma coordinates, under each section), from most rostral (left) to most caudal (right). Outlines of major structures are shown, and there is some overlap between nuclei delineations due to the collapsing process. Unit CFs are given in ranges and are colour coded from low frequency (red) to high frequency (violet). **B:** Computer generated semi-opaque surface model of the VCLL showing the same distribution of units as in (A) but visualised in three dimensions. The viewing aspect of the reconstruction is taken from rostral (left), dorsal (middle) and lateral (right). Orthogonal orientation arrows represent 500 μm and are colour coded (dorsal – green, lateral – red and rostral – blue).

Merchán and Berbel's (1996) findings using tract-tracing following injections of BDA, as well as combination injections of horseradish peroxidase (HRP) and biocytin combined with 3D computer reconstructions, supported a dorsoventral helicoidal distribution of neurons and processes. In addition, they found a concentric topography with respect to the tonotopic map of the IC. The helicoids were arranged in isofrequency laminae, whereby neurons from the central helicoidal laminae send projections to ventromedial high frequency regions of the IC and peripheral helicoidal laminae neurons project to dorsolateral low-frequency portions of the IC. When viewing sections of the VCLL, the individual coils of the helicoids appear as horizontal bands. When reconstructed in 3D, the true nature of the helicoidal structure becomes apparent. These horizontal bands are reminiscent of c-Fos immunoreactive horizontal bands that have been observed after pure tone stimulation (rat: Friauf, 1992). Merchán and Berbel hypothesised that their horizontal bands could therefore correspond to the isofrequency planes indicated by the Friauf (1992) study. In addition, their helicoidal model may account for the multiple tonotopic representations found in Covey and Casseday's (1991) bat study. They also noted a similar concentric pattern of fibrodendritic laminae, which seems to be present in the VNLL of cats, which might indicate that their findings for the projection of VNLL to CNIC in the rat are common to other mammals.

Malmierca et al. (cat; 1998) proposed a new 'complex mosaic' arrangement with interdigitating clusters of neurons throughout the VCLL, each representing projections to different frequency-specific regions of the IC. These data were based on computer-assisted 3D reconstructions of retrograde-labelled cells and terminal fibres, following focal injections of BDA in different frequency band regions of the IC (Figure 5). These authors challenged the idea of a single frequency gradient and the recently published helicoidal arrangement in the VNLL (rat: Merchán and Berbel, 1996). They also found an overall medial to lateral, high to low frequency gradient. The authors claimed that their findings were compatible with the electrophysiological studies in cat (Aitkin et al., 1970a) and rabbit (Batra and Fitzpatrick, 1997) even though Aitkin et al.'s (1970a) study suggested a dorsoventral tonotopic gradient not a mediolateral one. Malmierca et al. (1998) suggested that given the oblique angle of Aitkin et al.'s electrode penetrations with respect to the orientation of the VCLL, they were in fact traversing the nucleus from dorsolateral to ventromedial and thus the recorded high to low sequence of CFs may reflect a mediolateral rather than dorsoventral distribution. Similarly, Malmierca et al.'s (1998) reasoning for drawing comparisons with the rabbit was based on Batra and Fitzpatrick (1997) recordings of single units with CFs < 2kHz in the medial region of the VCLL. Malmierca et al. (1998) also describe their findings as compatible with previous anatomical studies, in particular those of Whitley and Henkel's (1984). They found that their smallest, medial injection on the edge of the VNLL, which produced labelling in the lateral part of the CNIC, could be interpreted as evidence for mediolateral tonotopicity (cat: Whitley and Henkel, 1984).

Kelly et al. (1998b) performed two studies to investigate the topography of the rat's lateral lemniscal nuclei. Although the studies tended to concentrate on the DNLL and the emerging theory of a concentric onion-like frequency representation, the VNLL was also examined. They found distinct bands in the INLL and VNLL when retrograde tracer was injected into the low frequency region of the ipsilateral IC. They were considering the INLL and VNLL as a single nucleus, much like Merchán and Berbel (1996) (see above). However, Kelly et al. (1998b) retained the terms INLL and VNLL to distinguish between different positions along the lemniscal pathway. A similar injection into middle and high frequency areas of the IC resulted in a more even distributions throughout the INLL and VNLL with less evidence of banding. Injections into IC regions representing frequencies above ~20kHz showed no evidence of banding in the VNLL or INLL. The difference was not due to inconsistent spread of tracer as other auditory brainstem nuclei showed highly localised patterns of high and low frequency labelled areas following the same injections. The findings of Kelly et al. (1998b) therefore support, in part, the findings by Merchán and Berbel (1996) of a banded pattern of labelling, but only for frequencies below 20 kHz.

**Table 3. Topographic organisation in the VCLL determined by tracing and 2-DG activation studies in non-echolocating species.**

| Author(s)/Year | Species | Topography | Techniques |
|---|---|---|---|
| Whitley and Henkel (1984) | Cat | Widespread divergent projection to IC with specific variations | Anterograde / autoradiographic tracing from VCLL to IC |
| Merchán and Berbel (1996) | Rat | Concentric Helicoid. Peripheral – Central; Low – High frequency | Retrograde tracing from IC to VCLL; 3D reconstructions |
| Malmierca et al. (1998) | Cat | Complex but orderly mosaic of frequency representations. Medial – Lateral; High – Low frequency | Retrograde tracing from IC to VCLL; 3D reconstructions |
| Glendenning and Hutson (1998) | Cat | No Evidence Found. Randomly distributed clusters after trracing. Widespread activation of 2-DG | Triple injections (into high, middle and low frequency regions of IC) and retrograde tracing from IC to VCLL. 2-DG with tonal stimulation in high middle or low frequency ranges |
| Langner et al. (2006) | Gerbil | Low – High; Dorsal – Ventral. Helical periodicity map | 2-DG activation. Retrograde tracing from IC to VCLL |
| Benson and Cant (2008) | Gerbil | Topographic organisation from: CN to VCLL- high frequencies central, low frequencies lateral and caudal; VCLL to IC - relationship between frequencies axid of IC and medial-lateral position in VCLL | Anterograde (from CN) and retrograde from (IC) tracing of focal injections of BDA. |

The bands of labelling in the VNLL found in the Kelly et al. (1998) study and the Merchán and Berbel (1996) study are reminiscent of the findings of other researchers that used c-fos activation following pure tone stimulation (rat: Friauf, 1992) or retrograde tracing from the IC (cat: Roth et al., 1978; Glendenning et al., 1981). The laddering of afferent projections from the contralateral CN to the VNLL, similar to those found by Merchán and Berbel (1996) and Kelly et al. (1998) in the rat (from efferent projections to the IC), has also been reported in the rat (Friauf and Ostwald, 1988; Kandler and Friauf, 1993). It has been suggested that the banding may be caused by periodic ladder-rung like collaterals being given off by ascending fibres from the CN to the IC and passing through the VCLL (rat: Merchán and Berbel, 1996). This implies that the topography indicated by the banding of CN inputs is reflected in bands of VNLL cells that project to a specific frequency region in the IC.

In an attempt to uncover topography, Glendenning and Hutson (cat; 1998) used a combination of 2-DG (followed by tonal stimulation at high, middle or low frequencies) or retrograde triple labelling (injected into high, middle and low frequency regions of the IC) techniques to visualise any potential spatial maps of frequency. Both methods yielded well-organised tonotopically arranged cell labelling in brainstem nuclei with the exception of the VCLL. Retrograde labelling revealed clusters of neurons randomly distributed throughout the VCLL. 2-DG was activated throughout the VCLL, in support of the retrograde transport. This finding is consistent with the anterograde tracing studies of Whitley and Henkel (cat: 1984) which found widespread divergent projections from the VCLL to the IC. Glendenning and Hutson (1998) concluded that there is no apparent orderliness of the cat VCLL afferents or efferents with respect to frequency.

Recent studies in the gerbil (Langner et al., 2006; Benson and Cant, 2008) have examined the connections from the CN through the VCLL to the CNIC. Both studies have demonstrated a topography in these afferent and efferent connections. Langner et al. (2006) suggested a helical organisation best fitted their 2-DG activation and retrograde tracing data. Benson and Cant (2008) concluded that a lateral to medial distribution in the VCLL is topographically related to the established frequency axis of the IC. They recommend future electrophysiological studies would be wise to consider a horizontal rather than the more traditional dorso-ventral approach to uncover potential tonotopic maps arising from this pattern of connectivity. They also described a concentric pattern of connections from frequency specific regions of the CN to the centre (high frequency) or periphery (low frequency) of the VCLL. Their results are compatible with previous descriptions of VCLL topography in other species (rat: Merchán and Berbel, 1996; opossum: Willard and Martin, 1983; mouse: Willard and Ryugo, 1983; cat: Warr, 1982) and lends strong support to the case for a clear topography in the afferents and efferents to and from the VCLL.

## Tonotopic and Topographic Organisation of the Echolocating Bat VCLL

In the bat, the situation is somewhat different and both topography and tonotopicty of the VCLL has been described after anatomical tracing studies, but with limited electrophysiological confirmation. Covey and Casseday (Covey and Casseday, 1995; 1986; 1991) found frequency gradients within the VCLL (INLL and VNLL) of the big brown bat. The columnar area of the VNLL (VNLLc) was organised with projections from low frequency neurons located dorsally and projections from high frequency cells ventrally, but other areas of VNLL and INLL were not as well organised. Covey and Casseday (1986) studied tonotopicity within the VCLL of echolocating bats, using a combination of retrograde labelling, anterograde labelling and electrophysiology. They recorded the CFs of neurons at the tracer injection sites in the AVCN and the IC to provide an indication of the frequency of the anterogradely or retrogradely labelled cells in the columnar region of the VNLL. The labelled cells were not entirely located within the columnar region; however, this is the area that they concentrated on since its connections seemed more precisely organised than other nuclei of the lateral lemniscus. They found an orderly progression of dorsal to ventral, low to high frequencies in the columnar area, VNLLc. Their findings appeared to agree with the Aitkin et al. (1970a) study in the cat. However, the results in the bat are more complicated than a simple dorsoventral distribution of CFs. Anterograde and retrogradely labelled cells in the VNLLc were arranged in "sheets" that were aligned orthogonally to the lemniscal fibres. The thickness, extent and orientation of these sheets were determined by the tonotopic range of the injection site as opposed to the amount of tracer injected. In other words, a large

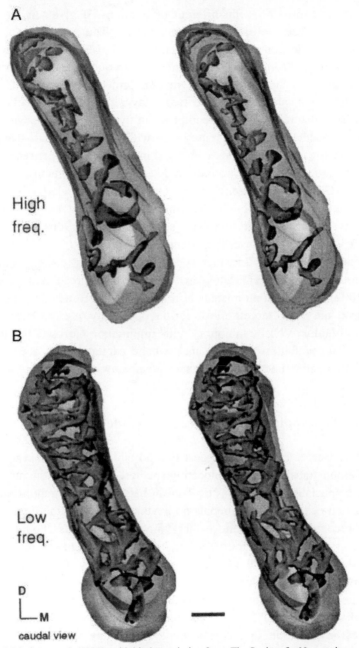

- Modified from Malmierca et al. (1998): with kind permission from The Society for Neuroscience

Figure 5. Stereo-images of 3D distribution of retrograde label within the VCLL of the rat following injections into high and low frequency regions of the IC.

Computer generated stereo pairs showing the VCLL viewed from the caudal aspect. Retrogradely labelled clusters are shown as DARK shaded fragments within the solid VCLL surface. **A:** Shows labelled clusters which are mainly located adjacent to the rostrolateral surface following focal injections of BDA into high frequency regions of the IC. **B:** Shows labelled clusters, which are more widely distributed following focal injections of BDA into low frequency regions of the IC. To visualise the 3D image for each pair the viewer must cross their eyes such that the stereo pairs merge into a single image with the illusion of depth. Scale bar is 500 µm. D: dorsal, M: medial.

injection and a small injection with different orientations, if given in the same frequency range, will produce sheets of similar characteristics. The precise relationship between tonotopicity and the projection sheets was explained by Covey and Casseday (1986) in terms of divergent projections from a point within an isofrequency contour within the AVCN forming a sheet in the columnar area, that in turn projected (converged) to another sheet within the IC, thus maintaining the same frequency representation as the original AVCN source. The authors also referred to the compression that must be occurring in the system to allow the entire frequency range to be represented within the very small space of the VNLLc. Two possible scenarios arise from this compression: first, each sheet represents a relatively broad range of frequencies, and second, only selected frequencies are represented by individual sheets (Covey and Casseday, 1986). There was also a relative 'over-representation' of the 25 – 50 kHz range within the IC which corresponded to the range of frequency modulated (FM) echolocation in the bats studied. Whether this over-representation is occurring at the VNLLc or at a lower level remains unknown.

In tracing studies of the VCLL, the ascending projections to the ipsilateral IC imply a haphazard tonotopic arrangement; they are uneven, widespread and patchy (Oertel and Wickesberg, 2002). This apparent mismatch in frequency representations between the VCLL projection neuron and the IC targets allows for the possibility of cross-frequency interactions. In the bat, broadly tuned VNLLc inhibitory units impinge on narrowly tuned IC targets. This pattern of wideband inhibition acting on narrowband excitation has been observed in other species and is of potential functional importance (see below).

## Evaluation of Tonotopic and Topographic Models

Merchán and Berbel (rat: 1996) suggest two possibilities given that a clear tonotopicity has yet to be demonstrated in non-echolocating species, particularly the rat. First, that VNLL tonotopicity is a specialisation that has evolved in bats to support echolocation in some way or second, that non-echolocating mammals do have some kind of tonotopic arrangement that has yet to be recognised. They believe that tonotopicity in rats should not be ruled out. However, there are a third and/or fourth possibility worth stating here: that tonotopicity is not necessary for the function of the VCLL or, more specifically, that broadly tuned elements (that do not support a tonotopic arrangement) are *necessary* for the VCLL's function.

Several topographical organisation schemes have been proposed and evidence given to support each of them. Typically, when evaluating conflicting scientific arguments, one looks for the simplest explanation that can account for all the variables without introducing unnecessary complications (Occam's razor). In this case, the helicoidal models are certainly more complex than single gradients, multiple gradients or lack of tonotopicity. However, the various, seemingly incongruent observations across species (isofrequency banding, multiple gradients, mediolateral as well as dorsoventral frequency arrangements) may be explained by a helicoidal configuration. Ultimately, whether the tonotopic or topographic model is one of a continuous distribution, a multiple representation, a helicoid, a 3D cluster of interdigitating laminae, a combination of these, a disparate ensemble of these models in different species, or simply none at all, is a matter for future studies to attempt to determine.

## CONNECTIONS OF THE VENTRAL NUCLEUS OF THE LATERAL LEMNISCUS

### Ascending Auditory Afferents to the VCLL

In response to sound, early studies considered the VCLL to be a monaural structure (cat: Aitkin et al., 1970a; Brugge et al., 1970b; Guinan et al., 1972b) and believed that the major projections to the VCLL were from the contralateral VCN and ipsilateral SOC. However, binaural units within the VCLL and bilateral projections to the VCLL from several brainstem nuclei, including the VCN and SOC, were subsequently identified (Batra and Fitzpatrick, 2002b; guinea pig: Schofield and Cant, 1997; cat: Glendenning et al., 1981; rabbit: Batra and Fitzpatrick, 1999).

The most comprehensive attempt to identify all the ascending afferents to the NLL was performed by Glendenning et al. (cat: 1981) and became the benchmark for subsequent studies. The researchers used anterograde degeneration, retrograde HRP techniques and auto-radiographic analysis to trace the ascending afferents to the various nuclei of the lateral lemniscus. The present review will concentrate on the projections to the 'monaural' nuclei (VCLL), omitting the DNLL. The aim of their study was not to specify which cell classes gave rise to specific inputs, but rather to provide an indication of which nuclei project to the VCLL. Recall the subdivisions proposed by Glendenning et al. (1981) included the INLL as a separate nucleus, and for now the INLL and VNLL will be discussed separately. At the time of the study it was already well established that the main route of fibres to the VNLL was from the contralateral VCN via the trapezoid body and then rostral via the lateral band of the contralateral lateral lemniscus (rat: Browner and Webster, 1975; monkey: Strominger and Strominger, 1971; cat: Warr, 1966; van Noort, 1969; Warr, 1969, 1972; Brunso-Bechtold and Thompson, 1978). In addition, a few fibres had been traced from the CN via the dorsal acoustic stria to the contralateral VNLL (cat: van Noort, 1969; Warr, 1969; Osen, 1972; Warr, 1972; Adams and Warr, 1976). HRP bolus injections restricted to the VNLL showed retrogradely labelled cells almost exclusively in the VCN (almost 90% of labelled cells) with three times as many cells in the AVCN compared to the PVCN. Only five out of nine hundred and ninety-four cells were labelled in the DCN. These findings confirmed the earlier work in other animals using a variety of techniques (rat: Browner and Webster, 1975; monkey: Strominger and Strominger, 1971; cat: Stotler, 1953; Harrison and Warr, 1962; Warr, 1966; van Noort, 1969; Warr, 1969, 1972). This domination of direct projections from the CN to neurons of the VNLL is what set it apart from the DNLL. In cats, a small, unique dorsomedial region of the VNLL also seemed to receive substantial projections from the ipsilateral VCN via the trapezoid body (cat: Glendenning, 1981). This supported reports of ipsilateral input from the VCN in other species, although the segregation of ipsilateral and contralateral projections may not be as clear as in cats (rat: Browner and Webster, 1975; monkey: Strominger and Strominger, 1971; guinea pig: Schofield and Cant, 1997; cat: Warr, 1969). There have been previous reports of minor projections from the SOC to the VNLL, but far less than was present in the DNLL (cat: Stotler, 1953; Elverland, 1978). The earlier studies generally agreed that the LSO alone projects bilaterally to the NLL (various species: Niemer and Cheng, 1949; rat: Browner and Webster, 1975; cat: Stotler, 1953; van Noort, 1969; Elverland, 1978; bat: Zook and Casseday, 1979). The MSO was found to be the source of strictly ipsilateral ascending projections, some of which terminated in the VNLL (cat: Elverland, 1978). In addition, the LSO was found not to project to the VNLL, although ascending bilaterally. Glendenning et al. (1981) agreed with these previous findings and noted that the majority of nuclei of the SOC contribute to the projections to the VNLL, including the MNTB, MSO, LSO and the periolivary nuclei. The primary contributors are the MNTB, VNTB and other periolivary nuclei, which make up 90% of the afferents from the SOC (Glendenning et al., 1981).

Tracing studies have also provided evidence of cross-bridges, which are collaterals of ascending fibres that traverse the nuclei laterally (ladder-like rungs), from SOC projections that turn at right angles to the primary ascending axons travelling to the IC (cat: van Noort, 1969; Elverland, 1978). Glendenning et al. (1981) stated that further investigation was required to address the issue of cross-bridges, however, after ablations of the CN or SOC the degenerating anterograde material showed thin bridges between the medial and lateral bands of the lateral lemniscus, passing through the NLL. These degenerating bridges were larger and more obvious after SOC ablations than CN ablations (Glendenning et al., 1981). 'Cross-bridged cells' have previously been noted by Roth et al. (cat; 1978) after HRP injections in the IC. Glendenning et al. (1981) postulated that the horizontal cells described by Adams (cat; 1979) may provide a substrate for the cross-bridges. They go on to suggest that there may be a connection between their own findings of cross-bridged degenerating fibres, Adams' horizontal cells and Roth et al.'s HRP labelled horizontal bridges (cat: Roth et al., 1978; Adams, 1979; Glendenning et al., 1981). Cross bridges have implications in sound processing as they provide a means for convergence of input from the SOC and CN onto cells at many levels of the NLL.

HRP injections into the INLL result in labelled cells throughout the AVCN (large and multipolar cells), as well as most of the PVCN (excluding the OCA). These injections also labelled many cells in the LNTB, the ventral part of the trapezoid body and the MNTB, but not the MSO or LSO (bat: Zook and Casseday, 1987). In contrast, similar injections into the VNLL of bats do label cells in the octopus cell region of the PVCN (Zook and Casseday, 1979). Cat studies (Glendenning et al., 1981) support the findings in bat, in that, for the most part, the projections to the INLL are very similar to those of the VNLL, and arise mainly from the AVCN. However, there are nonetheless differences in the projection patterns to INLL and to VNLL. In particular, the projection from the SOC to the INLL is different to the projection from the SOC to the VNLL or DNLL; the INLL receives major projections from the MNTB, and, in the bat, from the LNTB as well (bat Zook and Casseday, 1987; cat: Glendenning et al., 1981). Although previous studies did not find a projection to the INLL from the contralateral NLL, Glendenning et al. (1981) did find a very sparse projection (1%-2%) from the contralateral DNLL. However, the INLL may yet be distinguished from the DNLL by the absence of a larger (13%) commissural projection between DNLLs (cat: Glendenning, 1981).

### Sources of Excitatory and Inhibitory inputs to the VCLL

All principal cell groups of the VCN project to the VNLL: small and large spherical bushy cells, globular bushy cells, octopus cells and type I multipolar (T stellate) cells (for review see: Cant and Benson, 2003). In a study on rat, the synaptic physiology of the VNLL was investigated by examining synaptic potentials of VNLL neurons in response to electrical stimulation of the lateral lemniscus ventral to the VNLL (Wu, 1999). The author suggested that, although inhibitory post-synaptic potentials (IPSPs) are present and somewhat obscure the excitatory post-synaptic potentials (EPSPs), some of the short latency, large amplitude and short duration EPSPs observed in cells with an onset response to stimulation (see below) may be from octopus cells in the PVCN (Wu, 1999). This study also found medium-sized bead-like boutons in the VNLL that probably originated from bushy or stellate (multipolar) cells in the AVCN and PVCN which send thin axons through the VNLL en route to the IC (see also; various species: Schwartz, 1992; rat: Friauf and Ostwald, 1988; mouse: Iwahori, 1986; guinea pig: Schofield and Cant, 1997; bat: Covey, 1993a). Presumably these smaller synaptic connections would result in the lower amplitude and longer latency EPSPs recorded in the Wu (1999) study. Since the AVCN projection to the IC is excitatory (cat: Oliver, 1987), and the VNLL receives collaterals from this projection, it is likely that the AVCN provides excitatory inputs to cells in the VNLL as well, probably using glutamate or aspartate as a neurotransmitter (rat: Zhao and Wu, 2001; guinea pig: Suneja et al., 1995).

Zhao and Wu (2001) suggested that the source of EPSPs in the rat VNLL was probably from octopus, bushy and stellate (multipolar) cells in the VCN. EPSPs recorded from stellate I cells in the VCLL generated only one suprathreshold action potential (AP) and were short in duration. In comparison, EPSPs recorded from stellate II and elongate cells were much longer and generated many APs. The short EPSPs may be due to low input resistance or may be due to the influence of IPSPs truncating the EPSPs. Further study involving pharmacological manipulation was recommended to clarify this issue (Zhao and Wu, 2001).

Both bushy and stellate cells in the VNLL receive inhibitory projections which lead to IPSPs that were recorded by Zhao and Wu (2001). IPSPs in the VCLL may be originating from cells in the ipsilateral MNTB and periolivary nuclei (cat: Warr and Beck, 1996; Elverland, 1978; Glendenning et al., 1981; Spangler et al., 1985; bat: Vater and Feng, 1990; Huffman and Covey, 1995). Collaterals of glycinergic (guinea pig: Helfert et al., 1989) projections from the MNTB principal neurons bound for the LSO and GABAergic neurons from VNTB and LNTB (rat: Moore and Moore, 1987; guinea pig: Helfert et al., 1989; González-Hernández et al., 1996; gerbil: Roberts and Ribak, 1987; cat: Adams and Mugnaini, 1990; bat: Vater et al., 1992; Winer et al., 1995) are other possible sources of IPSPs in the VCLL (Zhao and Wu, 2001). Another possible source of IPSPs within the VCLL is from internal intrinsic projections (further discussion below). The presence of synaptic potentials mediated by many different neurotransmitters, both excitatory and inhibitory (AMPA, NMDA, GABA$_A$, Glycine) in individual cells of the VCLL further supports an integrative and processing role rather than simple relay of signals within the auditory system (rat: Irfan et al., 2005).

## Major Ascending Efferents from the VCLL

### The VNLL is a Major Source of Inhibition to the IC

The DNLL projects bilaterally to the CNIC, whilst the VNLL primarily projects ipsilaterally to the CNIC in many mammalian species (rat: Beyerl, 1978; Druga and Syka, 1984; Tokunaga et al., 1984; Tanaka et al., 1985; Coleman and Clerici, 1987; opossum: Willard and Martin, 1983; mouse: Willard and Ryugo, 1983; mole: Kudo et al., 1990; guinea pig: Shneiderman et al., 1993; Nordeen, 1983; ferret: Moore, 1988; cat: van Noort, 1969; Roth et al., 1978; Adams, 1979; Brunso-Bechtold et al., 1981; Glendenning et al., 1981; Glendenning and Masterton, 1983; Saint Marie and Baker, 1990; Hutson et al., 1991; bat:

Schweizer, 1981; Zook and Casseday, 1982a, b; Frisina et al., 1989). Retrograde tracing studies indicate that 25-50% of the projections to the IC originate from the VNLL (mole: Kudo et al., 1990; ferret: Moore, 1988; cat: Roth et al., 1978; Brunso-Bechtold et al., 1981; bat: Ross et al., 1988; Ross and Pollak, 1989). Nearly 68% of the glycinergic projections to the IC (identified with retrograde labelling of tritiated glycine) are from the VNLL (cat: Saint Marie and Baker, 1990) and, coupled with the high proportion of glycinergic and GABAergic cells identified within the VNLL (rat: Moore and Moore, 1987; Aoki et al., 1988; Campos et al., 2001; Riquelme et al., 2001; gerbil: Roberts and Ribak, 1987; Saint Marie and Baker, 1990; bat: Vater et al., 1992; Winer et al., 1995), provides strong evidence for the VNLL being the major source of inhibitory input to the IC. The extent of the terminations within the IC also suggest that the VNLL is well placed to widely influence IC responses (guinea pig: Schofield and Cant, 1997).

In addition to the projection to the CNIC, sparse projections from the dorsal VNLL to the external cortex of the IC, medial geniculate body, DNLL, dorsomedial periolivary region and the VNTB have been described (chinchilla: Morest et al., 1997; cat: Kudo, 1981; Whitley and Henkel, 1983, 1984; Kudo and Nakamura, 1988). A projection from giant multipolar cells of the VNLLv to the auditory thalamus is interesting as it appears to bypass the IC, and this sub-collicular projection has been described in cats (Henkel, 1983) and some species of bats (Casseday et al., 1989). There are also some minor projections to the superior colliculus (rat: Tanaka et al., 1985; cat: Kudo, 1981; bat: Casseday and Covey, 1983). Some recent studies have identified small numbers of cholinergic neurons within the VCLL (guinea pig: Motts et al. 2008; goldfish: Giraldez-Perez et al., 2009) and have proposed that acetylcholine may play a role in auditory processing. However, the source of these cholinergic projections and their precise circuitry within the auditory brainstem remains unknown.

Few studies have explicitly investigated the INLL's projections separately from the VNLL. However, it has been suggested that the INLL projects to both the contralateral and ipsilateral CNIC in the cat (Brunso-Bechtold et al., 1981). Unlike the VNLL, the INLL has been identified as an excitatory structure (cat: Saint Marie et al., 1997).

## Intrinsic Projections of the VCLL

Adams (1979) described a population of oval cells in the ventral VNLL of the cat that were not stained by retrograde HRP label following widespread injections in the IC. He believed that these oval cells projected internally within the VCLL. The oval cells were described as having large endbulbs and resembled the principle cells of the MNTB (Adams, 1979). They received a thick axon input which originated from octopus cells of the PVCN (guinea pig: Schofield and Cant, 1997; cat: Adams, 1997). Other studies have also described both bushy and stellate cells in the middle and ventral zones of the VNLL that project to other cells within the VNLL (rat: Zhao and Wu, 2001; cat: Whitley and Henkel, 1984), typically as collaterals or descending branches of an ascending projection to the IC (Zhao and Wu, 2001). The local projections typically terminate in bouton terminals within the ventral part of the VCLL and most likely form inhibitory circuits (Zhao and Wu, 2001). The nature and function of these intrinsic projections within the VCLL have been described as "the missing key piece in this puzzle" (Merchán et al., 1997 p. 214). Nayagam et al. (2005, 2006) recently proposed a function for these inhibitory VNLL interneurons. They suggested that this intrinsic circuit within the VCLL was activated by octopus cells of the contralateral PVCN and provided fast inhibitory control of action potential timing in the VCLL, and by extension, the IC as well. This circuit will be described in more detail below.

## Input from the Octopus Cell Area and Calyceal Synapses in the VCLL

### Characteristics of Input to the VCLL from Octopus Cells

VNLL neurons receive convergent excitatory input from a variety of cell types within the contralateral CN (rat: Zhao and Wu, 2001; cat: Glendenning et al., 1981), including a predominantly exclusive projection (with the occasional collateral to the SOC) from the OCA of the contralateral CN (guinea pig: Schofield and Cant, 1997; cat: Adams, 1997, Smith et al., 2005). Octopus cells respond to the onsets of sounds with exquisitely timed responses (cat: Godfrey et al., 1975; Rhode and Smith, 1986), termed onset-ideal ($O_I$). This response pattern is a result of the detection of synchrony in auditory nerve fibre inputs representing a wide range of CFs (Oertel et al., 2000; mouse: Golding et al., 1995). Consequently, octopus cells are very broadly tuned to sound stimulus frequency and often it is not possible to distinguish a CF for these cells. The function of these cells is unknown, although they seem well suited to encode onsets, transients, and temporal features of complex, periodic stimuli (Oertel and Wickesberg, 2002).

### Characteristics of Calyceal Synapses in the VCLL Of Mammals

Some afferent projections to the VNLL terminate in specialised calyceal synapses. Similar large synaptic connections known as 'endbulbs of Held', are described in the AVCN (cat: Ibata and Pappas, 1976; Ryugo and Sento, 1991), others known as 'calyces of Held' have been found in the MNTB (cat: Morest, 1968; rat: Lenn and Reese, 1966; various species: Morest and Jean-Baptiste, 1975). First described by Held (1893), this specialisation in some subcollicular neurons is essentially a secure synapse that typically leads to faithful one-to-one transmission of input to output (cat: Adams, 1997). This synapse allows the precise timing information contained in nerve fibre discharges to be preserved within the AVCN, thereby allowing a faithful representation of the original auditory stimulus. Studies on the AVCN and the MNTB calyces have shown that one AP in the presynaptic axon generates one AP in the postsynaptic cell (cat: Guinan and Li, 1990). However, this does not necessarily lead to the conclusion that the postsynaptic cell faithfully reflects the primary input, as it is possible that other sources may modify the output (gerbil: Kopp-Scheinpflug et al., 2002; bat: Vater et al., 1997).The calyx consists of a large and complex terminal which envelops a high proportion of the post-synaptic cell and may incorporate multiple synapses (Adams, 1997).

Stotler (cat; 1953) first described large calyces in the VNLL and Pfeiffer (cat; 1966) first reported their physiological properties, discovering by means of extracellular recordings that the post-synaptic APs would faithfully follow the pre-synaptic potentials with a fixed delay of approximately 0.5 msec. This discovery of VCLL cells that receive a calyx-like synapse is important as it allows insight into the properties of the cell from which the projection originated (by examining the pre-synaptic potentials in single-cell recordings). Furthermore, the fact that the VCLL contains calyces suggests that it plays an important role in coding auditory timing information.

Subsequent to the discovery in cats, specialised calyceal synaptic endings have been described now in the VCLL of many mammalian species. Typically these calyceal endings are not distributed throughout the VCLL, but in subregions of the VNLL (guinea pig: Schofield and Cant, 1997) and are known to provide a substrate for fast, robust synaptic signal transmission to cells that receive them (bat: Vater et al., 1997).

In echolocating bats there have been several studies that have indicated that VNLLc neurons receive large putatively excitatory synaptic endings that resemble endbulbs of Held (Zook and Casseday, 1985; Covey and Casseday, 1986; Vater and Feng, 1990; Covey, 1993a; Huffman and Covey, 1995; Vater et al., 1997). The study by Vater et al. (1997) in bat attempted to determine, firstly, if the large synaptic terminals in the VNLLc were indeed typical of calyces and, secondly, what other types of inputs did VNLLc cells receive and how were the synapses on these cells organised? In this study, the authors used similar criteria for distinguishing calyx-like endings as have been used in the MNTB (for calyces of Held) and in the CN (for endbulbs of Held). The criteria are three fold: 1) very large boutons containing sparsely distributed round type vesicles with multiple active zones; 2) an asymmetric synapse whereby the postsynaptic membrane density is more prominent than the presynaptic membrane density within the active zones; 3) an enlarged extracellular space in the elongated zone of apposition between the calyx and the postsynaptic cell (Vater et al., 1997).

Vater et al. (1997) found that calyx-like endings can contact both the soma of a particular cell and the surrounding dendrites of other cells, and this was a robust organisational feature of the VNLLc of bats. Small round vesicle boutons may represent extensions of a calyx-like ending, and may be found in locations around the soma and on dendritic profiles (Vater et al., 1997). The more symmetrically organised flattened and pleomorphic vesicles have also been observed in perisomatic locations and on dendritic profiles. In this way, VNLLc neurons may receive input from a wide range of frequencies, albeit with some amount of delay introduced for the non-somatic transmission. It has been hypothesised that the VNLLc neurons of bats do not simply reflect the response properties of their inputs but are able to extract even greater timing resolution over a wide frequency range by modifying the inputs (Vater et al., 1997).

### *Source of VCLL Calyces*

VCLL calyces are the terminals of thick myelinated axons, which, are likely to contribute to rapid neural propagation (guinea pig: Schofield, 1995; Schofield and Cant, 1997). These fibres can innervate multiple targets, and equally a single recipient cell may receive input from two afferent thick fibres (Vater et al., 1997). In non-echolocating species, the source of the thick axon projection that ends in these calyces has been identified by several studies as the octopus cells of the PVCN. Using anterograde and retrograde transport, Schofield and Cant (1997) correlated the distal segments of thick axons with octopus cells of the PVCN. The electrophysiological signatures of cells that gave rise  to the calyces in the VNLL matched those of octopus cells (various species: Rhode and Greenberg, 1992; cat: Godfrey et al., 1975) in the CN. The fact that both octopus cells and endbulbs are calretinin positive (octopus cells are the only CN cell type that are calretinin positive), strengthens the case. A similar circuit appears to be present in the human VNLL as well (Adams, 1997) and provides further support for the suggestion that octopus cells are the origin of the calyces in the VNLL (rat: Wu, 1999; Zhao and Wu, 2001; guinea pig: Schofield and Cant, 1997; cat: Warr, 1966; van Noort, 1969; Warr, 1969).

There have been other possible sources suggested for the thick axon projection to the VCLL. In big brown bats the calyces in the VNLL arise from both the AVCN and PVCN (Huffman and Covey, 1995). Covey and Casseday (bat: 1986), as well as Vater and Feng (bat: 1990), proposed that the endbulbs originated from large multipolar cells. However, in cat (Osen, 1972; Adams and Warr, 1976; Adams, 1993) and horseshoe bat (Vater and Feng, 1990), the calyceal endings originated purely from the PVCN and were probably from octopus cells or large multipolar cells that are known to precisely encode the onset of sound. In contrast, results from Huffman and Covey (1995), as well as Vater and Braun (1994) (also in bat), did not show that the calyces originated from octopus cells.

## Neurons Receiving Calyces in the VCLL

A study by Schofield and Cant (guinea pig; 1997) identified the VNLL cells with calyces as globular cells (mouse: Willard and Ryugo, 1983; cat: Adams, 1979; bat: Zook and Casseday, 1985; Vater and Feng, 1990). Adams (cat and human; 1997) also described the projection of octopus cells to globular bushy cells of the contralateral VNLL by using anterograde filling of axons, immunostaining for calretinin, and making single unit electrophysiological recordings. He found converging lines of evidence that, coupled with the results from other studies, supported the claim that the terminations of the axons of octopus cells were calyces of Held and that these endbulbs terminate upon globular bushy cells of the VNLL.

In a study in rat brain slices (Zhao and Wu, 2001), it was suggested that synapses similar to calyces of Held are found on VNLL bushy cells. By providing a large synaptic current when activated by APs originating from the VCN, these terminals can provide secure and faithful transmission of signals through the VNLL even when the receiving cell's input resistance is low. Zhao and Wu (2001) believe that this configuration might be significant for preserving the fine temporal structure of auditory stimuli.

In mice and bats, globular cells are segregated from other cell types (mouse: Willard and Ryugo, 1983; bat: Zook and Casseday, 1985; Covey and Casseday, 1986; Vater and Feng, 1990). In some species, globular/bushy cells tend to be preferentially distributed ventrally within the VCLL (Schofield and Cant, 1997). There have been no reports of calyceal synapses within, or thick axon projections to, the INLL. Furthermore, octopus cells are not known to innervate the ipsilateral VNLL of any species. Therefore, VNLL cells receiving octopus cell input respond exclusively to stimulation of the contralateral ear.

In summary, at least in non-echolocating species, octopus cells give rise to thick myelinated axons that terminate in large calyx-like synapses on globular cells of the VNLL, akin to endbulbs of Held in other auditory nuclei (Schofield and Cant, 1997; Adams, 1997). Given that nerve propagation velocity in myelinated axons (saltatory conduction) is known to be a function of axon diameter, and given the secure nature of calyceal connections, these characteristics suggest that this pathway provides fast and faithful transmission of neural signals (Zhao and Wu, 2001; Batra and Fitzpatrick, 1999). The presence of a specialised circuit of this nature suggests that the VNLL may be important in conveying and processing timing information.

# RESPONSE PROPERTIES OF VCLL NEURONS

There are relatively few electrophysiological studies of the VCLL in non-echolocating animals. Of the studies that exist, mainly extracellular responses have been recorded in response to acoustic stimulation in the rat (Zhang and Kelly, 2006a, b), rabbit (Batra and Fitzpatrick, 1997, 2002a, b; Batra, 2006; Batra and Fitzpatrick, 1999), and cat (Aitkin et al., 1970a; Aitkin et al., 1970b; Guinan et al., 1972b; Guinan et al., 1972a). Intracellular responses to current injection have been recorded in slice preparation (rat: Wu, 1999; Zhao and Wu, 2001). Responses to complex stimulation such as frequency or amplitude-modulated tones have been studied to a limited extent (Zhang and Kelly, 2006b; Batra, 2006; Huffman et al., 1998a, b) but are beyond the scope of this chapter. To date, there have been only two studies that have investigated the intracellular neural responses to acoustic stimulation *in vivo* (Nayagam et al. 2005, 2006).

## Frequency Tuning Properties of VCLL Neurons

There is a great deal of convergence that occurs within the VNLL; many cells within the structure have been described as coincidence detectors (various species: Oertel and Wickesberg, 2002), and although this endows the cells with greater temporal accuracy it comes at the expense of frequency acuity (bat: Covey and Casseday, 1991). Therefore, it would be expected that many VNLL cells would be broadly tuned.

### Tuning Properties of VCLL Neurons in Echolocating Bats

Covey and Casseday (1991) recorded frequency tuning curves (TCs) from neurons in the monaural nuclei (INLL, VNLLc and VNLLm) of echolocating big brown bats. Their results showed that the TCs of units located in the VNLLc were much broader than units found in the other monaural NLL. The TCs of VNLLc cells were asymmetrical and resembled broad-band filters with steep upper cut-offs and shallow lower cut-offs. The TCs of neurons in the INLL and the VNLLm were typically more symmetrical V-shaped responses with similar upper and lower slopes. However, on average, all the monaural NLL in bat showed broader TCs than other neurons at the midbrain level. In particular, the neurons of the VNLLc were not well suited to frequency encoding (Covey and Casseday, 1991). However, another study in the mustache bat found that the INLL contained neurons that detected and responded optimally to combinations of sound (Portfors and Wenstrup, 2001). Recently, Xie et al. reporting on the response properties of neurons in the INLL of the Mexican free-tailed bat described mainly broadly tuned neurons with no surround inhibition or inhibition dependent properties (bat: Xie et al., 2005). Clearly, even within the bat genus, there are many species-specific differences in the response properties and specialisations of VNLL and INLL cells.

### Tuning Properties of VCLL Cells in Non-Echolocating Species

Studies performed on rabbits to determine the frequency TCs of neurons in the lateral lemniscus have provided contradictory findings. Metzner and Radtke-Schuller (1987) found no increased frequency selectivity in the VCLL compared to neurons at lower auditory levels, while Batra and Fitzpatrick (1999) observed a range of tuning  selectivity when the isofrequency contours of responses recorded at a range of intensities and frequencies were mapped in unanaesthetised preparations (Batra and Fitzpatrick, 1999). Neurons that responded to acoustic stimuli with an onset type response typically had broad frequency tuning, a finding compatible with inputs from broadly tuned, onset cells of the CN. On the other hand, neurons that responded with sustained and transient responses tended to be more narrowly tuned. Tuning of short latency, sustained neurons tended to be narrower for higher frequency units. In the rat, Zhang and Kelly (2006a) recently reported on the tuning properties of VCLL units. They found a majority (55%) of extracellularly recorded units had V- or U-shaped frequency TCs with discernable CFs. They also found many units with more complex multipeaked (37%) or other (8%) tuning curve (TC) patterns. However, it must be remembered that in extracellular electrophysiological studies, it is difficult to differentiate neural responses from fibres of passage, and it is possible that some of these data may in fact reflect responses from ascending lemniscal fibres. In a subset of their sample (17/96 units) Zhang and Kelly (2006a) used the AMPA ($\alpha$-amino-3-hydroxy-5-methyl-4-isoxazolepropionic acid) antagonist NBQX (2,3-dihydroxy-6-nitro-7-sulfamoyl-benzo[f]quinoxaline-2,3-dione) to differentiate neural responses from fibres. The authors do not explicitly state whether or not this sample of 'definite' units differed in any way from the larger sample of 'assumed' cells. However, the synaptic antagonist, NBQX, did substantially reduce both monaural and binaural responses under all stimulus conditions.

Figure 6 shows intracellular threshold tuning curves recorded by Nayagam et al. (2006) from 9 VCLL neurons in response to suprathreshold best frequency tones. These neurons responded with predominantly single peaked V-shaped tuning curves as well as some multi-peaked curves similar to the descriptions from Zhang and Kelly (2006a).

## Classification of Response Types of VCLL Neurons

For the most part, it is possible to classify the neuronal response types found in the NLL using the same categories established in the CN (cat: Pfeiffer, 1966; Blackburn and Sachs, 1989); for review of VCN response types, see Rhode and Greenberg (1992). As the VCN is a principal input to the VCLL, it is interesting to consider to what extent the response types in the VCN are reflected in the VCLL. Table 4 provides a list of common synonymous terms used in various studies to describe responses of cells in the VCLL to pure tone and noise bursts.

**Table 4. Table of synonymous descriptors (grouped horizontally) used to label VCLL neural responses to tone and noise bursts.**

| Synonymous Terms | | |
|---|---|---|
| Onset | Phasic | On |
| Regular | Chopper | Multimodal |
| On-Pause | Pauser | Notch |
| Adapting | Primary-Like | Sustained |

*Response Types in Echolocating Species*

In echolocating bats, the most comprehensive electrophysiological study that addressed the response properties of monaural lateral lemniscal neurons was performed by Covey and Casseday (1991). In this study, the authors reported on the firing patterns and the classification they assigned based on responses to pure tones at the unit's CF and 20 dB above threshold. In summary, Covey and Casseday (1991) categorised neurons into 'phasic', 'choppers', 'tonic', 'primary-like' and 'pausers'; the phasic neurons could be further divided into two types, constant-latency and variable-latency.

Phasic constant-latency neurons usually fired one action potential (AP) per stimulus, tightly locked to the stimulus onset, whereas the phasic variable-latency neurons fired between one and three APs per stimulus at the onset, but with as much as several milliseconds variance in first spike latency. The constant-latency and the variable-latency types were clearly segregated in the monaural NLL of echolocating bats. The constant-latency neurons were almost exclusive to the columnar region (making up 95% of the population in this area), whereas the variable latency units were found in the INLL and the VNLLm, where they represented about 20-30% of the population.

The choppers that were classified in the Covey and Casseday (1991) study responded throughout the duration of the stimulus with regularly timed APs (regular interspike intervals; ISIs) and with tight locking of the first AP to the time of stimulus onset. They were mostly 'fast' choppers with ISIs of less than 2.5 ms (Tsuchitani, 1988a, b). The choppers were located in the VNLLm and INLL but not in the VNLLc.

The tonic neurons showed a constant high rate of discharge throughout the duration of the stimulus, with practically no adaptation even with long duration stimuli (of over 50 msec). The first AP of the tonic neurons was not locked to the onset of the sound, and the APs sometimes had regular ISIs (as regular as a chopper response) and sometimes did not. A few of the tonic neurons became more chopper-like and the first AP became more synchronised to the stimulus onset as the stimulus sound pressure level (SPL) was increased. These tonic neurons were only found in the INLL and VNLLm.

Another response type identified in the bat was a primary-like response that resembled the responses found in the auditory nerve (cat: Kiang et al., 1965a, b). These responded throughout the stimulus duration, but with a diminishing firing rate after the initial transient 'on' response. These units were rare, with less than 5% of the population in each of the three monaural nuclei.

The last response type identified by Covey and Casseday (1991) was the pauser response, which discharged initially then underwent a period of inactivity before resuming a lower level of sporadic discharge for the remainder of the stimulus. Again, these neurons were rare, making up less than 4% of the population of the VNLLm and the INLL. They were not found at all in the VNLLc.

Therefore, in the big brown bat at least, there are several different response types in the monaural NLL. Most of the neurons (59%) in these nuclei had monotonic rate-level functions (firing rate increased or remained level over increasing SPL), and the majority of the non-monotonic cells were choppers. The response types in the INLL and the VNLLm were mixed. However, between these two structures was a region, the VNLLc, that was almost entirely populated with one type of neuron (distinct both physiologically and cytoarchitecturally), and these neurons showed a phasic constant-latency response.

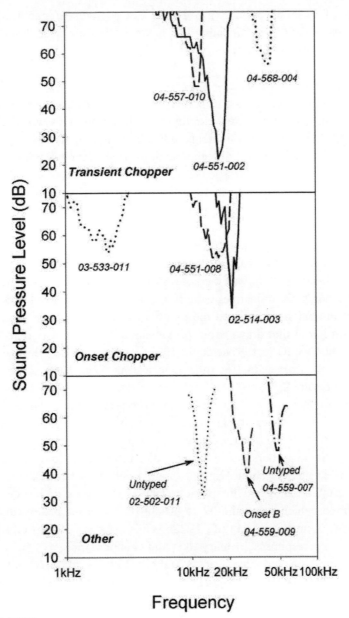

- Nayagam et al. (2006)

Figure 6. Intracellular threshold tuning curves from nine VCLL neurons.
Response type to suprathreshold characteristic frequency (CF) tones is indicated in the bottom left of each panel or by arrows. Numbers next to each plot provide the cell's ID.

In the INLL of the Mexican free-tailed bat, four response types were described by Xie et al. (2005) in response to CF tone bursts, sustained chopper, primary like, onset chopper and onset. All these responses were monotonic, unselective for species-specific calls, and unresponsive to blocking inhibition with the exception on one unit which was highly influenced by inhibition.

Given that VNLL and INLL in particular is highly developed in bats and dolphins it is likely that it plays a prominent role in echolocation, such as the extraction of spectral and temporal features of a stimuli, or delay processing. The spatial segregation of response types is an interesting feature of the echolocating bat, however, has not been described to the same extent in other non-echolocating species.

### Response Types in Non-Echolocating Species

Other species may share, at least in part, the neuron types and segregation that is most evident in echolocating bats (cat: Glendenning et al., 1981; bat: Covey and Casseday, 1991). Table 5 summarises the results of prominent studies investigating neural responses to acoustic stimulation in the VCLL of various non-echolocating species (excluding rats).

Aitkin et al. (1970a) found that the response patterns in the VCLL of cats were similar to the responses from the DNLL. They recorded sustained activity (sometimes with pauses in firing) as well as single APs at stimulus onset, in response to pure tones. In many cases, the firing patterns were both frequency and SPL dependent. Of the 17 units they studied for monotonicity, all but two were monotonic. These findings fit with those of Covey and Casseday (1991) in echolocating bats. Aitkin et al. (1970a) concluded that the timing and the extent of APs in a discharge train was the net result of excitatory and inhibitory inputs acting on the neuron. Further, these influences were frequency and SPL dependant and the balancing of excitation and inhibition determined the number of APs fired for a given stimulus. This conclusion was similar to that drawn from previous studies in the CN (cat: Greenwood and Maruyama, 1965) and the IC (cat: Rose et al., 1963), and was subsequently echoed in several VCLL electrophysiological studies in other species(rat: Wu, 1999; Zhao and Wu, 2001; rabbit: Batra and Fitzpatrick, 1999).

Response types found in the rabbit VNLL in more recent studies have, for the most part, been in agreement with the types of responses found in other species; however, there has been some debate over the proportions of neurons displaying different patterns (Batra and Fitzpatrick, 1999). Some authors attribute these disparities to the use of anaesthesia, which influences discharge patterns (rabbit: Kuwada et al., 1989; cat: Brownell et al., 1979; Ritz and Brownell, 1982; rabbit: Batra and Fitzpatrick, 1999). The types of responses found in the rabbit are: sustained, which were similar to sustained responses observed in the VCLL in other species such as cat (Guinan et al., 1972b; Guinan et al., 1972a) and bat (Covey and Casseday, 1991); onset responses; primary-like; and chopper types.

The neurons in Batra and Fitzpatrick's (rabbit: 1999) study were classified as either phasic or sustained based on their responses to tone bursts at CF at 60–80 dB SPL. Phasic neurons were separated into onset or transient sub-types based on the shape of the post-stimulus time histogram (PSTH). Phasic-onset neurons were characterised by ongoing firing rates (between 35–75 ms after stimulus onset) less than 25 APs per second, whereas phasic-transient responses gave an initial (between 0–35 ms) discharge rate greater than twice the driven sustained response (cat: Aitkin et al., 1970a). The sustained neurons were separated into three sub-types based on PSTH shape: long-latency, short-latency, and strongly adapting. Long-latency status was given if the latency was more than 7 ms greater than the median of the other neurons of similar CFs in the sample. Most of the neurons were located in the VNLLm and VNLLl, with VNLLm containing mainly onset neurons and VNLLl mainly short latency sustained neurons.

Table 6 summarises the results of studies that have investigated the neural responses in the rat VCLL. The intracellular brain slice study of Wu (1999) categorised rat VCLL neurons into two types, I and II, that displayed different intrinsic membrane properties. They found that type I cells had linear current-voltage relationships; they fired several APs in response to depolarising current injections. Type I cells were sub-classified, based on their discharge patterns, into three distinct classes: regular, adaptation and onset-pause. Type II cells have non-linear current-voltage relationships and only fired one AP at the onset of depolarising injections; they were referred to as onset cells (1999).

Extending Wu's (1999) findings, Zhao and Wu (2001) used whole cell patch-clamp recordings from rat VCLL neurons in brain slice preparations to examine the membrane properties and synaptic responses of single cells. The physiological results were correlated with cytoarchitectural and morphological findings derived from iontophoretically-injected Neurobiotin-filled neurons (see below). Following depolarising current injection, they found that VCLL neurons could be classified into one of five distinct groups: onset, regular, adapting, bursting, and onset-pause. Non-linear type II neurons showed onset responses of one to three small spikes at the onset of depolarisation elicited by positive current injection (up to 1 nA). Regular responses were observed in 19% of neurons and showed a continuous train of APs with almost regular ISIs. Adapting units (20%) were similar to the regular cells, in that they fired continuous trains of spikes. However, in response to low intensity current, there was a delay of 65-75 ms between the onset of current injection and the generation of the first AP; as the current level was increased, this delay was reduced. At lower current levels adapting neurons showed variable ISIs but at higher current levels the ISIs were regular.

**Table 5. Electrophysiological studies of neuron response type in the VCLL of non-echolocating species (excluding rats).**

| Author(s)/Year | Species | Technique/Stimulus | Response Type | % in VCLL | Location |
|---|---|---|---|---|---|
| Aitkin et al. (1970a) | Cat | Extracellular recordings *in vivo* / pure tones at CF | n = 17 | | |
| | | | Onset | - | - |
| | | | Sustained | - | - |
| | | | Pauser | - | - |
| Guinan et al. (1972b; 1972a) | Cat | Extracellular recordings *in vivo* / pure tones at CF | n = 25 | | |
| | | | *Onset/Phasic (n = 6)* | 24 | - |
| | | | *Sustained (n = 17)* | | - |
| | | | Primary-Like | 8 | - |
| | | | Pauser | 4 | - |
| | | | Chopper - Transient | 24 | - |
| | | | Chopper - Sustained | 32 | - |
| | | | *Long Latency (n = 1)* | 4 | - |
| | | | *Inhibition (n = 1)* | 4 | - |
| Batra and Fitzpatrick (1999) | Rabbit | Extracellular recordings *in vivo* (unanaesthetised) / pure tones at CF | n = 160 | | |
| | | | *Phasic / Onset (n = 86)* | | VNLLm |
| | | | Onset | 49 | |
| | | | Transient | 5 | |
| | | | Offset | 16 | |
| | | | *Sustained (n = 74)* | | VNLLl |
| | | | Short-Latency | 38 | |
| | | | Long Latency | 16 | |
| | | | Strongly Adapting | 2 | |
| | | | *Inhibited (n = 10 / 175)* | 6 | |

Percentages and sample do not necessarily sum to 100%, as some responses form intersecting sets and different samples are represented.

**Table 6. Electrophysiological studies of neuron response type in rat VCLL.**

| Author(s)/ Year | Species | Technique/Stimulus | Response Type | % in VCLL | Location | Morph- ology | Binaural Type |
|---|---|---|---|---|---|---|---|
| Wu (1999) | Rat | Intracellular recordings *in vitro* / current injection | n = 54 | | | | |
| | | | Onset (type II) | 23 | - | Bushy | |
| | | | Regular (type I) | 32 | - | - | |
| | | | Adapting (type I) | 20 | - | - | |
| | | | Onset-pause (type I) | 29 | - | - | |
| Zhao and Wu (2001) | Rat | Whole cell patch clamp *in vitro* / current injection | n = 59 | | | | |
| | | | Onset (non-linear) | 27 | ventral | Bushy | |
| | | | Regular (linear) | 19 | ventral | Stellate I | |
| | | | Adapting (linear) | 20 | mainly dorsal | Stellate II | |
| | | | Bursting (linear) | 27 | Through-out | Elongate | |
| | | | Onset-pause (linear) | 7 | ventral | Stellate I | |
| Zhang and Kelly (2006a) | Rat | Extracellular recordings *in vivo* / pure tones at CF | n = 99 | | | | n = 96; EI (60.4%), EI (13.5%), EE/EI (13.5%), E0 (12.5%)† |
| | | | *Onset (n = 33)* | | | | |
| | | | Phasic | 13 | - | - | |
| | | | Phasic Burst | 11 | - | - | |
| | | | Phasic Burst with High Spon | 12 | - | - | |
| | | | Double Burst | 2 | - | - | |
| | | | *Sustained (n = 55)* | | | | |
| | | | Primary Like | 33 | - | - | |
| | | | Pauser | 8 | - | - | |
| | | | Late Response | 7 | - | - | |
| | | | Irregular Sustained | 7 | - | - | |
| | | | *Other (n = 6)* | | | | |
| | | | Fast Adapting | 6 | - | - | |
| Nayagam et al. (2005, 2006) | Rat | Intracellular recordings *in vivo* / pure tones at CF | n = 24 | | | | |
| | | | Pauser (n = 3) | 13 | Through-out | | EI (66%), E0 (33%) |
| | | | Onset Ideal (n=2) | 8 | VNLL only | | E0 |
| | | | Onset Chopper (n = 5) | 21 | INLL only | | EI (40%), E0 (40%), EI (20%) |
| | | | Transient Chopper (n = 6) | 25 | Through-out | Stellate II | E0 (33%), EE (33%), EI (33%) |
| | | | Onset-A (n = 3) | 13 | Through-out | Bushy | EE (50%) E0 (50%) * |
| | | | Onset-B (n =5) | 21 | Through-out | Stellate I | E0 (80%) ** |

Percentages and sample sizes do not necessarily sum to 100%, as some responses form intersecting samples and different samples are represented. Values are rounded to the nearest integer. † 96 E0, EI, EE and combined EE/EI responses were recorded but not correlated with response type. * Only two of the three Onset-A cells in this study were presented with binaural stimuli. ** Only four out of the five Onset-B cells were presented with binaural stimuli.

Bursting trains of discharges were seen in 27% of the neurons arising from a hump of depolarisation that lasted longer than 100 ms at low current levels. Following the burst was a period of regular sustained firing at higher current levels. Finally, the onset-pause type of response was seen in 7% of neurons. A small amount of current produced a single spike at the onset of depolarisation, which became sustained firing as the current was increased. However, a period of inactivity after the first spike remained. Higher currents elicited an initial short train of spikes, followed by a pause, before settling into sustained firing. In all types of responses, except the onset class, the firing frequency and the strength of the current injection were proportional (Zhao and Wu, 2001).

A recently published study by Zhang and Kelly (2006a) comprehensively investigated extracellular VCLL responses to monaural and binaural tone bursts in the rat (Figure 7). They used micro-iontophoretic injection of an AMPA receptor antagonist NBQX to deactivate local synapses at the recording site to help establish whether the recording was from a cell or fibre. However, this technique was only used in 17 out of 96 neurons and it is unknown whether these 'proven' cells differed in any significant way to the larger sample of 'assumed' cells. However, the fact that all units showed a decreased firing rate when presented with the drug suggests that this study was recoding from cells and not fibres of passage. In response to 100 ms contralateral tone bursts 20 dB SPL above threshold at CF they sorted 99 neurons into 9 types based on temporal firing patterns. They divided their 9 types into 3 main categories: onset, sustained and other. Within the onset category, they described phasic (n = 13), phasic burst (n = 11), phasic burst with high spontaneous rate (SR) (n = 12), and double bursts (n = 2). The sustained category contained primary-like (n = 33), pauser (n = 8), late response (n = 7), and irregular sustained (n=7). The 'other' category contained fast adapting (n = 6) responses that, although they could have been classified as onset, were considered as a special group and excluded from further onset versus sustained analysis. They concluded that onset and sustained cells were not segregated within the VCLL, although they only examined the distribution of neurons in the dorsoventral plane and did not distinguish between various classes of onset neurons. They found that onset units, when compared with sustained units, had shorter average first spike latencies (onset mean FSL: 8.3 ms; sustained mean FSL: 14.8 ms) and a higher degree of temporal acuity (onset mean FSL standard deviation; SD: 0.59 ms; sustained mean FSL SD: 4.2 ms). Sustained neurons became less tightly locked to the onset of the stimulus with increasing stimulus level; however, onset neurons maintained their low jitter at various stimulus levels.

Intracellular recordings by Nayagam et al. (2006) have distinguished several classes of neurons based on their responses to noise and tone burst. Six response types were determined based on the single and average responses to CF tones. Intracellular recordings allow classification to be made based not only on AP times and pattern, but also on the synaptic events, membrane profile and, if filled with a neuronal dye, the cellular morphology as well. The 24 contralaterally excited responses determined in this study were termed onset ideal (n = 2), onset chopper (n = 5), onset-A (n = 3), onset-B (n = 5), transient chopper (n = 6) and pauser (n = 3). Within these six intracellular types, the first four were varieties of onset response separated by subtle yet distinct differences in their membrane profiles.

In response to broadband noise stimulation a complex range of responses was observed intracellularly. These noise responses did not consistently correlate with the responses to tones; however, it was observed that onset neurons with ongoing depolarised membranes in response to tones would typically respond with sustained firing when presented with noise.

Onset ideal units responded at a shorter latency compared to all other types and were only responsive to contralateral stimulation. Following their precisely-timed onset AP, a period of hyperpolarisation was observed, which may serve to prevent later arriving EPSPs from evoking APs (Figure 8). These onset ideal responses may be a result of a thick axon projection (ending with a calyceal synapse) from the OCA of the contralateral CN (Nayagam et al., 2005). A future study could be designed to visualise synapses on the somas of physiologically characterised and dye filled neurons, particularly the onset ideal cells. This would prove that the onset ideal responses are indeed from bushy cells with calyx-like synapses.

Onset chopper neurons showed a characteristic second AP discharged at a regular inter-spike interval, in response to CF tones. These cells also had a short and narrow distribution of FSLs. Onset-A cells were distinguished by a negatively graded membrane potential throughout the stimulus and a bushy cell morphology, whereas onset-B neurons showed stable depolarisation and a stellate cell morphology. Onset-A neurons had a longer and wider distribution of FSL compared with onset-B cells. Presumably, onset ideal, onset-A and onset-B type responses would be difficult to differentiate based only on extracellular recordings and response pattern; they may have been considered as one class of cell with a wide distribution of FSLs.

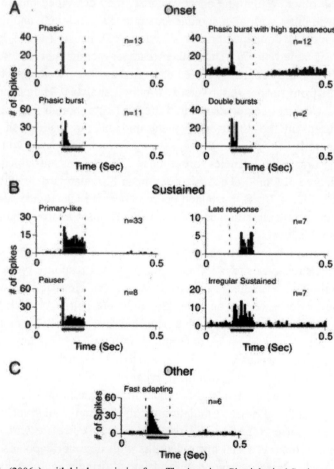

- Zhang and Kelly (2006a): with kind permission from The American Physiological Society.

Figure 7. Extracellularly recorded temporal response patterns of rat VCLL neurons.
Post-stimulus time histograms (PSTHs) representing the number of spikes occurring in 5 ms time bins before, during, and after presentation of a 100 ms CF tone burst 20 dB SPL above cell threshold. Figure shows nine extracellular response subtypes of three major response groups. A: Responses of onset units. B: Responses of sustained units. C: Response of other unit. Spike counts are based on 20 repetitions of the stimulus. Dashed vertical lines and black bars below the x-axes of the lower histograms of section A, B, and C indicate the limits of the tone presentation.

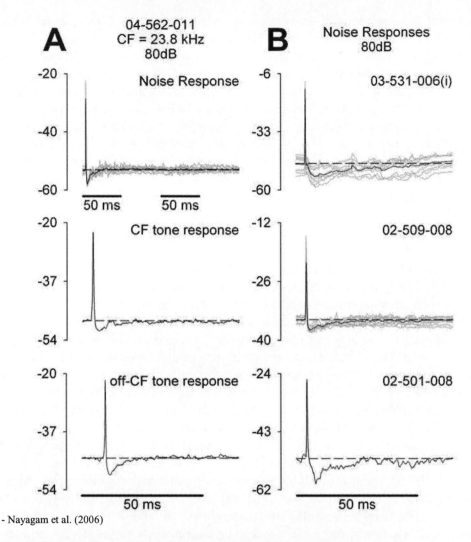

- Nayagam et al. (2006)

Figure 8. Intracellular responses to noise and tones of onset ideal neurons.
**A:** Response from a onset ideal neuron showing the similarity in intracellular profile between noise and tone stimuli. Top panel shows 10 trace overlay (grey) and average response (black) to contralaterally and ipsilaterally presented 80 dB RMS noise (contralateral and ipsilateral stimuli were offset by 100 ms). Lower panels show single trace responses to contralaterally presented CF (middle) and off-CF (bottom) tones presented at 80 dB SPL. **B:** 10 trace overlay and average responses (top, middle) and single trace responses (bottom) from three onset ideal neurons with similar intracellular profiles to noise and to the cell shown in (A). Horizontal dashed lines show resting membrane potential (RMP) and thick horizontal bars show stimulus duration.

Nayagam et al.'s (2006) intracellular responses to CF tones are comparable to extracellular *in vivo* responses from the VNLL of other non echolocating species (Aitkin et al., 1970a; Guinan et al., 1972b; Batra and Fitzpatrick, 1999). These studies have described onset, regular, sustained, and chopping response. Batra and Fitzpatrick (1999) described neurons that were suppressed below spontaneous rate after the initial onset peak. This may correspond with onset ideal units from the Nayagam et al. (2006) study. They also found at least one other class of onset cell, preferentially distributed within the medial limb of the VNLL that did not appear to be innervated by octopus cells. They concluded that the VNLL contains multiple populations of onset neurons, consistent with the Nayagam et al. (2006) study. Transient chopper neurons from the Nayagam et al. (2006) study may also correspond with the chopper neurons described in previous extracellular studies, although transient chopper neurons in the present study had a wider distribution of FSLs. The Nayagam et al. (2006) study did not record any neurons that chopped throughout the stimulus within the VCLL, however, this response type was observed in the DNLL (data not shown).

The dynamic range of onset responses in the Nayagam et al., (2006) study was narrower than that of pauser and transient chopper responses, consistent with the extracellular findings of Batra and Fitzpatrick (1999). The neurons presented in this study all showed latencies that decreased with increasing stimulus level or proximity to CF. This result is also in agreement with *in vivo* extracellular studies of the VCLL (Batra and Fitzpatrick, 1999). Although phasic and sustained offset (including offset chopper) responses to noise were observed, these types were not classified in response to CF tones.

Nayagam et al.'s (2006) intracellular responses to acoustic stimuli *in vivo* are similar in many ways to intracellular responses to current injection *in vitro* within the VCLL (Wu, 1999; Zhao and Wu, 2001). Both techniques found different response classes, some with onset, some with sustained and some with pauser profiles, but in response to current injection there was more sustained activity (regular, adapting). Additional circuitry (particularly the inhibitory projections to the VNLL) is most likely the reason for the reduction in sustained spike rate *in vivo*. The illustrated contour plots (see below), showing broadly tuned onset components and narrowly tuned sustained components, as well as a mixture of excitation and inhibition off-CF, supports the notion of convergent input streams. Additionally, in most cells, different responses to noise and tones were observed, suggesting that specific mechanisms are activated for broad and narrow band stimulation.

Powerful, short-duration inhibition before the first AP was recorded from units with both onset and long duration firing patterns and is thought to be activated by octopus cells in the contralateral CN (Nayagam et al., 2005) (see below). Long duration inhibition was also seen in response to both contralateral and ipsilateral stimuli, sometimes in conjunction with excitation but sometimes without any excitation present (I0 and 0I response types). These long duration IPSPs may be the result of ascending projections from the MNTB, other nuclei within the SOC (Glendenning et al., 1981) or even intrinsic circuitry (Zhao and Wu, 2001; Whitley and Henkel, 1984).

Of the 6 response classes to CF tones described by Nayagam et al. (2006), evidence was found for a preferential spatial distribution of two of these types; onset ideal units were only located within the VNLL and onset chopper units were localised to the INLL. The dorsal part of the VCLL (INLL) contained a greater proportion of cells that responded with excitation to stimulation of the contralateral ear and inhibition from ipsilateral stimulation.

The proportion of neurons from Nayagam et al.'s (2006) study for which the rate of AP discharge was a non-monotonic function of SPL (~9%) was comparable with the proportion reported by Aitkin (1970a) (~12%) and suggests a level-dependant inhibitory input, despite the lack of visible IPSPs in the intracellular traces. Aitkin (1970a) suggested that the mechanism causing non-monotonicity within the VNLL is activated before or along with the excitatory process. Given that the two neuronal types in Nayagam et al.'s (2006) sample that showed non-monotonic responses (transient chopper and onset-A) had long FSLs with a wide distribution, it is conceivable that they received projections from local inhibitory neurons with a shorter FSL. Intrinsic connections within the VNLL have been described previously as local collaterals of ascending axons and are believed to be inhibitory (Zhao and Wu, 2001).

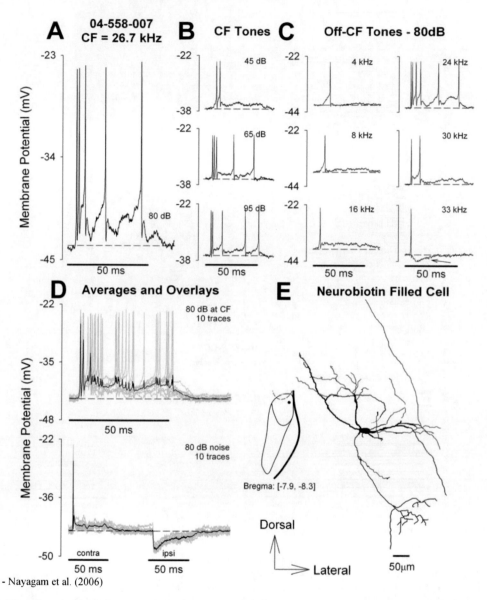

- Nayagam et al. (2006)

Figure 9. Morphology and intracellular responses of a transient chopper neuron.
**A:** Single trace in response to a contralaterally presented CF tone at 80 dB SPL. **B:** Single traces showing responses to CF tones at 3 SPLs. **C:** Single traces in response to a range of off-CF tones at 80 dB SPL. Arrow indicates membrane hyperpolarisation to a high frequency tone. **D:** Overlay of 10 traces (grey) and average response (black) to contralaterally presented 80 dB SPL CF tone (top) and contralaterally and ipsilaterally presented 80 dB RMS noise (bottom; contralateral and ipsilateral stimuli offset by 100 ms). Horizontal dashed lines show RMP and thick horizontal bars show stimulus duration. **E:** Morphology of recorded transient chopper neuron revealed by Neurobiotin labelling. The presumed axon is indicated by 'a'. Inset shows neuron's location (black dot) within the VCLL.

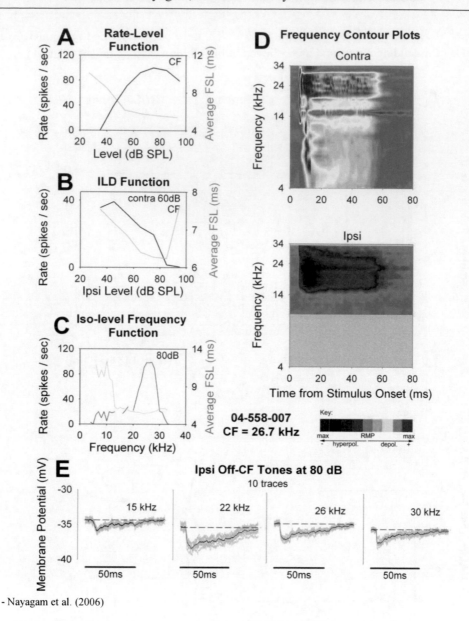

- Nayagam et al. (2006)

Figure 10.Intracellular responses to tones of a transient chopper neuron
Same cell as shown in Figure 9. **A:** Rate-level function (black) and average FSL (grey) at CF in steps of 10 dB SPL. **B:** ILD function showing the firing rate in response to a range of ipsilateral CF tone SPLs presented concurrently with an 60 dB SPL contralateral CF tone (black), and average FSL of the ILD function (grey). **C:** Iso-level frequency function (black) and average FSL (grey) at 70 dB SPL (data collected in steps of 1 kHz). Breaks in the frequency function were due to corrupted results at 15 and 19 kHz. **D:** Frequency contour plots showing changes in MP, as a colour gradient, with respect to frequency (incremented in 1 kHz steps) and time from the contralateral (top) and ipsilateral (bottom) stimulus (50 ms, 70 dB SPL) onset. The change in MP is indicated by the colour spectrum in the key; RMP is shown as green, whilst red indicates more positive MPs and blue indicates more negative MPs. The range of depolarisation shown does not encompass the entire AP height (range from RMP to maximum depolarisation / hyperpolarisation shown = +/- 4 mV). Grey area in bottom panel represents data not collected. **E:** 10 trace overlay (grey) and average response (black) to various ipsilaterally presented off-CF tones at 80 dB SPL. Horizontal dashed line is RMP and dark horizontal bar indicates stimulus duration.

Figure 9 and Figure 10 give examples of the sort of intracellular electrophysiological data recorded by Nayagam et al. (2006). The examples given are from a transient chopper neuron in response to CF (Figure 9A,B) and off-CF (Figure 9C) tones as well as averaged noise and tones (Figure 9D). This particular transient chopper showed an increased firing rate and decreased FSL with increasing SPL; however was sightly non-monotonic at high SPLs (Figure 9A). Off-CF, the onset component of this cell's response was dominant and broadband, whilst the ongoing depolarisation was limited to around CF (Figure 9C, Figure 10D). In response to 80dB noise, this cell showed an EI response (Figure 9D, bottom traces). E0 (n = 2) and EE (n = 2) responses to noise were also seen in transient chopper units (binaural responses in the VCLL are discussed below). Ipsilaterally, strong inhibition was seen at stimulus onset that gradually decayed throughout the 80 dB noise or tone stimulus. There was no evidence of mixed excitation with inhibition during the ipsilateral response (Figure 9D, bottom traces, Figure 10E). The bandwidth of the ipsilaterally-evoked inhibition was greater than the contralaterally-evoked and sustained excitation, and the latency of the inhibition was longer with that of the excitation (6.3 ms ipsilateral inhibition vs. 5.6 ms contralateral excitation). Supra-threshold contour plots show the average ipsilateral response plotted across the same frequency range as the contralateral excitation (Figure 10D).

In the contralateral response plot, more negative contours at 15 kHz and 19 kHz are caused by an artefact and are not indicative of membrane hyperpolarisation, unlike the true hyperpolarisation seen in Figure 10D, top panel at 32 – 34 kHz. When contralateral and ipsilateral tones were combined, the resultant firing rate was suppressed. Total suppression of firing occurred when ipsilateral CF tones were ~20 dB higher than contralateral CF tones (Figure 10B). This cell was iontophoretically filled with Neurobiotin and a digital reconstruction of the cell showing its dendritic morphology and location in relation to the VCLL and the lateral lemniscus tract is presented in Figure 9E. This cell had a small number of large dendrites that travel ~0.2 – 1 mm away from the soma before branching sparsely, consistent with the stellate morphology described by Zhao and Wu (2001). There was a tendency for the dendrites to be aligned with the lateral lemniscus fibre tract. Reconstructions of recorded cells may be used to correlate the physiological responses with the cell's morphology (discussed in more detail below). Data from other the 5 intracellular response types were presented in a similar fashion, for more details refer to Nayagam et al. (2006).

Mean FSL to 80 dB noise (Figure 11, white box plots) and CF tones (Figure 11, filled box plots) was calculated for each of Nayagam et al.'s (2006) 6 intracellular CF response types .All neurons had FSLs between 3.3 and 31 ms and in all cases the mean CF tone latency was less than the mean noise latency (Figure 11). Onset ideal neurons showed the shortest latency responses and the distribution of their FSLs was narrow. Onset ideal neurons had similar mean FSL for noise and tones (noise: 4.4 ms, tones: 3.9 ms). Onset chopper neurons also had similar latencies for noise and tones (noise: 6 ms, tones: 5.9 ms). Onset-A cells showed the longest mean latency and had a large spread of FSLs (9.6 ms) particularly in response to noise. Transient chopper neurons were the only type with a very wide distribution (27.3 ms).

All electrophysiological studies have described a heterogeneous neural population that responds to noise and tones with a variety of response patterns. The major classes of response are similar to those described in other auditory structures, such as onset, sustained and chopping. In studies that investigated binaural responses, the VCLL was consistently found to contain a range of cells that responded with a complex range of binaural interactions. More recent investigations, have also found evidence of inhibitory influence on spike timing within the VCLL, and this will be discuss further below.

## Powerful, Fast Inhibition before First Action Potential in the VCLL

Nayagam et al. (2005) proposed a novel mechanism to explain their observation of powerful and fast inhibition acting on some of the cells in the ventral VCLL (VNLL). In order to understand this proposed mechanism, it is important to recall three key findings. Firstly, the specialised calyx-like endings in the ventral VCLL (VNLL) are thought to play an important role in understanding the function of this nucleus. The neurons receiving calyx-like endings receive more secure input (various species: Morest, 1968) and respond to acoustic transients across a broader frequency bandwidth (various species: Oertel et al., 2000; Oertel and Wickesberg, 2002) with shorter latency than the other neurons of the VNLL (cat: Pfeiffer, 1966; bat: Covey and Casseday, 1986). Secondly, the ventral VCLL (VNLL) is known to contain cells that are immunoreactive for glycine (Saint Marie and Baker, 1990; Saint Marie et al., 1997, Irfan et al., 2005), and is thus considered to be a major source of inhibition to the IC. VCLL cells receive input from all major cell types of the CN via ladder-rung like collaterals from the ascending lemniscal pathway to the IC. Particularly important is a projection from the OCA of the PVCN to bushy cells of the ventral VCLL. This thick-axon projection terminates in large, secure, calyx-like synapses capable of conveying the precisely timed and broadly tuned excitatory onset ideal responses of octopus cells to the inhibitory VCLL target cells. Thirdly, within the VCLL are intrinsic connections, which have been described as collaterals of ascending axons from VCLL cells to the IC (Wu, 1997; Zhao and Wu, 2001).

The intracellular observation of broadly tuned, powerful, pre-spike onset inhibition from onset and sustained cells of the VNLL (Figure 12 A,B,C) suggested the involvement of the OCA and the thick axon projection to the VCLL (Nayagam et al. 2005). However, the octopus cell projection to the VNLL is excitatory, not inhibitory, so it cannot be the source of this fast inhibition. Nayagam et al. (2005) proposed that the fast inhibition was from another VNLL neuron that was itself activated by octopus cell input. This possibility was consistent with previous descriptions of local circuits within the VCLL. Examination of response latencies (Figure 12, D,E) verified that a cell group existed within the VNLL that met the requirements of the proposed local circuit: a cell group that responded to noise and tones with an ideal onset response (Figure 8). These onset ideal cells responded only to contralateral stimulation and were found only in the ventral part of the VCLL (VNLL). These characteristics were consistent with octopus cell input (Figure 13 a,a1).

It was found that fast onset inhibition delayed the first AP of the cell from which it was recorded (Figure 13 b1). A downstream effect of a delayed population of inhibitory VCLL onset and sustained responses (Figure 13 b2,b3) would be expected in the IC. IC cells receiving sustained excitation from the CN, combined with delayed onset inhibition or sustained inhibition from the VCLL would be expected to show pauser and onset responses respectively (Figure 13 c1,c2), both of which have been observed (Nayagam et al. 2005).

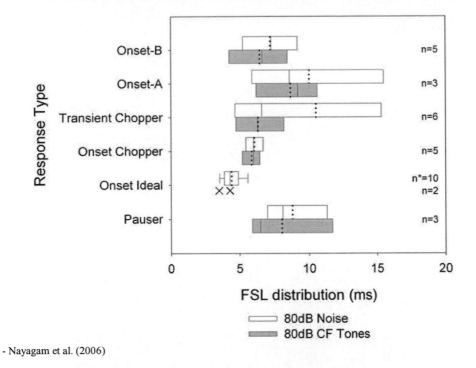

- Nayagam et al. (2006)

Figure 11. Intracellular first spike latency distribution of VCLL response types
Box plots showing mean (vertical dotted lines), median (vertical solid line), $25^{th}$ percentile (left box border) and $75^{th}$ percentile (right box border) FSL for the 6 VCLL response types. FSL to 80 dB RMS noise (unshaded boxes) and 80 dB SPL CF tones (shaded boxes) are shown. Crosses indicate FSLs for two responses; due to the small sample size box plot not shown. Asterisk indicates the onset ideal sample included 8 units that were classified according to their noise response. Whiskers shown for onset ideal noise sample indicate $10^{th}$ and $90^{th}$ percentile.

Furthermore, as the local fast inhibitory circuit in the VCLL is likely to be a collateral of an ascending projection to the IC, fast pre-spike inhibition would also be expected in the IC target of this projection (Figure 13 d1); this has indeed been observed (or predicted) in several studies (Adams, 1997; Carney and Yin, 1989; Kuwada et al., 1997; Nayagam et al., 2005; Smith et al., 1993)

## Correlation between Physiology and Morphology of Neurons in the VCLL

The most detailed attempt to correlate firing patterns with morphology in non-echolocating species was the rat study by Zhao and Wu (2001). As detailed above, they found two distinct morphological types, bushy and stellate. Stellate cells were subdivided into three types (I, II or elongate) based on their somatic and dendritic morphologies. Zhao and Wu (2001) found that bushy cells tended to have onset firing patterns and non-linear current-voltage relationships. Stellate I cells showed regular or onset-pause responses, whereas stellate II had adapting responses and elongate cells displayed burst patterns. shows the *in vitro* intracellular responses to current injection recorded by whole cell patch clamp in rat VCLL neurons correlated, where possible, with the cell's morphological type (refer Figure 3).

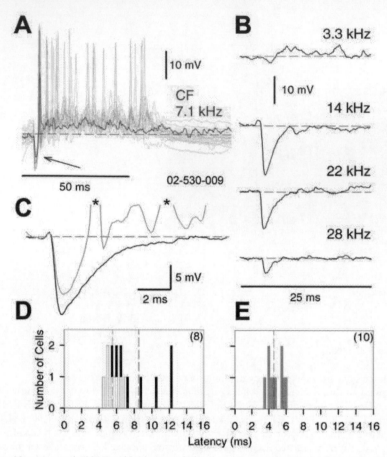

Figure 12. Onset inhibition in VNLL neurons.
**A:** *In vivo* intracellular responses recorded from a VNLL neuron to contralaterally presented noise bursts (80 dB RMS; 20 trace overlay, grey) and a CF tone burst (80 dB SPL; single trace, red). Horizontal dashed line indicates the mean RMP (-47 ± 4 mV). The arrow indicates membrane hyperpolarisation and the horizontal bar indicates stimulus duration. **B:** Single traces to off-CF tone bursts. Horizontal bar indicates time scale from stimulus onset. **C:** Spontaneous IPSPs were also observed in this cell (black trace) and are compared to the onset component of a single noise response (grey trace). Asterisks indicate truncated APs. **D:** Distribution of latencies of first AP (black bars) and maximum hyperpolarisation (white bars) for cells with onset inhibition. **E:** FSL distribution of VNLL $O_I$ neurons. Vertical dashed lines indicate the average of each sample. Bin widths are 0.25 ms.

Bushy cells in the VNLL with their onset firing patterns and non-linear current-voltage relationship have been compared to VCN bushy cells (rat: Zhao and Wu, 2001; mouse: Wu and Oertel, 1984) and to principal cells in the MNTB (rat: Banks and Smith, 1992; Zhao and Wu, 2001; Wu and Kelly, 1991). These cells all share lower membrane input resistance when the cell is excited and non-linear current-voltage relationships. It has been proposed that these properties are useful for maintaining and conveying the precise timing of synaptic inputs. Lower membrane resistance makes for faster repolarisation, shortening the excitation and preventing temporal summations, hence allowing the cells to reflect precisely the firing patterns of their afferents. These properties are invaluable for effective encoding of temporal information (Oertel, 1997; Zhao and Wu, 2001; Oertel, 1983, 1991). Bushy cells in the VNLL also resemble bushy cells in the VCN and principal cells in the MNTB morphologically with round to oval somas and profuse dendritic trees in spatially restricted areas (Zhao and Wu, 2001). Bushy cells in the rat VNLL closely resemble bushy cells found in the big brown bat (Covey and Casseday, 1991). The onset pattern produced by these cells also matches the onset responses found in VNLL cells of cat (Aitkin et al., 1970a; Guinan et al., 1972b; Adams, 1997), rabbit (Batra and Fitzpatrick, 1999) and rat (Wu, 1999). The small, oval (putative bushy) cells located ventrally in the VCLL are thought to be the recipients of a calyx-like synapse and the targets of a thick axon projection from the OCA of the contralateral PVCN (guinea pig: Schofield and Cant, 1997).

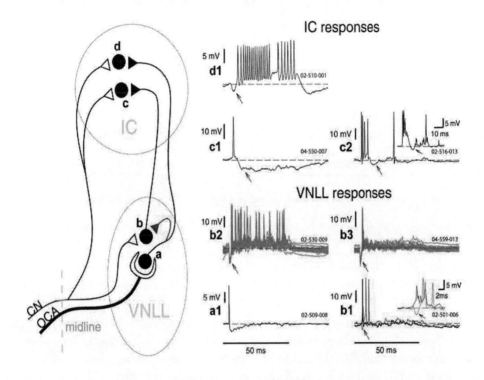

- Modified from Nayagam et al. (2005): with kind permission from The American Physiological Society.

Figure 13. Pathways mediating fast inhibition within the VNLL and IC.
**a:** VNLL neuron receiving input from the OCA via a thick axon projection ending in a calyx. **a1:** Intracellular response of a VNLL $O_I$ cell. **b:** VNLL neuron receiving onset inhibition via a collateral (red) of an ascending axon. **b1:** VNLL cell with intermittent onset inhibition. Red trace is a response when inhibition was present and the black trace is a response when it was absent. Inset: shows the average response (first 15 ms from stimulus onset) with (n=3) and without (n=7) inhibition. **b2, b3:** Overlayed traces (n=20) of onset inhibition in two VNLL cells showing a sustained and onset response, respectively. **c:** An IC neuron receiving delayed inhibition from a VNLL cell with onset inhibition. **c1:** An IC neuron that receives delayed and *sustained* inhibition from a VNLL cell (as in b2) would be expected to exhibit a phasic response. **c2:** An IC neuron that receives delayed and *onset* inhibition from a VNLL cell (as in b3) would be expected to exhibit a pauser response. Inset shows the average response (30 stimulus presentations; first 50 ms from stimulus onset). Pause in AP firing is between 11.7 and 19.4 ms. **d:** An IC neuron receiving input from a VNLL $O_I$ cell (as in a1) would be expected to show onset inhibition (d1) similar to that observed within the VNLL. Horizontal dashed lines indicate RMPs that were -29, -52, -47, -43, -56, -52 and -26 mV for traces shown in a1, b1-b3, c1, c2 and d1, respectively. Traces shown in a1, b1, c1, c2, and d1 (excluding insets) are responses to a single stimulus presentation. In all cases, stimuli were 80 dB noise bursts. Inhibitory projections are shaded and excitatory projections are unshaded. Arrows indicate membrane hyperpolarisation. All traces correspond with neurons in the circuit diagram with the equivalent letter.

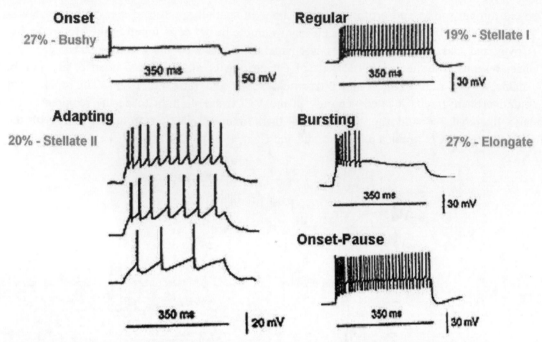

- Modified from Zhao and Wu (2001): with kind permission from John Wiley and Sons, Inc.

Figure 14. Correlation of *in vitro* intracellular responses to current injection with cellular morphology. Responses to intracellular injections of depolarising current of cells in the VCLL of the rat. Three current levels are presented for the adapting neuron. Correlation of response type with neuronal morphology is indicated where possible. The proportion of the VCLL sample made up by each cell type is shown as a percentage. The resting membrane potentials (RMPs) of onset, regular, adapting, bursting, and onset-pause were -57.5 ± 1.3 mV, -56.5 ± 1.9 mV, -58.9 ± 2.1 mV, -59,6 ± 1.3 mV, and -55.0 ± 1.3 mV, respectively.

Regular and onset-pause firing patterns were observed in stellate I cells by Zhao and Wu (2001). In other nuclei, regular cells and the onset-pause cells have different ion conductances on the cell membrane (rat: Kanold and Manis, 1999). However, these regular and onset-pause cells do share some similarities, including the timing of the first spike, as well as the frequency of responses to positive current injection (Zhao and Wu, 2001). These findings of Zhao and Wu (2001) are supported by *in vivo* studies in other species. Most VNLL neurons in bat (Metzner and Radtke-Schuller, 1987; Covey and Casseday, 1991), cat (Guinan et al., 1972b; Guinan et al., 1972a) and rabbit (Batra and Fitzpatrick, 1999) responded to tone bursts with sustained, regular (chopper) discharge patterns. This corresponds nicely with the regular stellate I cells in the rat. A pause in the response was also reported in bat (Metzner and Radtke-Schuller, 1987; Covey and Casseday, 1991), however, whether it is a direct result of the membrane properties identified in the rat, or as a result of other *in vivo* effects, needs further study (Zhao and Wu, 2001).

Stellate II cells were characterised by linear current-voltage relationships and adapting firing patterns (Wu, 1999; Zhao and Wu, 2001). Although they showed sustained firing throughout the duration of the stimulus (like stellate I cells) they did have slight, but definite, differences when compared with the stellate I cells. In response to lower intensity current, stellate I cells fired APs with obvious adaptation. The first spike was often delayed from the onset of stimulus. However, the authors speculate that stellate II neurons encode intensity rather than timing, because the discharge rate was proportional to the strength of the stimulus.

These cells have wide dendritic trees (see above) and it was speculated that these arbours may be used to integrate information across a broader range of ascending lemniscal fibres than stellate I cells (Zhao and Wu, 2001).

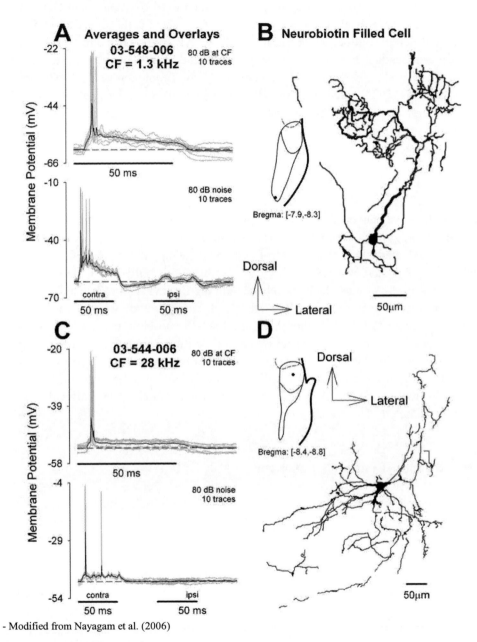

- Modified from Nayagam et al. (2006)

Figure 15. Morphology and intracellular responses of onset-A and onset-B neurons.
**A,C:** Overlay of 10 traces (grey) and average response (black) to contralaterally presented 80 dB SPL CF tones (top) and contralaterally and ipsilaterally presented 80 dB RMS noise (bottom; contralateral and ipsilateral stimuli offset by 100 ms). Horizontal dashed lines show RMP and thick horizontal bars show stimulus duration. **B,D:** Morphology of recorded onset-A and onset-B (respectively) neurons revealed by Neurobiotin labelling. The presumed axons are indicated by 'a'. Discontinuities within a given process have been indicated by dashed lines. Insets show neurons' location (black dot) within the VCLL.

The elongate cells in the VNLL of rats were not found in the *in vitro* intracellular study by Wu (1999) but were identified by Zhao and Wu (2001). Zhao and Wu (2001) postulated that a clue to their function may lie with the cartwheel cells of the DCN first encountered by Hirsch and Oertel (mouse; 1988) and subsequently identified by Zhang and Oertel (mouse; 1993), as well as by Manis et al. (guinea pig: 1994). Cartwheel cells generate a slow wave of $Ca^{2+}$ dependant depolarisation, on which bursts of $Na^+$ APs ride (Zhao and Wu, 2001). These $Na^+$ and $Ca^{2+}$ dependant burst responses are also found in the auditory thalamus (various species: Steriade et al., 1993; rat: Tennigkeit et al., 1996; Tennigkeit et al., 1998; guinea pig: Jahnsen and Llinas, 1984). Zhao and Wu (2001) suggested that similar dual ion channels may mediate the burst response in the elongate cells of the VNLL. Whether these channels are indeed sodium and calcium is yet to be determined. This type of response is consistent with the transient phasic neurons reported in rabbit (Batra and Fitzpatrick, 1999), which responded with bursts of four or more non-chopping APs. The dendritic arbours of this type of unit were orthogonal to the lemniscal pathway implying a possible basis for integration across a wide range of inputs (Zhao and Wu, 2001).

In the rat, Nayagam et al. (2006) correlated three physiological response types with cellular morphology by combining intracellular *in vivo* recordings with Neurobiotin injections. They classified Neurobioton-filled cells using the cytoarchitectural criteria established by Zhao and Wu (2001). Two of the three cells filled, a stellate II / transient chopper and an onset-A / bushy cell, correlated with the findings from Zhao and Wu (2001).

However, the third cell (an onset-B / stellate I) did not correlate with the regular response found by Zhao and Wu (2001; Figure 9, Figure 15). It is possible that the regular sustained firing to current injection *in vitro* is mitigated by additional neural inhibition *in vivo*. The bushy cell described by Nayagam et al. (2006) did not appear to receive calyx-like synaptic connections based on its intracellular response profile, therefore it appears that only a subset of bushy cells within the VCLL are the recipients of the thick-axon, calyceal terminating projection from the OCA.

## Binaural Responses of VCLL Neurons

*In vivo* electrophysiological studies of the DNLL have been conducted in the cat (Aitkin et al., 1970a; Brugge et al., 1970a, b) and echolocating bat (Covey and Casseday, 1995; Metzner and Radtke-Schuller, 1987; Covey, 1993a; Markovitz and Pollak, 1993, 1994; Yang and Pollak, 1994a, b; Yang et al., 1996) and these studies agree that the DNLL is a binaural nucleus. In contrast, the VCLL has been considered to be a monaural structure because its inputs originate primarily from the contralateral CN (cat: Aitkin et al., 1970a; Glendenning et al., 1981; bat: Covey and Casseday, 1991). However, there have been relatively few studies that have recorded VCLL neural responses to bilaterally presented sounds to confirm this assertion. Although all studies tend to agree that most VCLL cells are excited by stimulation of the contralateral ear, some studies have shown that a proportion of VCLL cells are responsive to input from the ipsilateral ear (rabbit: Batra and Fitzpatrick, 1997; cat: Aitkin et al., 1970a; Guinan et al., 1972b; rabbit: Batra and Fitzpatrick, 1999; rat: Nayagam et al., 2006). Binaural responsiveness is assessed by whether there are responses to stimulation of both or either ear and sensitivity to interaural disparities are typically assayed by introducing ILDs or ITDs. In the big brown bat, Covey and Casseday (1991) found no evidence for binaural responses in the VNLLc and VNLLm nuclei. However, they found a small number of binaural cells in the INLL but not enough to exclude the INLL from being included in the 'monaural' complex. There have been reports of both forms (ITD and ILD) of binaural sensitivity in the VCLL of non-echolocating mammals. However, there are significant differences between mammalian species with respect to the existence and the extent of binaural units within the VCLL (Zhang and Kelly, 2006a).

It is possible that there is a distinct population of neurons in the medial VNLL (VNLLm) of rabbits that is sensitive to ITDs (Batra and Fitzpatrick, 1997), supporting the anatomical evidence that the medial part of the VCLL is specialised for binaural processing (Glendenning et al., 1981; Henkel and Spangler, 1983)[3]. Zhang and Kelly (2006a) have recently reported widely distributed cells responsive to ILDs throughout the VCLL of the rat.

There are a handful of *in vivo* electrophysiological studies in the VNLL of non-echolocating animals that have identified binaural responses (rat: Zhang and Kelly, 2006a; Nayagam et al., 2006; rabbit: Batra and Fitzpatrick, 1997; Batra and Fitzpatrick, 2002a, b; cat: Aitkin et al., 1970a; Guinan et al., 1972b; Guinan et al., 1972a; rabbit: Batra and Fitzpatrick, 1999). Batra and Fitzpatrick (1997) found 21 neurons that were sensitive to ITDs of low frequency tones (less than 2kHz), although some had CFs of up to 5.5kHz. The locations of the neurons were reconstructed and found to lie in the medial portion of the VCLL of rabbits or in the adjacent reticular formation. Five of the neurons were visualised with tracer dye and found to be within the low cell density, medial part of the VNLL. Most of the neurons responded to the onset of binaural stimulation at the most favourable ITD. The responses would vary cyclically with a period equal to that of the tone when the ipsilateral stimuli was progressively delayed or advanced with respect to the contralateral stimuli. Most of the neurons studied did not produce onset responses to ipsilateral stimulation and did not follow dynamic changes in ITD produced by a binaural-beat stimulus. However, there were some (6/14) neurons that did respond weakly to an ipsilateral stimulus and about a third of the neurons responded (although sometimes poorly) to dynamic changes in ITD (Batra and Fitzpatrick, 1997).The difference between the binaural responses from their study and those found in the SOC suggested that the ITD sensitivity recorded in the VCLL originated from a unique population of the SOC or there was a substantial transformation in the VCLL. It is unlikely that the VCLL ITD sensitivity is a direct result of converging phase-locked inputs (Batra and Fitzpatrick, 1997).

Batra and Fitzpatrick (1997) found that many neurons were influenced by ipsilateral, as well as contralateral stimulation. The two major types of binaural interactions were ILD of the type E0/I, and sensitivity to ITDs. E0/I type responses were exhibited by both onset and sustained type neurons, whereas ITD sensitivity was mostly limited to onset cells. Binaural cells were located throughout the VCLL, but there appeared to be a preference for cells receiving inhibition, and ITD sensitive neurons, to be located medially and around the boundary of the nucleus. Monaural and transient neurons were more likely found in ventral VNLL (referred to as VNLL1). Batra and Fitzpatrick (1999) described many VCLL E0/I neurons that were unresponsive to ITDs. At least some of these cells were located in the marginal ventral VNLL (VNLL1). This supports findings of Aitkin et al. (1970a) who found

---

[3] Glendenning et al. (1981) refer to this region as the lateral tegmentum, whilst Schofield and Cant (1997) refer to it as the VNLLa. It is not the same as the multipolar region of the VNLL in bats or the middle VNLL used by Adams (1979) (see above).

that binaural neurons appeared to be present only at the margins of the nucleus. The idea that the binaural and monaural neurons may be at least partially segregated provides some reconciliation between different studies. Aitkin et al. (cat: 1970a) found few (11%) binaural neurons in the cat VCLL, whereas Guinan et al. (cat: 1972b) found over 60%. It is possible that the two studies sampled different populations, and therefore arrived at different estimates of the number of binaural neurons (Batra and Fitzpatrick, 1999).

In the rat, there has been two published studies that have investigated responsiveness to binaural stimulation (Zhang and Kelly, 2006a; Nayagam et al., 2006). In the Zhang and Kelly study, a substantial proportion (87%) of tested units responded with some form of binaural ILD sensitivity. The majority of interactions (59%) were excited by contralateral stimulation and inhibited by ipsilateral stimulation. Binaural cells were found distributed throughout the dorsoventral extent of the VCLL. However, Zhang and Kelly (2006a) did not examine the spatial distribution of binaural types within the structure, but rather the relationship between the dorsoventral position and the strength of the binaural suppression.

Nayagam et al (2006) found that the VCLL exhibited a diverse and complex suite of binaural and inhibitory inputs. Figure 16A,B,C presents example intracellular responses showing E0, EI and EE types. Their intracellular data show that a number of cells that would appear as E0 extracellularly actually received some concurrent contralateral inhibition, either notch, short or long duration. This inhibition, observed as IPSPs, is only visible in intracellular recordings and had not been reported previously. EE units tested in their study showed evidence of complex EE/EI interactions at different ILDs. This finding is consistent with results of previous extracellular studies (Zhang and Kelly, 2006a). However, due to the complex nature of binaural excitatory and inhibitory interaction, Nayagam et al's (2006) classifications were simplified. They reported binaural type for 137 intracellularly recorded VCLL neurons in response to 80 dB SPL bilateral noise bursts (separated by 100 ms). All binaural types (E0, EI, EE, I0, II, IE, 0E) were found within the VCLL. The proportion of each type is shown in Figure 16D. Almost all units (97%) responded to contralateral stimulation, mostly with excitation (83%). Contralaterally inhibited neurons, both monaural and binaural were located throughout the structure. However, of the contralaterally excited cells, the EI units were preferentially distributed within the INLL, while E0 and EE units were common throughout the VNLL and INLL. Roughly half of VCLL units tested (55%) received monaural inputs and the other half (45%) received binaural inputs. Within the VNLL, two thirds of units (67%) were monaural, while in the INLL the proportions were reversed with one third (35%) monaural (Figure 16E). The spatial distribution of the three forms of contralaterally excited responses (E0, EI and EE) is shown in 3D (Figure 17B) and collapsed into three coronal sections (Figure 17A). The various binaural interactions observed in VCLL neurons, as well as the variable response types to noise and tones, suggest convergence of excitatory and inhibitory inputs across a wide range of frequencies onto VCLL cells.

# FUNCTIONAL ROLE OF THE VCLL IN AUDITORY PROCESSING

Many possible functional roles have been suggested for the VCLL, however, the exact function of the VCLL remains poorly understood. Contemporary studies have suggested that the VCLL is a crucial integrative nucleus in the auditory brainstem, rather than a simple relay station (rat: Wu, 1999), and is a major source of inhibition to the IC (rat: Zhang et al., 1998; cat: Saint Marie and Baker, 1990). Several roles in auditory processing (various species: Oertel and Wickesberg, 2002; bat: Ross et al., 1988) have been proposed for the VCLL in various species, including a role in pitch perception (cat: Malmierca et al., 1998), temporal processing (bat: Covey and Casseday, 1991), pattern recognition (various species: Oertel and Wickesberg, 2002), a filter of time-variant signals (bat: Covey and Casseday, 1986) or multiple functions (cat: Glendenning and Hutson, 1998).

The observed responses in the VNLL of echolocating (Covey and Casseday, 1991) and non-echolocating species (Aitkin et al., 1970a; Adams, 1997; Guinan et al., 1972a) have been mainly onset, although the recent Zhang and Kelly (rat; 2006a) and Nayagam et al. (rat; 2006) studies found an increased population of sustained neurons. Batra and Fitzpatrick's (rabbit; 1997) study also described neurons with onset responses in the VNLL that may be sensitive to ITDs. These findings led to the conclusion that the VNLL may be involved in the localisation of acoustic transients (rabbit: Batra and Fitzpatrick, 1997). This certainly seems likely in the echolocating bat, where the specialised needs of echolocation have led to an anatomically and physiologically specialised auditory pathway.

The lemniscal nuclei of bats are significantly different to the VCLL of non-echolocating species. The lemniscal nuclei of bats are divided into monaural and binaural regions and contain highly segregated cell types that perform different roles in sound processing. Covey and Casseday (bat; 1986) suggested a possible frequency-to-time converter role for the NLL. They viewed the entire network from the AVCN, through the various VCLL nuclei to the IC, as a means to provide the IC with a set of delays of the AVCN output (Covey and Casseday, 1986). In 1991, Covey and Casseday described a monaural subdivision of the VCLL, termed VNLLc, which contained cells capable of responding very accurately to the onset of contralateral stimulation with a constant latency over a wide range of frequencies and intensities. These cells were not found in the rest of the complex, leading to the conclusion that the VNLLc was suited to precisely encode timing, particularly with respect to onsets and acoustic transients. The rest of the structure contained cells with sustained or chopper responses and thus it was concluded that these other areas were responsible for coding the ongoing properties of a sound.

Three transformations occur within the brainstem of echolocating species that have a bearing on the processing of time-distributed information. These are: 1) a conversion of excitatory to inhibitory signals, 2) changes in the temporal response pattern, often from sustained to onset, and 3) a large increase in the range of response latencies. These transformations occur multiple times within segregated processing streams of the bat brainstem and create increasingly complex and diverse response properties at each successive level before ultimately converging at the IC (Covey and Casseday, 1999; Covey, 2003).

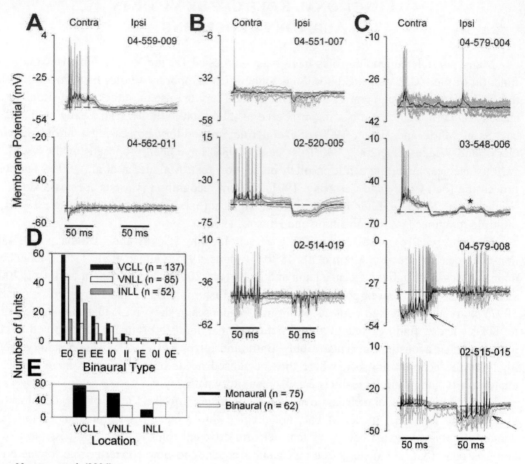

- Nayagam et al. (2006)

Figure 16. Intracellular binaural responses types to noise in the VCLL.
**A-C:** In vivo intracellular recordings from VCLL neurons to contralateral and ipsilateral 50 ms, 80 dB RMS noise bursts (10 trace overlay shown in grey; 10 trace average shown in black). All traces shown are from VCLL neurons that were excited by contralateral stimulation. Horizontal dashed lines indicate RMP and dark horizontal bars indicate duration of contralateral (left) and ipsilateral (right) stimuli that were offset by 100 ms. A: Examples of responses from cells that were not influenced by ipsilateral noise stimulation (E0), showing sustained (top) and onset (bottom) firing patterns. B: Examples of responses that were inhibited by ipsilateral stimulation (EI) with inhibitory post-synaptic potentials (IPSPs) of varying duration and temporal summation properties (top traces, medium duration; middle traces, long duration; bottom traces, short duration). Different contralateral responses were observed for EI units, including onset (top), sustained (middle) and chopper (bottom) patterns. C: Examples of various responses that were excited by ipsilateral stimulation (EE). Ipsilateral excitation was transient (top traces), continuous (middle traces) or delayed (bottom trace). EE units showed a variety of contralateral response patterns including onset (top two traces), delayed (third trace) and chopper (bottom trace). Asterisk shows excitatory post-synaptic potentials (EPSPs) in the absence of action potentials (APs). Arrows show APs generated during underlying long-duration inhibition. **D:** Distribution of VCLL units across 8 binaural categories showing differences in binaural type distribution between the ventral and intermediate nuclei of the lateral lemniscus (VNLL and INLL respectively). **E:** Proportion of monaural (E0, I0, 0I and 0E) and binaural (EI, EE, II, IE) units in the VCLL, VNLL and INLL.

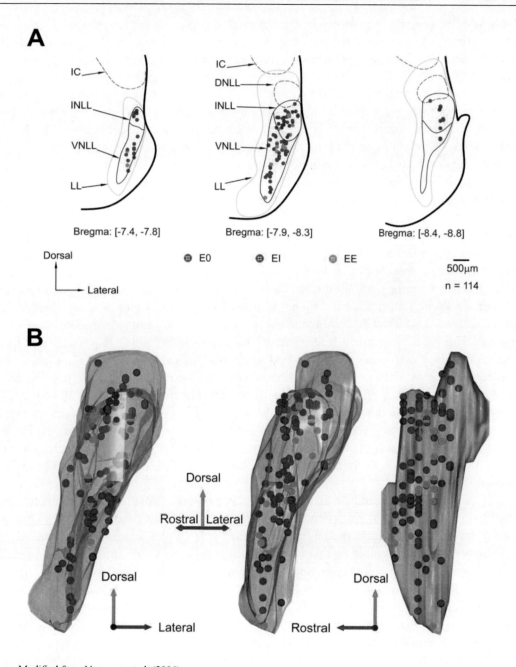

- Modified from Nayagam et al. (2006)

Figure 17. Spatial distribution of intracellular unit's binaural type within the VCLL.
Only units that were excited by contralateral stimulation (E0, EI and EE; key provided bottom of panel A) are shown. Format the same as Figure 4. The viewing aspects of the 3D reconstructions in (B) are rostral (left), oblique between rostral and lateral (middle) and lateral (right). Each orthogonal orientation arrow is 500 μm, although the central panel's rostral and lateral orientation axes are 2D representations of 3D objects that are projecting "out of the page" at 45 degrees to the page surface and therefore appear shorter than the other axes.

Bat studies (Covey and Casseday, 1999; Covey, 2003) provide neural models which show that convergence of these three separate processing streams creates the potential for IC neurons to filter temporal features of sound including tuning for duration, direction of frequency sweeps, modulation rate, and interstimulus intervals (gap detection). The ability to discriminate these temporal features of sound is a critical part of echolocation. However, these features are not exclusive to the realm of navigating caves or hunting insects. Processing animal vocalisations in non-echolocating species, or comprehending human speech requires the ability to discriminate the same temporal features mentioned above.

Findings from studies in non-echolocating species, suggest that despite the differences in the setup of the lemniscal nuclei, the basic ingredients for performing the three transformations in the brainstem are preserved. Furthermore, the three transformations may all occur within the VCLL: 1) The VNLL receives excitatory input from the CN and sends inhibitory projections to the IC. 2) Response patterns are altered in the VCLL, via either membrane properties of VCLL neurons or convergence of inhibition and excitation. Indeed, several classes of onset responses within the VCLL were described by Nayagam et al. (2006) that, with the exception onset ideal cells, showed differing responses to noise versus tones. 3) Fast, pre-spike inhibition has been shown to actively delay the output of a subset of VCLL and IC responses which will contribute to the increase in the range of response latencies of IC neurons. The VCLL contains a heterogenous neural population and it is possible that these three transformations occur in segregated processing streams within the structure that converge at the IC. These functions proposed in echolocating species do not require a tonotopic arrangement of the VCLL, in line with the results from Nayagam et al. (rat; 2006). However, they also do not require binaurally responsive neurons. Several recent studies in non-echolocating species (Nayagam et al., 2006; Zhang and Kelly, 2006a; Batra and Fitzpatrick, 1997; Guinan et al., 1972b) have reported binaurally responsive neurons within the VCLL and thus it is likely that, at least in these species, the VCLL performs additional functional processing.

A recent study by Langner et al. (gerbil; 2006) found that the transfer functions of neurons in the IC changed from comb filters at sound onset into band-pass filters after the initial phase. They postulated that the inhibition (precisely synchronised to the signal periodicity) that is responsible for this mechanism was from the VCLL. Furthermore, these IC neurons were tuned to modulation frequencies and arranged in periodicity maps. There is significant feedback from the IC, through the VCLL (rat: Caicedo and Herbert, 1993; guinea pig: Malmierca et al., 1996), to the SOC and CN (cat: Whitley and Henkel, 1984). Thus, it was expected that the VCLL would show some evidence for the periodotopy found in the IC. Using 2-DG activation as well as retrograde tracing of BDA from the IC, they found evidence for a helical periodicity map with 7 to 8 turns (compatible with the findings of Merchán and Berbel, 1996) of a low to high, dorsal to ventral pitch representation within the VCLL. However, this finding has not been validated by electrophysiological studies.

Based predominantly on tracing studies performed by Merchán and Berbel (1996) in the rat as well as new tracing studies in the cat, Merchán et al. (1997) proposed a processing rationale for the VCLL that is in line with the general organisational principal of the auditory system: i.e. an orderly spatial representation of tonal frequency. They suggested that the VCLL processes information on a frequency-frame basis, preserving the cochlea's spectral decomposition of the input signal. However, Nayagam et al. (2006), using 3D reconstructions of intracellular response locations, found no evidence to support an orderly tonotopic distribution within the VCLL. The apparent lack of tonotopicity within the VCLL described by the Nayagam et al. (2006) and other studies (Glendenning, 1981; Guinan et al., 1972a,b; Kelly et al., 1998a; Zhang and Kelly, 2006a) suggests a role that is removed from direct processing of frequency. If these neurons are involved in frequency processing, then it is possibly through an indirect means such as influencing sideband inhibition in IC neurons. There is a crucial difference, which has been largely overlooked between tonotopicity and topography. A nucleus may send or receive topographically ordered projections with respect to the tonotopicity of the target or source, but this does not lead inexorably to a tonotopic arrangement within that nucleus.

Batra and Fitzpatrick (1997) described a population of neurons in the medial VCLL of the rabbit that was sensitive to ITDs. These neurons responded with onset responses and obviously had low CFs. They were located in a region that had previously been described in the cat as the lateral tegmentum (Glendenning et al., 1981), however Batra and Fitzpatrick believed that the ITD sensitive cells in their study lay within the boundaries of the lateral lemniscal tract in the rabbit. The authors claimed that the ITD sensitivity of these neurons was a feature that was not created by bilateral convergence of phase-locked inputs but rather transmitted from the SOC. The VCLL has already been shown to contain a large proportion of onset responses (Aitkin et al., 1970a; Guinan et al., 1972b; Adams, 1997; Covey and Casseday, 1991; Guinan et al., 1972a) and has been implicated to play a role in processing acoustic transients (Covey and Casseday, 1991). Batra and Fitzpatrick concluded that these features combined with ITD sensitivity, which provides insight into the location of a stimulus along the azimuth, suggests that the nucleus plays a role in localising acoustic transients.

The recent electrophysiological investigation of the VCLL by Nayagam et al. (2006) did not test low CF neurons for ITD sensitivity. Typically, if a neuron were creating ITDs through bilateral convergence of phase-locked inputs then it would be affected by monaural contralateral as well as monaural ipsilateral stimulation. Even if not driven to discharge, synaptic inputs following monaural contralateral and ipsilateral stimulation would alter the membrane potential and this would be visible in intracellular traces. However, in the Batra and Fitzpatrick (1997) study, ITD sensitivity was not generated within the VCLL but rather transmitted from the SOC. In this situation, ITD sensitive neurons cannot be identified based on their synaptic inputs following monaural contralateral and ipsilateral stimulation. However, reconstructions of the location of neuron's CFs within the VCLL, by Nayagam et al. (2006), provided no evidence for an increased distribution of low CF cells in the medial part of the structure. This finding suggests that in the rat VCLL, ITD sensitive neurons, if they exist, are not localised to a medial portion of the nucleus. This does not rule out the possibility of ITD sensitive cells in the rat VCLL performing a role in localising acoustic transients as proposed in the rabbit. It is likely that species specific differences in hearing ranges and parcellation may underlie the different functional observation between studies.

Oertel and Wickesberg (2002), by a process of elimination, speculated that the VCLL is involved in processing the transient and temporal features of auditory stimulus. In reaching this working hypothesis, the authors considered the ubiquitous presence of the VNLL across all mammalian species as well as reptiles and birds. This suggests that this nucleus plays a fundamental role in localising or recognising sound. Given that the VCLL had mainly been described as a monaural structure, the authors focused on the recognition and interpretation of the temporal patterns within natural and complex sounds (Oertel and Wickesberg, 2002), as this is a function that depends on monaural rather than binaural cues. One of the temporal patterns that the VCLL may be well suited to encode, is the detection of the interval between acoustic transients. This is useful for encoding periodic sounds, such as low-frequency tones, harmonic complexes, and click trains, which are modelled by repeated acoustic transients. These signals produce coincident firing of a wide frequency range of auditory nerve fibres. Octopus cells have biophysical specialisations which allow them to detect and sum this coincident firing, and transmit the periodic signal to the VCLL (Golding et al., 1995; Oertel et al., 1990; Golding et al., 1999). This interpretation is in line with the current descriptions of the VCLL and the prominent projection it receives from octopus cells that are well suited to convey the accurate timing of onset and pattern information.

The intrinsic circuitry of the VCLL proposed by Nayagam et al. (2005) suggests that the cells receiving octopus cell input send fast onset inhibition, via local collaterals, to other cells in the VCLL in order to delay the VCLL's inhibitory output to the IC. How this fits with the role that the octopus cell projection may play in the detection of acoustic transients is unclear. The fact that the pathway terminates on the bushy cells of the VCLL suggests that the signals encoding acoustic transients are converted to play another role. It is possible that the fast inhibitory local circuit is one of many parallel processing channels stemming from the octopus cell projection to the VCLL. However, the proportion of VCLL cells described by Nayagam et al. (2005) that received fast onset inhibition (14.3%) was roughly equivalent to the proportion of cells with $O_I$ responses (proposed octopus cell targets; 17.9%), suggesting a one to one relationship. If each octopus cell activates a fast inhibitory circuit, then it is unlikely that parallel processing streams performing other functions stem from the cells receiving octopus cell input in the ventral VCLL.

Oertel and Wickesberg (2002) ruled out a role for the VCLL in localising sound in the horizontal plane based on the fact that many older studies had shown the lemniscal nuclei to be predominantly monaural structures. However, given data from Nayagam et al. (2006) and other recent studies (Zhang and Kelly, 2006a; Batra and Fitzpatrick, 2002b) showing that the VCLL contains a high proportion of binaural units responsive to interaural level and time cues, a role in azimuth localisation may be worth reconsidering. Given Nayagam et al.'s (2006) finding of an increased proportion of ILD sensitive neurons in the excitatory INLL, APs signalling azimuth may be separated from APs signalling onset, which stem from inhibitory VNLL cells.

From an anatomical perspective, functionality would depend, in part, on which tonotopic model one assumes to be correct. Malmierca et al.'s (cat; 1998) 3D mosaic arrangement of interdigitating clusters of neurons suggests a situation whereby disparate frequency specific regions of the CNIC receive inputs from compartments within the VCLL that share large interfaces, creating a diversity of neuronal properties. This is similar to the relationship between the cerebral cortex and the pontine nuclei (Malmierca et al., 1998). The functional implications of this would seem to depend on the spatial relationship of the dendritic arbours to the cluster borders.

Given the mosaic organisation of the VCLL revealed in Malmierca et al.'s (cat; 1998) study, these authors proposed a role for the VCLL in pitch perception based on temporal features of the stimulus. This is in line with evidence suggesting that pitch perception requires not only spectral (Goldstein, 1973) but also temporal (Moore and Rosen, 1979; Shofner et al., 2005) information. Their proposal was founded on a model initially described by (Licklider, 1951) and refined by (Meddis and Hewitt, 1991). In this model, the summation of autocorrelated neural responses across frequency-selective channels was described as a mechanism for pitch perception based on extraction of both temporal and spectral information from an auditory signal. This model had three requirements, which are: 1) delayed versions of the input signal, 2) convergence of the delayed signal onto single cells, and 3) convergence between frequency channels. Malmierca et al. (1998) suggest that the VCLL is capable of satisfying these three requirements via: 1) Multiple ladder-rung like collaterals of the long lemniscal fibres creating delay lines along the dorsoventral axis of the VCLL. 2) Local collaterals with ventral neurons supplying convergent input on successively more dorsal neurons (cat: Whitley and Henkel, 1984). 3) The spatially specific, but still interdigitating clusters of frequency representation creating cross-frequency interactions. However, this proposal suffers from at least two setbacks. Firstly, the output of the ventral VCLL is inhibitory; this is not accounted for by the model. Secondly, recent studies have shown that response latency is unaffected by position along the dorsoventral axis of the VCLL (Zhang and Kelly, 2006a) and thus the requirement for delayed versions of the input signal is not satisfied in this way.

Results from Nayagam et al. (2006) suggest that a modified version of Malmierca et al.'s (1998) proposal may still satisfy the requirements of the model. This modification would involve altering the site of integration, from the VCLL to the IC, with the VCLL acting as a pre-processor setting up the appropriate timings and inputs. In this way, the three model requirements may still be met via: 1) Delays of the original input signal created by the fast onset inhibition described in Nayagam et al. (2005) and observed in the IC of this and previous studies (see above). 2) Convergence of the delayed signal on single cells at the level of the IC via inputs and intrinsic circuitry. 3) The lack of tonotopicity within the VCLL together with the organised topography of its inputs and outputs, described by some tracing studies, combining to create cross-frequency interaction in the VCLL. This proposal is supported by data from Nayagam et al. (2006); it accounts for the inhibitory nature of the structure and it brings together seemingly disparate results from anatomical and electrophysiological studies. Once again, this proposal only utilises a subset of the response types and properties observed in the VCLL, and therefore, it is likely that if the VCLL is involved in timing based pitch perception, it is only one of many functional roles performed by the nucleus.

The lack of a clearly demonstrable tonotopicity within the VCLL contrasts with the basic organising principle of the auditory brainstem, and may give a clue as to its function in temporal processing (Oertel and Wickesberg, 2002; Glendenning and Hutson, 1998). Onset ideal cells within the VCLL are broadly tuned and are a crucial part of the local neural circuitry activated by octopus cell input. Components of this circuit have been described in many species and it is particularly prominent in humans. The onset of a natural sound is an important acoustic event resulting in broadband activation of coincidence detecting neurons such as octopus cells. Onset responses may provide a reference point for the ongoing frequency component processing of a stimulus. Powerful broadband onset inhibition within the VCLL is well placed to control the timing of subsequent APs, whilst remaining independent of APs signalling other frequency-dependant parameters of the stimulus. Nayagam et al. (2005) have proposed that the onset ideal cells are recipients of octopus cell input and provide a source of powerful, fast, pre-spike onset inhibition in VCLL cells, and probably IC cells as well. Additionally, they suggested that this onset inhibition is capable of mediating the timing of the inhibitory output of the VNLL to the IC (Nayagam et al., 2006). When viewed across a neural population, the onset inhibition within the VCLL could coordinate the VCLL's inhibitory output to the IC. This presumably creates a population of IC neurons that respond to a spectrally complex stimuli with onsets that occur within a narrower time window than they would without the VCLL circuitry (Nayagam et al., 2006).

## CONCLUSION

At a perceptual level, the binding of a distributed signal within the sensory system into a cohesive conscious thought is a crucial but poorly understood aspect of neural processing. The activity of various auditory neurons, coding different properties of many distinct but concurrent sounds, is combined to create a unified perception of a listeners' auditory environment. Identifying the neural correlates of this conscious experience is one of the great challenges that face neuroscientists, and is well beyond the scope of the current discussion. However, the neural circuitry proposed in Nayagam et al. (2005) may provide the basis for grouping or binding responses to different frequency components of an auditory signal at the level of the IC. A complex stimulus (such as human speech) with two or more spectral peaks excites neural populations in the brainstem tuned to those spectral peaks. The population response to the higher amplitude peak occurs with a shorter latency that the population response to the lower amplitude peaks. In a situation without the VCLL, these brainstem responses would result in an IC population with onsets that occur within a wide time-window. However, the addition of the inhibitory VCLL, in a parallel processing stream to the excitatory projections from the brainstem to the IC, dramatically alters the timing of IC responses to the spectrally complex stimulus. The onset of the complex stimulus, a broadband event, stimulates octopus cells of the PVCN, which in turn activate the inhibitory VNLL onset ideal cells. These onset ideal cells project to the IC, and send collaterals of this powerful, fast, and well-timed inhibitory projection to other cells of the VCLL. The resulting inhibition arrives at the IC target neurons before the excitation from the brainstem population responding to the higher amplitude spectral peak, and actively delays the IC's response to this component of the signal. The IC's response to the onset of later arriving lower amplitude peaks is unaffected. Similarly, delayed and later arriving inhibition from the other VCLL cells may refine the IC's onset responses by attenuating post-onset excitatory inputs. The overall result is a population of IC neurons which respond to a complex stimulus incorporating multiple spectral peaks, with onsets that are grouped into a narrower time-window and book-ended by inhibition from the VCLL (Nayagam et al., 2006).

This mechanism may be viewed as time-domain binding of the various neural responses to different features of a complex frequency domain signal. The advantage of this setup is that it allows parallel processing streams to de-compose and examine different temporal and spectral components of an input signal and yet retain the ability to re-integrate this information into a perceptually unified entity. This feature-binding role of the VCLL does not require tonotopic organisation and is consistent with previous suggestions that the VCLL is involved in processing timing. The fine-tuning of first spike timing by onset-evoked inhibition provides an explanation of how the IC might re-integrate its multitude of inputs, following stimulation with complex sounds such as human speech.

Humans have an increased proportion of globular cells in ventral VNLL compared to other terrestrial mammals. We have a greater projection from the OCA to the ventral VCLL and more calyces on bushy cells of the VCLL (Adams, 1997). Therefore, the powerful onset inhibition described by Nayagam et al. (2005), and the entire neural circuit responsible for adjusting spike timing in the VCLL and IC must play an important and enhanced function in humans, once again suggesting a role in interpreting temporal patterns within natural sounds like speech. In humans, the fact that there does not seem to be an equivalent of an INLL suggests that this nucleus may perform a role that is redundant in humans. However, the lack of a clearly distinguishable INLL does not exclude the possibility that the circuits that make up the INLL in other species are incorporated into the VNLL of humans. Additionally, the high proportion of globular cells with large calyx-like inputs in human VNLL (Adams, 1997) implies the kind of processing that requires a specialised and fast neural circuit is more important in humans than in other species. The various roles proposed for the VCLL are not mutually exclusive and it is possible, if not likely, that the VCLL plays multiple roles in auditory processing.

## ACKNOWLEDGMENTS

The authors would like to thank the Bionic Ear Institute, the Department of Otolaryngology, The University of Melbourne, Dame Elisabeth Murdoch and the International Brain Research Organisation for financial support of this work. We would also like to thank the scientists and publishers who have kindly allowed reproduction of their original figures.

## REFERENCES

Adams JC (1979) Ascending projections to the inferior colliculus. *J Comp Neurol* 183:519-538.

Adams JC (1981) Cytology of the Nuclei of the Lateral Lemniscus. *Anatomical Record* 199:A6-A6.

Adams JC (1993) *Non-Primary Inputs to the Cochlear Nucleus Visualized Using Immunocytochemistry.* In: The Mammalian Cochlear Nuclei: Organization and Function (Merchán MA, ed), pp 133-141. New York: Plenum Press.

Adams JC (1997) Projections from octopus cells of the posteroventral cochlear nucleus to the ventral nucleus of the lateral lemniscus in cat and human. *Aud Neurosci* 3:335-350.

Adams JC, Warr WB (1976) Origins of axons in the cat's acoustic striae determined by injection of horseradish peroxidase into severed tracts. *J Comp Neurol* 170:107-121.

Adams JC, Mugnaini E (1990) Immunocytochemical evidence for inhibitory and disinhibitory circuits in the superior olive. *Hear Res* 49:281-298.

Aitkin LM, Anderson DJ, Brugge JF (1970a) Tonotopic organization and discharge characteristics of single neurons in nuclei of lateral lemniscus of the cat. *J Neurophysiol* 33:421-440.

Aitkin LM, Anderson DJ, Brugge JF (1970b) Frequency Organization and Response Characteristics of Single Neurons in Nuclei of Lateral Lemniscus of Cat. *Journal of the Acoustical Society of America* 47:59.

Aoki E, Semba R, Keino H, Kato K, Kashiwamata S (1988) Glycine-like immunoreactivity in the rat auditory pathway. *Brain Res* 442:63-71.

Bajo VM, Merchán MA, Lopez DE, Rouiller EM (1993) Neuronal Morphology and Efferent Projections of the Dorsal Nucleus of the Lateral Lemniscus in the Rat. *J Comp Neurol* 334:241-262.

Banks MI, Smith PH (1992) Intracellular recordings from neurobiotin-labeled cells in brain slices of the rat medial nucleus of the trapezoid body. *J Neurosci* 12:2819-2837.

Batra R (2006) Responses of neurons in the ventral nucleus of the lateral lemniscus to sinusoidally amplitude modulated tones. *J Neurophysiol* 96:2388-2398.

Batra R, Fitzpatrick DC (1997) Neurons sensitive to interaural temporal disparities in the medial part of the ventral nucleus of the lateral lemniscus. *J Neurophysiol* 78:511-515.

Batra R, Fitzpatrick DC (1999) Discharge patterns of neurons in the ventral nucleus of the lateral lemniscus of the unanesthetized rabbit. *Journal of Neurophysiology* 82:1097-1113.

Batra R, Fitzpatrick DC (2002a) Processing of interaural temporal disparities in the medial division of the ventral nucleus of the lateral lemniscus. *J Neurophysiol* 88:666-675.

Batra R, Fitzpatrick DC (2002b) Monaural and binaural processing in the ventral nucleus of the lateral lemniscus: a major source of inhibition to the inferior colliculus. *Hearing Res* 168:90-97.

Benson CG, Cant NB (2008) The ventral nucleus of the lateral lemniscus of the gerbil (Meriones unguiculatus): organization of connections with the cochlear nucleus and the inferior colliculus. *J Comp Neurol* 510:673-690.

Berne RM, Levy MN, Stanton BA, Koeppen BM (1998) *Physiology*, 4 Edition: Mosby-Year Book, Inc.

Beyerl BD (1978) Afferent projections to the central nucleus of the inferior colliculus in the rat. *Brain Res* 145:209-223.

Blackburn CC, Sachs MB (1989) Classification of Unit Types in the Anteroventral Cochlear Nucleus - Pst Histograms and Regularity Analysis. *J Neurophysiol* 62:1303-1329.

Bourk TR, Mielcarz JP, Norris BE (1981) Tonotopic organization of the anteroventral cochlear nucleus of the cat. *Hear Res* 4:215-241.

Brawer JR, Morest DK, Kane EC (1974) Neuronal Architecture of Cochlear Nucleus of Cat. *J Comp Neurol* 157:251-300.

Brownell WE, Manis PB, Ritz LA (1979) Ipsilateral Inhibitory Responses in the Cat Lateral Superior Olive. *Brain Res* 177:189-193.

Browner RH, Webster DB (1975) Projections of the trapezoid body and the superior olivary complex of the Kangaroo rat (Dipodomys merriami). *Brain, Behavior And Evolution* 11:322-354.

Brugge JF, Anderson DJ, Aitkin LM (1970a) Sensitivity of Single Neurons in Dorsal Nucleus of Lateral Lemniscus of Cat to Binaural Tonal Stimulation. *Journal of the Acoustical Society of America* 47:77-&.

Brugge JF, Anderson DJ, Aitkin LM (1970b) Responses of Neurons in Dorsal Nucleus of Lateral Lemniscus of Cat to Binaural Tonal Stimulation. *J Neurophysiol* 33:441-&.

Brunso-Bechtold JK, Thompson GC (1978) Ascending Auditory Projections to Nuclei of Lateral Lemniscus as Demonstrated by Horseradish-Peroxidase. *Anatomical Record* 190:350-350.

Brunso-Bechtold JK, Thompson GC, Masterton RB (1981) HRP study of the organization of auditory afferents ascending to central nucleus of inferior colliculus in cat. *J Comp Neurol* 197:705-722.

Caicedo A, Herbert H (1993) Topography of Descending Projections from the Inferior Colliculus to Auditory Brain-Stem Nuclei in the Rat. *J Comp Neurol* 328:377-392.

Cajal RyS (1909) *Histologie du Systeme Nerveux de l'Homme et des Vertébrés*. In: Tome *I:* Instituto Ramon y Cajal, pp 774-838. Madrid.

Campos ML, De Cabo C, Wisden W, Juiz JM, Merlo D (2001) Expression of GABA(A) receptor subunits in rat brainstem auditory pathways: Cochlear nuclei, superior olivary complex and nucleus of the lateral lemniscus. *Neuroscience* 102:625-638.

Cant NB, Benson CG (2003) Parallel auditory pathways: projection patterns of the different neuronal populations in the dorsal and ventral cochlear nuclei. *Brain Research Bulletin* 60:457-474.

Casseday JH, Covey E (1983) Laminar projections to the inferior colliculus as seen from injections of wheat germ agglutinin-horseradish peroxidase in the superioir ollivary complex of the cat. *Soc Neurosci Abstr* 9:766.

Casseday JH, Kobler JB, Isbey SF, Covey E (1989) Central acoustic tract in an echolocating bat: an extralemniscal auditory pathway to the thalamus. *J Comp Neurol* 287:247-259.

Clopton BM, Winfield JA (1973) Tonotopic organization in the inferior colliculus of the rat. *Brain Res* 56:355-358.

Coleman JR, Clerici WJ (1987) Sources of projections to subdivisions of the inferior colliculus in the rat. *J Comp Neurol* 262:215-226.

Coleman JR, Campbell M, Clerici WJ (1982) Observations on tonotopic organization within the rat inferior colliculus using 2-deoxy-D[1-3H] glucose. *Otolaryngol Head Neck Surg* 90:795-800.

Covey E (1993a) Response Properties of Single Units in the Dorsal Nucleus of the Lateral Lemniscus and Paralemniscal Zone of an Echolocating Bat. *J Neurophysiol* 69:842-859.

Covey E (1993b) *The monaural nuclei of the lateral lemniscus: parallel pathways from cochlear nucleus to midbrain*. In: The Mammalian Cochlear Nuclei: Organization and Function (Merchan MA, Juiz JM, Godfrey DA, Mugnaini E, eds), pp 321-334. New York: Plenum Publishing Co.

Covey E (2003) Brainstem mechanisms for analyzing temporal patterns of echolocation sounds: a model for understanding early stages of speech processing? *Speech Communication* 41:151-163.

Covey E, Casseday JH (1986) Connectional Basis for Frequency Representation in the Nuclei of the Lateral Lemniscus of the Bat Eptesicus-Fuscus. *J Neurosci* 6:2926-2940.

Covey E, Casseday JH (1991) The Monaural Nuclei of the Lateral Lemniscus in an Echolocating Bat - Parallel Pathways for Analyzing Temporal Features of Sound. *J Neurosci* 11:3456-3470.

Covey E, Casseday JH (1995) *The lower brainstem auditory pathway*. In: Hearing by Bats (Popper AN, Fay RR, eds), pp 235-295. New York: Springer-Verlag.

Covey E, Casseday JH (1999) Timing in the auditory system of the bat. *Annu Rev Physiol* 61:457-476.

Druga R, Syka J (1984) Ascending and descending projections to the inferior colliculus in the rat. *Physiol Bohemoslov* 33:31-42.

Elverland HH (1978) Ascending and intrinsic projections of the superior olivary complex in the cat. *Exp Brain Res* 32:117-134.

Faingold CL, Anderson CAB, Randall ME (1993) Stimulation or Blockade of the Dorsal Nucleus of the Lateral Lemniscus Alters Binaural and Tonic Inhibition in Contralateral Inferior Colliculus Neurons. *Hearing Res* 69:98-106.

Flammino F, Clopton BM (1975) Neural responses in the inferior colliculus of albino rat to binaural stimuli. *J Acoust Soc Am* 57:692-695.

Friauf E (1992) Tonotopic Order in the Adult and Developing Auditory-System of the Rat as Shown by C-Fos Immunocytochemistry. *European Journal of Neuroscience* 4:798-812.

Friauf E, Ostwald J (1988) Divergent Projections of Physiologically Characterized Rat Ventral Cochlear Nucleus Neurons as Shown by Intra-Axonal Injection of Horseradish-Peroxidase. *Experimental Brain Research* 73:263-284.

Frisina RD, O'Neill WE, Zettel ML (1989) Functional organization of mustached bat inferior colliculus: II. Connections of the FM2 region. *J Comp Neurol* 284:85-107.

Fu XW, Brezden BL, Wu SH (1997a) Hyperpolarization-activated inward current in neurons of the rat's dorsal nucleus of the lateral lemniscus in vitro. *J Neurophysiol* 78:2235-2245.

Fu XW, Wu SH, Brezden BL, Kelly JB (1996) Potassium currents and membrane excitability of neurons in the rat's dorsal nucleus of the lateral lemniscus. *J Neurophysiol* 76:1121-1132.

Fu XW, Brezden BL, Kelly JB, Wu SH (1997b) Synaptic excitation in the dorsal nucleus of the lateral lemniscus: Whole-cell patch-clamp recordings from rat brain slice. *Neuroscience* 78:815-827.

Giraldez-Perez RM, Gaytan SP, Torres B, Pasaro R (2009) Co-localization of nitric oxide synthase and choline acetyltransferase in the brain of the goldfish (Carassius auratus). J *Chem Neuroanat* 37:1-17.

Glendenning KK, Masterton RB (1983) Acoustic Chiasm: Efferent projections of the lateral superior olive. *J Neurosci* 3:1521-1537.

Glendenning KK, Hutson KA (1998) Lack of topography in the ventral nucleus of the lateral lemniscus. *Microscopy Research and Technique* 41:298-312.

Glendenning KK, Brunso-Bechtold JK, Thompson GC, Masterton RB (1981) Ascending Auditory Afferents to the Nuclei of the Lateral Lemniscus. *J Comp Neurol* 197:673-703.

Glendenning KK, Masterton RB, Hutson KA, Nudo RJ (1990) Ventral nucleus of the lateral lemniscus: Nontonotopic organization. *Anat Rec Abstract* 226:37A.

Godfrey DA, Kiang NY, Norris BE (1975) Single unit activity in the posteroventral cochlear nucleus of the cat. *J Comp Neurol* 162:247-268.

Golding NL, Robertson D, Oertel D (1995) Recordings from slices indicate that octopus cells of the cochlear nucleus detect coincident firing of auditory nerve fibers with temporal precision. *J Neurosci* 15:3138-3153.

Golding NL, Ferragamo MJ, Oertel D (1999) Role of intrinsic conductances underlying responses to transients in octopus cells of the cochlear nucleus. *J Neurosci* 19:2897-2905.

Goldstein JL (1973) An optimum processor theory for the central formation of the pitch of complex tones. *J Acoust Soc Am* 54:1496-1516.

González-Hernández T, Mantolán-Sarmiento B, González-González B, Pérez-González H (1996) Sources of GABAergic input to the inferior colliculus of the rat. *J Comp Neurol* 372:309-326.

Greenwood DD, Maruyama N (1965) Excitatory and inhibitory response areas of auditory neurons in the cochlear nucleus. *J Neurophysiol* 28:863-892.

Guinan J, John J., Li RY-S (1990) Signal processing in brainstem auditory neurons which receive giant endings (calyces of Held) in the medial nucleus of the trapezoid body of the cat. *Hearing Res* 49:321-334.

Guinan J, John J., Norris BE, Guinan SS (1972a) Single auditory units in the superior olivary complex: II. Locations of unit categories and tonotopic organization. *Int J Neurosci* 4:147-166.

Guinan J, John J., Guinan SS, Norris BE (1972b) Single auditory units in the superior olivary complex. I. Responses to sound and classification based on physiological properties. *Int J Neurosci* 4:101-120.

Harrison JM, Warr WB (1962) A study of the cochlear nuclei and ascending auditory pathways of the medulla. *J Comp Neurol* 119:341-379.

Held H (1893) Die Zentrale Gehörleitung. *Arch Anat Physiol,* Anat Abt 17:201-248.

Helfert RH, Bonneau JM, Wenthold RJ, Altschuler RA (1989) GABA and glycine immunoreactivity in the guinea pig superior olivary complex. *Brain Res* 501:269-286.

Henkel CK (1981) Afferent sources of a lateral midbrain tegmental zone associated with the pinnae in the cat as mapped by retrograde transport of horseradish peroxidase. *J Comp Neurol* 203:213-226.

Henkel CK (1983) Evidence of sub-collicular auditory projections to the medial geniculate nucleus in the cat: an autoradiographic and horseradish peroxidase study. *Brain Res* 259:21-30.

Henkel CK, Edwards SB (1978) The superior colliculus control of pinna movements in the cat: possible anatomical connections. *J Comp Neurol* 182:763-776.

Henkel CK, Spangler KM (1983) Organization of the efferent projections of the medial superior olivary nucleus in the cat as revealed by HRP and autoradiographic tracing methods. *J Comp Neurol* 221:416-428.

Hirsch JA, Oertel D (1988) Intrinsic properties of neurones in the dorsal cochlear nucleus of mice, in vitro. *J Physiol* 396:535-548.

Huang CM, Fex J (1986) Tonotopic organization in the inferior colliculus of the rat demonstrated with the 2-deoxyglucose method. *Exp Brain Res* 61:506-512.

Huffman RF, Covey E (1995) Origin of Ascending Projections to the Nuclei of the Lateral Lemniscus in the Big Brown Bat, Eptesicus-Fuscus. *J Comp Neurol* 357:532-545.

Huffman RF, Argeles PC, Covey E (1998a) Processing of sinusoidally frequency modulated signals in the nuclei of the lateral lemniscus of the big brown bat, Eptesicus fuscus. *Hearing Res* 126:161-180.

Huffman RF, Argeles PC, Covey E (1998b) Processing of sinusoidally amplitude modulated signals in the nuclei of the lateral lemniscus of the big brown bat, Eptesicus fuscus. *Hearing Res* 126:181-200.

Hutson KA, Glendenning KK, Masterton RB (1991) Acoustic Chiasm .4. 8 Midbrain Decussations of the Auditory-System in the Cat. *J Comp Neurol* 312:105-131.

Ibata Y, Pappas GD (1976) The fine structure of synapses in relation to the large spherical neurons in the anterior ventral cochlear of the cat. *J Neurocytol* 5:395-406.

Irfan N, Zhang H, Wu SH (2005) Synaptic transmission mediated by ionotropic glutamate, glycine and GABA receptors in the rat's ventral nucleus of the lateral lemniscus. *Hear Res* 203:159-171.

Irvine DRF (1992) *Physiology of the auditory brainstem.* In: The Mammalian Auditory Pathway: Neurophysiology (Popper AN, Fay RR, eds), pp 153-231. New York: Springer-Verlag.

Ito M, vanAdel B, Kelly JB (1996) Sound localization after transection of the commissure of Probst in the albino rat. *J Neurophysiol* 76:3493-3502.

Iwahori N (1986) A Golgi study on the dorsal nucleus of the lateral lemniscus in the mouse. *Neurosci Res* 3:196-212.

Jahnsen H, Llinas R (1984) Voltage-dependent burst-to-tonic switching of thalamic cell activity: an in vitro study. *Arch Ital Biol* 122:73-82.

Kandel ER, Schwartz JH, Jessell TM (1991) *Principals of Neural Science*, 3 Edition: Appleton and Lange.

Kandler K, Friauf E (1993) Prenatal and Postnatal-Development of Efferent Connections of the Cochlear Nucleus in the Rat. *J Comp Neurol* 328:161-184.

Kanold PO, Manis PB (1999) Transient potassium currents regulate the discharge patterns of dorsal cochlear nucleus pyramidal cells. *J Neurosci* 19:2195-2208.

Kelly JB, Glenn SL, Beaver CJ (1991) Sound frequency and binaural response properties of single neurons in rat inferior colliculus. *Hear Res* 56:273-280.

Kelly JB, Buckthought AD, Kidd SA (1998a) Monaural and binaural response properties of single neurons in the rat's dorsal nucleus of the lateral lemniscus. *Hearing Res* 122:25-40.

Kelly JB, Liscum A, van Adel B, Ito M (1995) Retrograde labelling in the rat's dorsal nucleus of the lateral lemniscus from frequency specific regions of the central nucleus of the inferior colliculus. *Assoc Res Otolaryngol Abstr* 18:40.

Kelly JB, Liscum A, van Adel B, Ito M (1998b) Projections from the superior olive and lateral lemniscus to tonotopic regions of the rat's inferior colliculus. *Hearing Res* 116:43-54.

Kelly JB, van Adel BA, Ito M (2009) Anatomical projections of the nuclei of the lateral lemniscus in the albino rat (rattus norvegicus). *J Comp Neurol* 512:573-593.

Kiang NY, Pfeiffer RR, Warr WB, Backus AS (1965a) Stimulus coding in the cochlear nucleus. *Trans Am Otol Soc* 53:35-58.

Kiang NY, Pfeiffer RR, Warr WB, Backus AS (1965b) Stimulus Coding in the Cochlear Nucleus. *Ann Otol Rhinol Laryngol* 74:463-485.

Kidd SA, Kelly JB (1996) Contribution of the dorsal nucleus of the lateral lemniscus to binaural responses in the inferior colliculus of the rat: Interaural time delays. *J Neurosci* 16:7390-7397.

Kopp-Scheinpflug C, Dehmel S, Dorrscheidt GJ, Rubsamen R (2002) Interaction of excitation and inhibition in anteroventral cochlear nucleus neurons that receive large endbulb synaptic endings. *J Neurosci* 22:11004-11018.

Kudo M (1981) Projections of the Nuclei of the Lateral Lemniscus in the Cat - an Autoradiographic Study. *Brain Res* 221:57-69.

Kudo M, Nakamura Y (1988) *Organization of the lateral lemniscal fibers converging onto the inferior colliculus in the cat:* An anatomical review. In: Auditory Pathway, Structure and Function (Syka J, Masterton RB, eds), pp 171-183. New York: Plenum Press.

Kudo M, Nakamura Y, Tokuno H, Kitao Y (1990) Auditory brainstem in the mole (Mogera): nuclear configurations and the projections to the inferior colliculus. *J Comp Neurol* 298:400-412.

Kuwada S, Batra R, Stanford TR (1989) Monaural and Binaural Response Properties of Neurons in the Inferior Colliculus of the Rabbit - Effects of Sodium Pentobarbital. *J Neurophysiol* 61:269-282.

Langner G, Braun S, Simonis C, Benson CG, Cant NB (2006) New evidence for a pitch helix in the ventral nucleus of the lateral lemniscus in the gerbil. *Assoc Res Otolaryngol Abstr* 29:771.

Lenn NJ, Reese TS (1966) The fine structure of nerve endings in the nucleus of the trapezoid body and the ventral cochlear nucleus. *Am J Anat* 118:375-389.

Li L, Kelly JB (1992) Binaural Responses in Rat Inferior Colliculus Following Kainic Acid Lesions of the Superior Olive - Interaural Intensity Difference Functions. *Hearing Res* 61:73-85.

Licklider JC (1951) A duplex theory of pitch perception. *Experientia* 7:128-134.

Malmierca MS, Le Beau FEN, Rees A (1996) The topographical organization of descending projections from the central nucleus of the inferior colliculus in guinea pig. *Hearing Res* 93:167-180.

Malmierca MS, Rees A, Le Beau FEN, Bjaalie JG (1995) Laminar Organization of Frequency-Defined Local Axons within and between the Inferior Colliculi of the Guinea-Pig. *J Comp Neurol* 357:124-144.

Malmierca MS, Leergaard TB, Bajo VM, Bjaalie JG, Merchán MA (1998) Anatomic evidence of a three-dimensional mosaic pattern of tonotopic organization in the ventral complex of the lateral lemniscus in cat. *J Neurosci* 18:10603-10618.

Manis PB, Spirou GA, Wright DD, Paydar S, Ryugo DK (1994) Physiology and morphology of complex spiking neurons in the guinea pig dorsal cochlear nucleus. *J Comp Neurol* 348:261-276.

Markovitz NS, Pollak GD (1993) The Dorsal Nucleus of the Lateral Lemniscus in the Moustache Bat - Monaural Properties. *Hearing Res* 71:51-63.

Markovitz NS, Pollak GD (1994) Binaural Processing in the Dorsal Nucleus of the Lateral Lemniscus. *Hearing Res* 73:121-140.

Masterton RB, Imig TJ (1984) Neural mechanisms for sound localization. *Annu Rev Physiol* 46:275-287.

May PJ, Vidal PP, Baker R (1990) Synaptic organization of tectal-facial pathways in cat. II. Synaptic potentials following midbrain tegmentum stimulation. *J Neurophysiol* 64:381-402.

Meddis R, Hewitt MJ (1991) Virtual pitch and phase sensitivity of a computer model of the auditory periphery I: pitch identification. *J Am Soc Audiol* 89:2866-2882.

Merchán MA, Berbel P (1996) Anatomy of the ventral nucleus of the lateral lemniscus in rats: A nucleus with a concentric laminar organization. *J Comp Neurol* 372:245-263.

Merchán MA, Saldaña E, Plaza I (1994) Dorsal Nucleus of the Lateral Lemniscus in the Rat - Concentric Organization and Tonotopic Projection to the Inferior Colliculus. *J Comp Neurol* 342:259-278.

Merchán MA, Malmierca MS, Bajo VM, Bjaalie JG (1997) *The Nuclei of the Lateral Lemniscus Old Views and New Perspectives*. In: Acoustic Signal Processing in the Central Auditory System (Syka J, ed), pp 211-226. New York: Plenum Press.

Merzenich MM, Reid MD (1974) Representation of the cochlea within the inferior colliculus of the cat. *Brain Res* 77:397-415.

Metzner W, Radtke-Schuller S (1987) The Nuclei of the Lateral Lemniscus in the Rufous Horseshoe Bat, Rhinolophus-Rouxi - a Neurophysiological Approach. *Journal of Comparative Physiology a-Sensory Neural and Behavioral Physiology* 160:395-411.

Moore BC, Rosen SM (1979) Tune recognition with reduced pitch and interval information. *Q J Exp Psychol* 31:229-240.

Moore DR (1988) Auditory brainstem of the ferret: sources of projections to the inferior colliculus. *J Comp Neurol* 269:342-354.

Moore JK, Moore RY (1987) Glutamic acid decarboxylase-like immunoreactivity in brainstem auditory nuclei of the rat. *J Comp Neurol* 260:157-174.

Morest DK (1968) *The growth of synaptic endings in the mammalian brain: a study of the calyces of the trapezoid body.* Z Anat Entwicklungsgesch 127:201-220.

Morest DK, Jean-Baptiste M (1975) Degeneration and phagocytosis of synaptic endings and axons in the medial trapezoid nucleus of the cat. *J Comp Neurol* 162:135-156.

Morest DK, Kim JN, Bohne BA (1997) Neuronal and transneuronal degeneration of auditory axons in the brainstem after cochlear lesions in the chinchilla: Cochleotopic and non-cochleotopic patterns. *Hearing Res* 103:151-168.

Motts SD, Slusarczyk AS, Sowick CS, Schofield BR (2008) Distribution of cholinergic cells in guinea pig brainstem. *Neuroscience* 154:186-195.

Nayagam DAX, Clarey JC, Paolini AG (2005) Powerful, onset inhibition in the ventral nucleus of the lateral lemniscus. *J Neurophysiol* 94:1651-1654.

Nayagam DAX, Clarey JC, Paolini AG (2006) Intracellular responses and morphology of rat ventral complex of the lateral lemniscus neurons in vivo. *J Comp Neurol* 498:295-315.

Niemer WR, Cheng SK (1949) The ascending auditory system: A study of retrograde degeneration. *Anat Rec* 103:490.

Nolte J, Angevine JB (1995) *Human Brain: In Photographs and Diagrams,* 1 Edition: Mosby-Year Book, Inc.

Nordeen KW, Killackey, J. P., and Kitzes, L. M. (1983) Ascending auditory projections to the inferior colliculus in the adult gerbil, *Meriones unguiculatus. J, Comp Neurol* 214:131-143.

Oertel D (1983) Synaptic responses and electrical properties of cells in brain slices of the mouse anteroventral cochlear nucleus. *J Neurosci* 3:2043-2053.

Oertel D (1991) The role of intrinsic neuronal properties in the encoding of auditory information in the cochlear nuclei. *Curr Opin Neurobiol* 1:221-228.

Oertel D (1997) Encoding of timing in the brain stem auditory nuclei of vertebrates. *Neuron* 19:959-962.

Oertel D, Wickesberg RE (2002) *Ascending Pathways Through Ventral Nuclei of the Lateral Lemniscus and Their Possible Role in Pattern Recognition in Natural Sounds.* In: Integrative Functions in the Mammalian Auditory Pathway (Oertel D, Popper AN, Fay RR, eds), pp 207-237. New York; London: Springer.

Oertel D, Wu SH, Garb MW, Dizack C (1990) Morphology and physiology of cells in slice preparations of the posteroventral cochlear nucleus of mice. *J Comp Neurol* 295:136-154.

Oertel D, Bal R, Gardner SM, Smith PH, Joris PX (2000) *Detection of synchrony in the activity of auditory nerve fibers by octopus cells of the mammalian cochlear nucleus.* P Natl Acad Sci USA 97:11773-11779.

Oliver DL (1987) Projections to the inferior colliculus from the anteroventral cochlear nucleus in the cat: possible substrates for binaural interaction. *J Comp Neurol* 264:24-46.

Osen KK (1969) Cytoarchitecture of the cochlear nuclei in the cat. *J Comp Neurol* 136:453-484.

Osen KK (1972) Projection of the cochlear nuclei on the inferior colliculus in the cat. *J Comp Neurol* 144:355-372.

Paxinos G, Watson C (1998) *The Rat Brain In Stereotaxic Co-Ordinates*, 4th Edition, 4th Edition Edition. San Diego: Academic Press.

Paxinos G, Watson C (2005) *The Rat Brain in Stereotaxic Coordinates,* 5th Edition. The new coronal set. Burlington: Elsevier Academic Press.

Pfeiffer RR (1966) Classification of response patterns of spike discharges for units in the cochlear nucleus: tone-burst stimulation. *Exp Brain Res* 1:220-235.

Portfors CV, Wenstrup JJ (2001) Responses to combinations of tones in the nuclei of the lateral lemniscus. *J Assoc Res Otolaryngol* 2:104-117.

Rhode WS, Smith PH (1986) Encoding timing and intensity in the ventral cochlear nucleus of the cat. *J Neurophysiol* 56:261-286.

Rhode WS, Greenberg S (1992) *Physiology of the Cochlear Nuclei.* In: Auditory Research, Volume 2: The Physiology of the Mammalian Auditory Central Nervous System (Fay RR, Popper AN, eds).

Riquelme R, Merchán MA, Ottersen OP (1998) GABA and glycine in the ventral nucleus of the lateral lemniscus: an immunocytochemical and in situ hybridization study in rat. *Assoc Res Otolaryngol Abstr* 21:93.

Riquelme R, Saldaña E, Osen KK, Ottersen OP, Merchán MA (2001) Colocalization of GABA and glycine in the ventral nucleus of the lateral lemniscus in rat: An in situ hybridization and semiquantitative immunocytochemical study. *J Comp Neurol* 432:409-424.

Ritz LA, Brownell WE (1982) Single Unit Analysis of the Posteroventral Cochlear Nucleus of the Decerebrate Cat. *Neuroscience* 7:1995-2010.

Roberts RC, Ribak CE (1987) GABAergic neurons and axon terminals in the brainstem auditory nuclei of the gerbil. *J Comp Neurol* 258:267-280.

Rose JE, Greenwood DD, Goldberg JM, Hind JE (1963) Some Discharge characteristics of single neurons in the inferior colliculus of the cat: I. Tonotopic organization, relation of spike counts to intensity, and firing pattern of single elements. *J Neuophysiol* 26:294-320.

Ross LS, Pollak GD (1989) Differential ascending projections to aural regions in the 60 kHz contour of the mustache bat's inferior colliculus. *J Neurosci* 9:2819-2834.

Ross LS, Pollak GD, Zook JM (1988) Origin of ascending projections to an isofrequency region of the mustache bat's inferior colliculus. *J Comp Neurol* 270:488-505.

Roth GL, Aitkin LM, Andersen RA, Merzenich MM (1978) Some features of the spatial organization of the central nucleus of the inferior colliculus of the cat. *J Comp Neurol* 182:661-680.

Ryan AF, Furlow Z, Woolf NK, Keithley EM (1988) The spatial representation of frequency in the rat dorsal cochlear nucleus and inferior colliculus. *Hear Res* 36:181-189.

Ryugo DK, Sento S (1991) Synaptic connections of the auditory nerve in cats: relationship between endbulbs of held and spherical bushy cells. *J Comp Neurol* 305:35-48.

Saint Marie RL, Baker RA (1990) Neurotransmitter-Specific Uptake and Retrograde Transport of [H-3] Glycine from the Inferior Colliculus by Ipsilateral Projections of the Superior Olivary Complex and Nuclei of the Lateral Lemniscus. *Brain Res* 524:244-253.

Saint Marie RL, Shneiderman A, Stanforth DA (1997) Patterns of gamma-aminobutyric acid and glycine immunoreactivities reflect structural and functional differences of the cat lateral lemniscal nuclei. *J Comp Neurol* 389:264-276.

Saint Marie RL, Luo L, Ryan AF (1999) Spatial representation of frequency in the rat dorsal nucleus of the lateral lemniscus as revealed by acoustically induced c-fos mRNA expression. *Hearing Res* 128:70-74.

Saldaña E (1993) *Descending projections from the inferior colliculus to the cochlear nuclei in mammals*. In: The Mammalian Cochlear Nuclei: Organization and Function (Merchan MA, Juiz JM, Godfrey DA, Mugnaini E, eds), pp 153-165. Ney York: Plenum.

Saldaña E, Merchán MA (199*2) Intrinsic and Commissural Connections of the Rat Inferior Colliculus*. J Comp Neurol 319:417-437.

Schofield BR (1995) Projections from the cochlear nucleus to the superior paraolivary nucleus in guinea pigs. *J Comp Neurol* 360:135-149.

Schofield BR, Cant NB (1997) Ventral nucleus of the lateral lemniscus in guinea pigs: Cytoarchitecture and inputs from the cochlear nucleus. *J Comp Neurol* 379:363-385.

Schwartz IR (1992) *The superior olivary complex and lateral lemniscal nuclei*. In: The mammalian auditory pathway: neuroanatomy (Webster DB, Popper AN, Fay RR, eds), pp 117-167. New York: Springer-Verlag.

Schweizer H (1981) The connections of the inferior colliculus and the organization of the brainstem auditory system in the greater horseshoe bat (Rhinolophus ferrumequinum). *J Comp Neurol* 201:25-49.

Semple MN, Aitkin LM (1979) Representation of Sound Frequency and Laterality by Units in Central Nucleus of Cat Inferior Colliculus. *J Neurophysiol* 42:1626-1639.

Shneiderman A, Chase MB, Rockwood JM, Benson CG, Potashner SJ (1993) Evidence for a Gabaergic Projection from the Dorsal Nucleus of the Lateral Lemniscus to the Inferior Colliculus. *Journal of Neurochemistry* 60:72-82.

Shofner WP, Whitmer WM, Yost WA (2005) Listening experience with iterated rippled noise alters the perception of 'pitch' strength of complex sounds in the chinchilla. *J Acoust Soc Am* 118:3187-3197.

Smith PH, Joris PX, Yin TCT (1993) Projections of Physiologically Characterized Spherical Bushy Cell Axons from the Cochlear Nucleus of the Cat - Evidence for Delay-Lines to the Medial Superior Olive. *J Comp Neurol* 331:245-260.

Smith PH, Massie A, Joris PX (2005) Acoustic stria: anatomy of physiologically characterized cells and their axonal projection patterns. *J Comp Neurol* 482:349-371.

Spangler KM, Warr WB, Henkel CK (1985) The projections of principal cells of the medial nucleus of the trapezoid body in the cat. *J Comp Neurol* 238:249-262.

Steriade M, McCormick DA, Sejnowski TJ (1993) Thalamocortical oscillations in the sleeping and aroused brain. *Science* 262:679-685.

Stotler WA (1953) An experimental study of the cells and connections of the superior olivary complex of the cat. *J Comp Neurol* 98:401-431.

Strominger NL, Strominger AI (1971) Ascending brain stem projections of the anteroventral cochlear nucleus in the rhesus monkey. *J Comp Neurol* 143:217-242.

Suneja SK, Benson CG, Gross J, Potashner SJ (1995) Evidence for Glutamatergic Projections from the Cochlear Nucleus to the Superior Olive and the Ventral Nucleus of the Lateral Lemniscus. *J Neurochem* 64:161-171.

Swanson LW (1998) *Brain Maps: Structure of the Rat Brain,* 2nd edition, Second revised Edition Edition. Amsterdam: Elsevier Science B.V.

Syka J, Radionova EA, Popelar J (1981) Discharge characteristics of neuronal pairs in the rabbit inferior colliculus. *Exp Brain Res* 44:11-18.

Tanaka K, Otani K, Tokunaga A, Sugita S (1985) The Organization of Neurons in the Nucleus of the Lateral Lemniscus Projecting to the Superior and Inferior Colliculi in the Rat. *Brain Res* 341:252-260.

Tennigkeit F, Schwarz DW, Puil E (1996) Mechanisms for signal transformation in lemniscal auditory thalamus. *J Neurophysiol* 76:3597-3608.

Tennigkeit F, Schwarz DW, Puil E (1998) Modulation of bursts and high-threshold calcium spikes in neurons of rat auditory thalamus. *Neuroscience* 83:1063-1073.

Tokunaga A, Sugita S, Otani K (1984) *Auditory and non-auditory subcortical afferents to the inferior colliculus in the rat.* J Hirnforsch 25:461-472.

Tsuchitani C (1988a) The inhibition of cat lateral superior olive unit excitatory responses to binaural tone bursts. II. The sustained discharges. *J Neurophysiol* 59:184-211.

Tsuchitani C (1988b) The inhibition of cat lateral superior olive unit excitatory responses to binaural tone bursts. I. The transient chopper response. *J Neurophysiol* 59:164-183.

van Gehuchten A (1906) *Le System Nerveux de l'Homme.* Fourth Edition., 4 Edition.

van Noort J (1969) The anatomical basis for frequency analysis in the cochlear nuclear complex. *Psychiatr Neurol Neurochir* 72:109-114.

Vater M, Feng AS (1990) Functional organization of ascending and descending connections of the cochlear nucleus of horseshoe bats. *J Comp Neurol* 292:373-395.

Vater M, Braun K (1994) Parvalbumin, Calbindin D-28k, and Calretinin Immunoreactivity in the Ascending Auditory Pathway of Horseshoe Bats. *J Comp Neurol* 341:534-558.

Vater M, Covey E, Casseday JH (1997) The columnar region of the ventral nucleus of the lateral lemniscus in the big brown bat (Eptesicus fuscus): Synaptic arrangements and structural correlates of feedforward inhibitory function. *Cell and Tissue Research* 289:223-233.

Vater M, Habbicht H, Kossl M, Grothe B (1992) The Functional-Role of Gaba and Glycine in Monaural and Binaural Processing in the Inferior Colliculus of Horseshoe Bats. *Journal of Comparative Physiology a-Sensory Neural and Behavioral Physiology* 171:541-553.

Warr WB (1966) Fiber degeneration following lesions in the anterior ventral cochlear nucleus of the cat. *Exp Neurol* 14:453-474.

Warr WB (1969) Fiber degeneration following lesions in the posteroventral cochlear nucleus of the cat. *Exp Neurol* 23:140-155.

Warr WB (1972) Fiber degeneration following lesions in the multipolar and globular cell areas in the ventral cochlear nucleus of the cat. *Brain Res* 40:247-270.

Warr WB, Beck JE (1996) Multiple projections from the ventral nucleus of the trapezoid body in the rat. *Hearing Res* 93:83-101.

Whitley JM, Henkel CK (1983) A Subcollicular Projection to the Medial Geniculate-Nucleus from the Ventral Nucleus of the Lateral Lemniscus - a Hrp and Fluorescent Dye Study. *Anatomical Record* 205:A214-A215.

Whitley JM, Henkel CK (1984) Topographical organization of the inferior collicular projection and other connections of the ventral nucleus of the lateral lemniscus in the cat. *J Comp Neurol* 229:257-270.

Willard FH, Ryugo DK (1983) *Anatomy of the central auditory system.* In: The Auditory Psychobiology of the Mouse (Thomas C, ed), pp 201-304. Springfield, IL.

Willard FH, Martin GF (1983) The auditory brainstem nuclei and some of their projections to the inferior colliculus in the North American opossum. *Neuroscience* 10:1203-1232.

Winer JA, Larue DT, Pollak GD (1995) Gaba and Glycine in the Central Auditory-System of the Moustache Bat - Structural Substrates for Inhibitory Neuronal Organization. *J Comp Neurol* 355:317-353.

Wu SH (1999) Physiological properties of neurons in the ventral nucleus of the lateral lemniscus of the rat: Intrinsic membrane properties and synaptic responses. *J Neurophysiol* 81:2862-2874.

Wu SH, Oertel D (1984) Intracellular injection with horseradish peroxidase of physiologically characterized stellate and bushy cells in slices of mouse anteroventral cochlear nucleus. *J Neurosci* 4:1577-1588.

Wu SH, Kelly JB (1991) Physiological properties of neurons in the mouse superior olive: membrane characteristics and postsynaptic responses studied in vitro. *J Neurophysiol* 65:230-246.

Wu SH, Kelly JB (1995a) In vitro brain slice studies of the rat's dorsal nucleus of the lateral lemniscus .2. Physiological properties of biocytin-labeled neurons (vol 73, pg 794, 1995). *J Neurophysiol* 74:U11-U11.

Wu SH, Kelly JB (1995b) In-Vitro Brain Slice Studies of the Rats Dorsal Nucleus of the Lateral Lemniscus .1. Membrane and Synaptic Response Properties. *J Neurophysiol* 73:780-793.

Wu SH, Kelly JB (1996) In vitro brain slice studies of the rat's dorsal nucleus of the lateral lemniscus .3. Synaptic pharmacology. *J Neurophysiol* 75:1271-1282.

Xie R, Meitzen J, Pollak GD (2005) Differing roles of inhibition in hierarchical processing of species-specific calls in auditory brainstem nuclei. *J Neurophysiol* 94:4019-4037.

Yang LC, Pollak GD (1994a) The Roles of Gabaergic and Glycinergic Inhibition on Binaural Processing in the Dorsal Nucleus of the Lateral Lemniscus of the Moustache Bat. *J Neurophysiol* 71:1999-2013.

Yang LC, Pollak GD (1994b) Gaba and Glycine Have Different Effects on Monaural Response Properties in the Dorsal Nucleus of the Lateral Lemniscus of the Moustache Bat. *J Neurophysiol* 71:2014-2024.

Yang LC, Liu Q, Pollak GD (1996) Afferent connections to the dorsal nucleus of the lateral lemniscus of the mustache bat: Evidence for two functional subdivisions. *J Comp Neurol* 373:575-592.

Young ED (1998) *Cochlear Nucleus.* In: The Synaptic Organization of the Brain, 4 Edition (Shepherd GM, ed). New York: Oxford University Press.

Zhang DX, Li L, Kelly JB, Wu SH (1998) GABAergic projections from the lateral lemniscus to the inferior colliculus of the rat. *Hearing Res* 117:1-12.

Zhang H, Kelly JB (2006a) Responses of neurons in the rat's ventral nucleus of the lateral lemniscus to monaural and binaural tone bursts. *J Neurophysiol* 95:2501-2512.

Zhang H, Kelly JB (2006b) Responses of Neurons in the Rat's Ventral Nucleus of the Lateral Lemniscus to Amplitude-Modulated Tones. *J Neuophysiol* 96:2905-2914.

Zhang S, Oertel D (1993) Cartwheel and superficial stellate cells of the dorsal cochlear nucleus of mice: intracellular recordings in slices. *J Neurophysiol* 69:1384-1397.

Zhao M, Wu SH (2001) Morphology and physiology of neurons in the ventral nucleus of the lateral lemniscus in rat brain slices. *J Comp Neurol* 433:255-271.

Zook JM, Casseday JH (1979) Connections of the nuclei of the lateral lemniscus in the mustache bat, *Pteronotus Parnellii. Soc Neurosci Abstr* 5:34.

Zook JM, Casseday JH (1982a) Origin of ascending projections to inferior colliculus in the mustache bat, Pteronotus parnellii. *J Comp Neurol* 207:14-28.

Zook JM, Casseday JH (1982b) Cytoarchitecture of auditory system in lower brainstem of the mustache bat, Pteronotus parnellii. *J Comp Neurol* 207:1-13.

Zook JM, Casseday JH (1985) Projections from the cochlear nuclei in the mustache bat, Pteronotus parnellii. *J Comp Neurol* 237:307-324.

Zook JM, Casseday JH (1987) Convergence of ascending pathways at the inferior colliculus of the mustache bat, Pteronotus parnellii. *J Comp Neurol* 261:347-361.

Zook JM, DiCaprio RA (1988) Intracellular labeling of afferents to the lateral superior olive in the bat, Eptesicus fuscus. *Hear Res* 34:141-147.

In: Deafness, Hearing Loss and the Auditory System
Editors: D. Fiedler and R. Krause, pp.81-110

ISBN: 978-1-60741-259-5
©2010 Nova Science Publishers, Inc.

*Chapter 2*

# NOISE-INDUCED HEARING LOSS IN YOUTH CAUSED BY LEISURE NOISE

## *H. Keppler, B. Vinck and I. Dhooge*
Ghent University, Ghent, Belgium

## ABSTRACT

Excessive noise exposure can lead to metabolic and/or mechanical effects resulting in alterations of the structural elements of the organ of Corti. Besides occupational noise exposure, there are several sources of leisure noise exposure attributing to noise-induced hearing loss (NIHL). These leisure noise exposures include exposure to loud music or even participation in non-musical activities. The major sources of the former activities are attendance at discotheques, nightclubs and live concerts, and usage of personal music players. Recently, it was estimated that the prevalence of leisure noise in the UK has tripled since the early 1980s. Therefore, an increase in prevalence of NIHL in adolescents and young adults is assumed, especially in the mainstream media. Epidemiologic literature is, however, more equivocal. The lack of hearing deterioration is most likely explained by the fact that leisure noise exposure is insufficient to cause important hearing loss. Nevertheless, the effects of leisure noise exposure on the auditory system of young people is a cause for concern. The purpose of this chapter is to review the sources of leisure noise in relation to their contribution in life-time noise exposure of individuals and to present epidemiologic data regarding NIHL in young people caused by leisure noise. Differences in attitude of young people regarding leisure noise exposure and usage of hearing protection are discussed, as well as the importance of prevention and sensitization campaigns. Moreover, short- and long-term effects of several leisure noise sources are reviewed. Shortcomings in the current literature are stressed, and proposals for additional research regarding the usefulness of several audiological tests to detect minimal cochlear damage after exposure to loud leisure noise are pointed out.

# INTRODUCTION

The fact that excessive occupational noise exposure can lead to noise-induced hearing loss (NIHL) is well known. Besides occupational noise exposure, non-occupational noise exposure is also a cause for concern, especially in young people. The purpose of this chapter is to give insight in the prevalence of NIHL caused by leisure noise exposure, and the sources of leisure noise. Research regarding temporary and permanent auditory effects caused by listening to personal music players and attending discotheques, nightclubs or live concerts is discussed. Further, preventive strategies are suggested, and finally, the current legislation regarding leisure noise exposure is reviewed.

# PATHOPHYSIOLOGY AND DIAGNOSIS OF NOISE-INDUCED HEARING LOSS

Sound perception is based on mechanical sound energy reaching the middle ear, inducing movement of the stapes footplate into the oval window, and producing pressure changes in the perilymph of the cochlea. The traveling wave of the basilar membrane (BM) deflects the stereocilia of the hair cells which stretches the tip links and forces them to open ionic channels on the stereocilia. The resulting potassium influx depolarizes the hair cells of the organ of Corti, and consequently releases neurotransmitters generating action potentials in the cochlear nerve by which neural afferent information is transferred to the brainstem. The motile activity of the outer hair cells (OHCs) [Brownell, 1990] amplifies the sound-induced micro-mechanical movement of the BM, especially at low-input levels. Thereby the input for the inner hair cells (IHCs) is enhanced. This non-linear active process, i.e. the cochlear amplifier, is responsible for the high sensitivity, sharp frequency selectivity and wide dynamic range of the human auditory system [Norton, 1992].

Excessive noise exposure can lead to metabolic and/or mechanical changes resulting in alterations of the structural elements of the organ of Corti [Sliwinska-Kowalska & Jedlinska, 1998; Céranic, 2007; Talaska & Schacht, 2007]. Metabolic disturbances induce cell death through toxic reactions, while mechanical damage results in direct physical loss of the integrity of hair cells and surroundings cells [Talaska & Schacht, 2007]. Morphological changes may include buckling of the pillar bodies, decreasing the height of the organ of Corti and thereby uncoupling the OHC stereocilia from the tectorial membrane [Nordmann et al, 2000]. This temporary uncoupling could affect hair cell stimulation, and is sufficient to explain temporary threshold shift (TTS). It is suggested that TTS and permanent threshold shift (PTS) arise from a fundamentally different mechanism [Nordmann et al, 2000], and that a PTS cannot be predicted form the initial TTS [Melnick, 1991] as it might depend on the recovery or repair processes within the cochlea [Nordmann et al, 2000]. Morphological correlates of PTS are focal losses of hair cells and adjacent afferent nerve fiber degeneration [Nordmann et al, 2000].

There are biochemical events that accompany morphological changes in the cochlea leading to degeneration of the sensory cells and eventually to degeneration of the spiral ganglion [Talaska & Schacht, 2007]. Prolonged noise exposure results in an accumulation of calcium, saturating the calcium-binding capacities of the OHCs [Heinrich & Feltens, 2006].

The disturbance of calcium homeostasis can result in an overload of calcium in the mitochondria, excitotoxic neural swelling, and reduction of cochlear blood flow. Thereby, reactive oxygen species (ROS) enzymes are activated and free radicals are generated [Henderson et al, 2006]. Although ROS formation is not limited to hair cells, but also occur in other structures such as supporting cells and the stria vascularis, the primary damage is concentrated on the OHCs [Sliwinska-Kowalska & Jedlinska, 1998; Lucertini et al, 2002; Sliwinska-Kowalska & Kotylo, 2008]. This might suggest that OHCs have a lower antioxidant capacity, and might therefore be more susceptible to ROS [Talaska & Schacht, 2007]. The co-existence of apoptosis and necrosis involved in OHC damage causes eventually cell death [Hu et al, 2002] and this induces disturbed physiological pathways in other cochlear cell types [Heinrich & Feltens, 2006]. Apoptosis is an active process that eliminates injured cells which could spread lesion to neighboring cells. The morphological correlate is nuclear condensation and fragmentation [Hu et al, 2002]. Necrosis, however, is a passive process associated with cell swelling resulting in cell rupture. Eventually, it results in damage to surrounding cells or inflammatory responses [Henderson et al, 2006]. However, necrosis is found to account for only a small portion of this damage, and apoptosis persists even several days after noise exposure [Hu et al, 2002]. Therefore, the clinical utility of delayed interventions must be further explored, as well as the role of antioxidant prevention of NIHL in humans [Le Prell et al, 2007].

Long periods of continuous or intermittent noise exposure can lead to a slowly developing chronic hearing loss, or NIHL. By analogy with NIHL, hearing loss caused by music is sometimes referred as music-induced hearing loss. Typically, noise is an unwanted, unpleasant acoustic signal [Hausler, 2004]. However, instead of the term music-induced hearing loss, the term NIHL is mainly used because noise is referred as an excessive acoustic signal possibly causing hearing damage, whether unwanted or not.

According to the Position Statement of the American College of Occupational and Environmental Medicine (ACOEM) on NIHL in 2002 (ACOEM, 2002), NIHL can be defined as a sensorineural, mostly bilateral symmetrical hearing loss initially presented in the frequency range 3 to 6 kHz. NIHL almost never progresses to a profound hearing loss, but the rate of hearing loss is greatest during the first 10 to 15 years of exposure and does not progress after cessation of noise exposure. However, it was postulated that hearing loss is only detected as soon as a considerable amount of hair cells is damaged [Daniel, 2007]. This suggests that there might be a period of latent damage making it impossible to distinguish audiometrically between subjects whether exposed to noise or not [LePage, 1998]. Moreover, the risk of hearing loss is influenced by the noise exposure level, duration, number of exposures and individual susceptibility [Mills & Going, 1982].

Henderson et al (1993) states that there is a large variability in susceptibility to NIHL in demographic studies, as well as laboratory studies, which seemed to be caused by several factors. First, some of the variability could be explained by the interaction between noise exposure and other ototoxic agents exacerbating NIHL. Second, the role of auditory characteristics such as middle ear muscle reflex, efferent system and subject's history of noise exposure could attribute to the variability of NIHL, and to a smaller extent, non-auditory characteristics such as gender, eye color and smoking [Henderson et al, 1993].

The diagnosis of NIHL is based on audiometric evaluation in combination with a history of noise exposure [Alberti, 1998]. Besides the loss of hearing sensitivity, concomitant tinnitus and impaired speech discrimination can be present. The sensitivity of pure-tone audiometry for the early detection of NIHL however has been questioned. The ACOEM has recommended additional research on NIHL, including in the area of early indicators of hearing loss such as otoacoustic emissions (OAEs) (ACOEM, 2002). OAEs are low-level sounds reflecting the non-linear active processes of the cochlea [Norton, 1992], which were discovered by Kemp in 1978 [Kemp, 1978]. It is an non-invasive, objective technique that does not require active participation of the subject. OAEs represent an indication of the integrity of the OHCs, but their presence does not exclude hearing impairment (e.g. retrocochlear hearing loss). However, OAEs depend highly on normal middle ear function [Probst et al 1991]. Nevertheless, OAE amplitude reduction may reflect OHC damage due to noise exposure [Sliwinska-Kowalska & Kotylo, 2008]. So, OAEs are a promising tool in the detection of sub-clinical OHC damage and pre-clinical hearing loss, overlooked by pure-tone audiometry. This has mainly been established in industrial or military settings [Hotz et al, 1993; Kowalska & Sulkowski, 1997; Hall & Lutman, 1999; Desai et al, 1999; Konopka et al, 2001; Attias et al, 2001; Lucertini et al, 2002; Céranic, 2007; Sliwinska-Kowalska & Kotylo, 2008]. Two types of OAEs, transient evoked OAEs (TEOAEs) and distortion product OAEs (DPOAEs), are commonly used. In contrast to TEOAEs, DPOAEs have a more high-frequency response which makes them an ideal tool for detecting relatively high frequency-specific cochlear damage such as NIHL [Probst et al 1993]. However, some studies indicate that TEOAEs are more sensitive than DPOAEs in the detection of minimal cochlear alteration caused by excessive noise exposure [Plinkert et al 1995; Lapsley-Miller et al 2004].

## PREVALENCE OF NOISE-INDUCED HEARING LOSS CAUSED BY LEISURE NOISE

In the mainstream media, an increase in prevalence of NIHL in adolescents and young adults attributed to leisure noise exposure is postulated. General statements regarding hearing loss in the youngest generation are not uncommon ('more young people lose hearing', 'the deaf MP3 generation', etc.), but are usually based on possibilities or estimations. For example, in the United States, it was estimated that non-occupational noise exposure probably has a similar impact on the burden of adult hearing loss as occupational noise exposure which represents 5 to 10% of the burden [Dobie, 2008].

Two types of epidemiologic research can provide firm evidence; either cross-sectional studies or longitudinal data. However, there are methodological difficulties in the accurate estimation of the number of subjects exposed, and in obtaining a sample of young individuals with representative sound levels, patterns and duration of exposure [MRC Institute of Hearing Research, 1986]. Furthermore, the criteria used to define hearing impairment, and the used audiological techniques to measure slight deterioration in hearing, as well as numerous confounding factors in lifestyle regarding noise exposure (e.g. environmental noise) make the design of such research complicated. Finally, longitudinal studies require an adequate long-term planning, as well as identical methodological conditions.

Research regarding the prevalence of NIHL caused by leisure noise has revealed inconsistent results. There are some adequately performed studies that do not report an increase in prevalence of hearing loss caused by leisure noise.

First, the prevalence of hearing loss in 500 18-year-old males was 14%, which was comparable with the prevalence of hearing loss in the same age group in previous studies [Axelsson et al, 1994]. In 1998, the prevalence of hearing loss in 951 Swedish 18-year-old conscripts was estimated at 19.6% [Augustsson & Engstrand, 2006]. However, taking different techniques into account, the authors concluded that there is no increase in prevalence as compared with 30 years earlier [Persson et al, 1993].

Second, the Third National Health and Nutrition Examination Survey (NHANE III) [Niskar et al, 1998; Niskar et al, 2001], performed between 1988 and 1994, estimated the prevalence of a noise-induced threshold shift in children from 6 to 19 year old (n=5249). A noise-induced hearing threshold shift was defined as: (1) pure-tone thresholds at 0.5 and 1.0 kHz equal or better than 15 dB HL, (2) a difference of at least 15 dB between the poorest pure-tone threshold at 3.0, 4.0 or 6.0 kHz on the one hand and at 0.5 and 1.0 kHz on the other hand, and finally, (3) pure tone threshold at 8.0 kHz at least 10 dB better than the poorest threshold at 3.0, 4.0 and 6.0 kHz. It was stated that the prevalence of a noise-induced hearing threshold shift in at least one ear amounted to 12.5%, representing approximately 5.2 million children. In those children, the prevalence of noise-induced threshold shift was significantly higher in boys (14.8%) than in girls (10.1%). Further, it was observed that 12- to 19-year old children had a significantly higher prevalence of noise-induced threshold shift (15.5%) than 6- to 11-year-olds (8.5%). However, the median hearing thresholds of this oldest group of children can be compared with those of children aged 12 to 17 years from the Health Examination Survey of 1966 to 1970 [Holmes et al, 2004]. All median thresholds except at 1 kHz were better in children from the NHANE III, indicating better hearing conservation over the past 20 years. More importantly, the largest improvement was at frequencies 4 and 6 kHz, suggesting a decrease in hearing loss suggestive of noise exposure.

More recently, the prevalence of hearing loss was examined in US adults from 17 to 25 years entering an industrial workforce [Rabinowitz et al, 2006]. The criteria for an audiometric notch were defined identically as the noise-induced hearing threshold shifts by Niskar et al (2001). The prevalence of audiometric notches was 23.2% for the new-hires between 1985 and 1989, 17.2% between 1990 and 1994, 19.3% between 1995 and 1999, and 20.4% between 2000 and 2004. So, no increasing prevalence of audiometric notches, nor high frequency hearing loss (average hearing loss at 3, 4 and 6 kHz greater than 15 dB) was reported for hearing tests performed between 1985 and 2004.

There are, however, other studies reporting an increase in prevalence of hearing loss caused by leisure noise. Montgomery & Fujikawa (1992) evaluated hearing thresholds in almost 1500 students from second, eight and twelfth grade. The prevalence of hearing loss of second graders and eighth graders had increased compared to the prevalence of hearing loss ten years ago [Montgomery & Fujikawa, 1992]. However, the history of noise exposure was not investigated, and could therefore not been correlated with hearing loss. Similarly, a higher prevalence of impaired hearing, typically at high frequencies, was observed in children who started school in 1987 and 1997 than those who started in 1977 [Gissel et al, 2002].

Further, in an interdisciplinary long-term study the effects of leisure noise exposure on hearing were yearly evaluated during a four-year period in adolescents (aged 14 to 17 years) [Biassoni et al, 2005]. During the third year, adolescents were divided into two subgroups based on hearing threshold shifts: small versus larger shifts. The ears of adolescents in these subgroups were labeled as 'tough ears' or 'tender ears', respectively. The authors concluded that leisure activities associated with both subgroups could result in permanent hearing loss in adolescents with tender ears, but does not always cause hearing damage in tough ears.

Thus, literature is so far not conclusive concerning the possible increase in prevalence of NIHL caused by leisure noise. An extensive amount of literature investigated the relation between hearing loss and leisure noise exposure. Some found a high-frequency deterioration of hearing which was attributed to noise during leisure time [Litke, 1971; Lipscomb, 1972; Lees et al, 1985; Spaeth et al, 1993]. However, others found no or only slight correlation between hearing loss and leisure time noise exposure [Hanson & Fearn, 1975; Strauss et al, 1977; Axelsson et al, 1981a; Axelsson et al, 1981b; Carter et al, 1982; Carter et al, 1984; Bradley et al, 1987; Lindeman et al, 1987; Mercier & Hohmann, 2002]. A review by Zenner et al (1999), translated in Maassen et al (2001), indicated that the reason no correlation between music exposure and hearing loss was found, is based on methodological shortcomings such as averaging music exposure without dividing in subgroups with extreme exposure, testing non-suitable subgroups or no extreme groups with substantial (life time) exposure, and failing to obtain a control group without any music exposure. Furthermore, these authors stated:

> "We can conclude from the cited studies that the noise induced PTS, which has to be expected according to ISO 1999, has been sufficiently demonstrated empirically, and that there is a considerable risk for ear damage resulting from electronically amplified music.",

and they further estimated that:

> "If the reported music listening habits of the 15 year olds are constant for 10 years, it can be expected that this will result in 10% of young Germans having an average hearing loss of 10 dB or more at 3 kHz. To this music-induce hearing loss, a further 10 dB hearing loss has to be added in 25 year olds due to age and therefore it can be expected that 10% of the 25 year olds have hearing thresholds above 20 dB at 3 kHz." [Zenner et al, 1999; Maassen et al, 2001].

Thus, it seems that the majority of properly designed research was not able to demonstrate a clear impact of leisure noise on auditory function. The most likely explanation for this lack of hearing deterioration could be that leisure noise exposure is insufficient to cause widespread hearing loss. It is plausible that the pattern of exposure to leisure noise is less frequent compared to occupational noise exposure, and attributes only for a small period in life probably between five and ten years [Hetu & Fortin, 1995; Axelsson & Prasher, 1999; Smith et al, 2000]. Moreover, the individual behavior regarding use of hearing protectors might have changed [Rabinowitz et al, 2006] and/or there might be an alteration in noise exposure habits [Mostafapour et al, 1998] due to greater public awareness of the potential harmful effects of leisure noise exposure. However, it is also suggested that it is too soon to detect permanent effects of recent advances in technology [Morata, 2007], such as MP3 players. Finally, pure-tone audiometry is possibly not the most sensitive technique to detect subtle cochlear changes, and other measures – high-frequency audiometry, high-definition audiometry and OAEs – might reveal subclinical cochlear damage. For example, significant weakening of TEOAEs was found in adolescents more exposed to amplified music than the less exposed adolescents [Mansfield et al, 1999].

Besides hearing loss, there is a high prevalence of tinnitus reported in individuals with occupational NIHL [Axelsson & Prasher, 2000]. While there seems to be an increased awareness of noise exposure in occupational settings, it is plausible that the prevalence of tinnitus due to leisure noise exposure is on the rise. In subjects reporting tinnitus, the level of social noise exposure determines the audiological characteristics as measured with pure-tone audiometry, speech-in-noise test, and otoacoustic emissions [Davis et al, 1998]. Also, it was found that 8.7% of 1285 Swedish participants between 13 and 19 years reported tinnitus, and 17.1% reported noise sensitivity [Widen & Erlandsson, 2004]. Both symptoms were more common in older than younger adolescents which could be explained by the longer period of leisure noise exposure. Thus, subjective audiological symptoms including tinnitus and hypersensitivity to sound should be considered in the evaluation of temporary or permanent thresholds shifts because it might indicate subtle cochlear changes [Schmuziger et al, 2006]. Tinnitus is also found to be a more suffering symptom than hearing loss [Metternich & Brusis, 1999; Axelsson & Prasher, 1999]. Therefore, more research is needed to estimate the prevalence of non-occupational noise-induced permanent tinnitus.

In summary, there is a large amount of research concerning the impact of leisure noise exposure on hearing, especially during music-related activities. However, the majority of these studies are characterized with poor methodology which leads to inconsistent results regarding a correlation between these aforementioned activities and hearing damage, as well as an assumed increase in prevalence of hearing loss caused by these activities. Nevertheless, in our opinion, as long as firm evidence based on adequately executed research is lacking, caution is necessary. As such, more research is urgently needed to gain more insight.

## LEISURE NOISE ACTIVITIES

Generally, leisure noise exposure can be categorized into exposure to loud music or participation in non-musical activities. The major sources of music-related leisure noise are: (1) using personal music players (PMPs), (2) attendance at nightclubs or discotheques, (3) attendance at live concerts, (4) listening to home stereo/ radio's, and (5) playing a musical instrument, playing in a band or an orchestra [MRC Institute of Hearing Research, 1986; Clark, 1991; Meyer-Bisch, 1996; Jokitulppo et al, 1997; Mansfield et al, 1999; Smith et al, 2000; Jokitulppo & Bjork, 2002; Jokitulppo et al, 2006]. Loud music listening is possible in almost every surroundings; associated with activities at home, while driving or traveling by bike, bus, train or underground [Rice et al, 1987a; Wong et al, 1990].

Smith et al (2000) studied the prevalence and type of social noise in England in 18- to 25-year-olds. It was found that the prevalence of leisure noise since the early 1980s has tripled from 6.7% to 18.8%, whereas occupational noise has decreased from 8.9% to 3.5%. About 11% received significant noise exposure from nightclubs, 3% from Hi-fis, 2% from PMPs, and 0.6% from attendance at live concerts. Significant noise exposure was defined as a situation in which raised voices between two normal hearing people four feet apart holding an conversation are needed [Smith et al, 2000]. Jokitulppo & Björk (2002) investigated the noisy leisure-time of Finnish adults (25-58 years) and found that 58% listened to a home stereo/radio, 34% went to nightclubs/pubs, 9% used a portable stereo player, 7% attended at live concerts, and only a small amount played a musical instrument (7%), in a band (1%) or orchestra (1%) [Jokitulppo & Bjork, 2002]. In Argentina, participation of adolescents in musical leisure activities was found highest for attendance at discotheques, followed by attendance at live concerts, usage of PMPs and playing musical instruments [Serra et al, 2005].

Thus, the contribution of PMPs to the total social noise exposure seems to be less than the attendance of discotheques or nightclubs. Recently however, it was found that more than 90% of 1016 American students listened to some type of personal music system through earphones [Torre, III, 2008]. It seems plausible that the technical evolution since the introduction of the Sony Walkman to the MP3 players has contributed to the current popularity of PMPs. There has been a miniaturization of the devices, an improvement of the storage and battery capacity, and online availability of music and podcasts. Thus, it is not known if findings from other PMPs – personal cassette players (PCPs) or Compact Disc players (CD players) - apply directly to MP3 player use [Vogel et al, 2007]. For example, there was a 5 dB increase in averaged levels between CD players and MP3 players using the same measurement technique [Keith et al, 2008]. Therefore, the effects of PMPs and especially MP3 players on the auditory system of young people is a cause for concern. This concern is based on the close coupling of headphones to the tympanic membrane, the ability of such devices to generate high maximum output levels, and uncertainties regarding listening habits.

Besides these music-related leisure noise sources, there are other sources of leisure noise such as attending or participating in (motor) sport events, watching movies or going to the theatre, using home tools, shooting firearms, use of fireworks, and other noisy toys. Participation in non-musical activities is, however, less common than in musical activities [Biassoni et al, 2005], and the highest participation in non-musical activities is watching movies or going to the theatre (26%), and using home tools indoors (19%) [Jokitulppo & Bjork, 2002].

## 1. Personal Music Players

### 1.1. Listening habits

There is a large variation in listening habits of adolescents using PMPs, between studies, as well as within studies. This variation is seen in duration of use (years), listening time (hours per week) and listening levels. It can largely be explained by the studied population; either no representative population was studied [e.g. Williams, 2005], or there were differences in sociodemographic characteristics in subjects between studies. Moreover, differences in questions regarding using PMPs explain the inconsistencies between studies. For example, the listening time is sometimes referred to as listening during one single session [Zogby, 2006], or for a full day [Torre, III, 2008]. Thereby, adequate comparisons in listening habits between studies are difficult. With consideration of these shortcomings, there are, however, some tendencies regarding listening habits with respect of gender and age.

First, females spend less time listening to PMPs [Catalano & Levin, 1985; Rice et al, 1987a; Meyer-Bisch, 1996; Torre, III, 2008], and prefer to listen at less intensive output levels [Catalano & Levin, 1985; Smith et al, 2000; Williams, 2005; Torre, III, 2008].

Catalano & Levin (1985) found that females listened on average 8.04 hours per week, whereas the average for males was 13.97 hours per week. Rice et al (1987a) reported that males listened on average about one hour per week more to their personal cassette players than females. Moreover, there was a higher percentage of females only occasionally listening to PCPs (17.3%) than males (10.9%) [Meyer-Bisch, 1996]. Further, it was found that 25.2% of the females used a PCP for at least two hours per week, whereas in males this was 37.6%. Recently, Torre (2008) reported that 11.2% more females listened to PMPs less than one hour per day. In contrast, 5.4% more males listened between one and three hours, 4.6% more males between three and five hours, and finally, 1.2% more males listened longer than five hours per day as compared to females.

On average, males set their personal cassette player 7.5 dB higher than females [Smith et al, 2000]. The mean 8 hour, A-weighted equivalent continuous noise level was 75.3 dB for the females, and 80.6 dB for the males [Williams, 2005]. Also, medium volume setting of PMPs was preferred for most women, whereas men were more likely to listen at a very loud listening level [Torre, III, 2008].

Second, listening habits tend to changes during lifetime [Fearn & Hanson, 1984; West & Evans, 1990; Smith et al, 2000; Meyer-Bisch, 1996; Zogby, 2006; Zenner et al, 1999; Maassen et al, 2001].

The percentage of young people listening through headphones increased from 10%, 12% and 35% for the age groups 9 to 12 years, 13 to 16 years and 18 to 25 years, respectively [Fearn & Hanson, 1984]. In contrast, the use of PMPs decreased from 67% in younger (15-16 years) to 39% in older (19-23 years) exposed adolescents [West & Evans, 1990]. Moreover, the most frequent use of personal cassette player was reported to range between 13 and 19 years [Smith et al, 2000], and Meyer-Bisch (1996) mentioned less often usage of personal cassette players after the age of 28. The percentage of high school (14-18 years) students using an Apple iPod or another brand of MP3 player was three times higher than for adults (18-+70 years), indicating that usage declines with increasing age [Zogby, 2006].

Median PMP listening duration increased from 16 years, with a median of approximately one hour 20 minutes at the age of 19 years [Zenner et al, 1999; Maassen et al, 2001]. In 2006, the length of a typical session of PMP usage was reported to range between one and four hours for a larger amount of adults, and between 30 minutes and one hour for students [Zogby, 2006].

Median listening levels were above 90 dBA between the ages of 13 and 16 years, reaching a median level of almost 100 dBA at 14 years [Zenner et al, 1999; Maassen et al, 2001]. Moreover, the typical volume setting for a student listening to a PMP was more often loud, somewhat loud or very loud, whereas adults listen to PMPs more at medium, somewhat low, low or very low volume settings [Zogby, 2006].

Besides gender and age differences in the output level of PMPs, the preferred listening levels of these devices depend on several other factors, such as the presence of background noise, the type of music, the earphone style, and the type of personal music device.

First, it was found that the presence of background noise increases the preferred listening levels. The results depend on whether the measurements were performed in laboratory or field conditions. For example, Rice et al (1987b) found a signal-to-noise ratio (SNR) of approximately 5 dB in laboratory conditions, whereas in the field study no correlation was seen between listening levels and background traffic noise. In contrast, the preferred listening levels in laboratory conditions had on average a signal-to-noise ratio of 12 dB, and in the field condition 17 dB [Airo et al, 1996]. Recently, the mean SNR in 55 subjects ranging in age from 15 to 48 years was about 13 dB measured at public areas [Williams, 2005]. Finally, the increase in preferred listening levels of an MP3 player in 38 subjects from 20 to 36 years was on average 9.4 dB higher for street noise and 7.7 dB higher for multi-talker babble, as compared to the quiet condition [Hodgetts et al, 2007]. Thus, it is important to evaluate the preferred listening levels of PMPs in the presence of background levels as these potentially result in a higher risk to hearing-related symptoms. Furthermore, increasing the listening levels might pose users at risk by decreasing their ability to hear warning signals. As such, adolescents should be advised to adjust the volume control of PMPs in quiet conditions.

Second, the preferred listening levels might be dependent on the type of music. One study evaluated the preferred listening levels for four music samples and found a difference of 10 dB between the quietest and loudest average listening levels in 14 subjects (16-26 years) [Airo et al, 1996]. Maximum output levels for different types of music were investigated by Turunen-Rise et al (1991) and more extensively by Fligor & Cox (2004). In the former study, sound pressure levels ranged from 100 to 108 dBA for pop music, 103 dBA for light classical music, and 98 dBA for classical music [Turunen-Rise et al, 1991]. Fligor & Cox (2004) measured maximum output levels of CD players for eight different styles of music relative to white noise. Country, rock and adult contemporary music samples were similar to the output levels measured with white noise. However, the output levels of the other music samples were overestimated by the white noise output levels. These overestimations were 2.5 dB, 3.9 dB, 4.9 dB, 5.6 dB and 12 dB for rap/ R&B, pop music, classical music, dance music and jazz, respectively. Moreover, the temporal pattern of these genres were evaluated. It was noticed that the highest peak SPLs were seen during the 10-sec rock and pop music sample, whereas the highest continuous 10-sec average SPL was during the rock sample. Further, dance music revealed the highest number of peaks in the 10-sec sample within 3 dB of the highest peak, and the temporal pattern of the jazz music sample was least pronounced. The number of transients during the 10-sec dance music sample ranged from 28 to 60 depending on the combination CD player and headphone [Fligor & Cox, 2004].

Third, the earphone style determines the preferred listening levels of PMPs. Preferred listening levels were on average 1.3 dB higher for the supra-aural earphones than with semi-aural earphones [Airo et al, 1996]. Further, significant lower preferred listening levels were chosen for the over-the-ear headphone as compared to earbuds [Hodgetts et al, 2007]. This difference was 2.6 dB in quiet, 4.3 dB in presence of street noise and 3.8 dB with multi-talker babble. Also, it was reported that earbuds produce significant higher maximum output levels than supra-aural headphones, up to 7 dB [Fligor and Cox 2004]. MacLean et al (1992) found a 6.2 dB higher output level for the earbuds than for the supra-aural headphones. The differences might be explained by the physical coupling of the headphones, as well as their differences in operating characteristics [MacLean et al, 1992]. Finally, outputs level of a tight fit of earbuds and supra-aural headphones was on average 16 dB higher than those of a loose fitting [Keith et al, 2008]. Thus, the coupling of the ear- and headphone, as well as the geometry of the ear defines the noise exposure using PMPs.

### 1.2. Short- and long term auditory effects

Generally, temporary reduction in hearing sensitivity may be the result of listening to high output levels of PMPs during a short period (hours), while permanent hearing deterioration may be caused by listening to PMPs during a much longer period (years), even at lower listening levels. As mentioned previously, the exact relationship between TTS and

PTS is uncertain. However, it is assumed that in the long term temporary hearing shifts may result in permanent hearing reduction.

Short-term effects of listening to PMPs were investigated measuring hearing thresholds, and recently, also by OAEs before and after a listening session. Lee et al (1985) found significant TTSs of 10 dB in 6 of the 16 subjects, as well as a TTS of approximately 30 dB in one subject after listening to three-hour during music with output levels ranging from 80 to 104 dB SPL [Lee et al, 1985]. Turunen-Rise et al (1991) described median TTSs of less than 12 dB after one hour listening to two types of pop music at a preset listening level between 85 and 95 dBA in six subjects [Turunen-Rise et al, 1991]. Hellström (1991) evaluated TTSs after exposure to one hour modern music via PMPs at loud, but comfortable volume. The mean listening levels ranged from 91 to 97 dBA with mean TTS from 4.01 to 5.74 dB [Hellstrom, 1991]. Loth et al (1992) found an average TTS of 5 dB in 12 subjects after one-hour at preferred equivalent levels between 89 and 94 dBA [Loth et al, 1992]. Pugsley et al (1993) reported no significant larger deterioration in hearing after listening to a PMP during one hour in 30 subjects than in the control group of 15 subjects [Pugsley et al, 1993]. Hellström et al (1998) exposed 21 subjects to music via PCP at a loud, but comfortable level. Subjects were divided in three groups depending on their listening pattern. The average equivalent listening levels were 91.4 dBA, 91.9 dBA and 97.1 dBA with mean TTSs 15.7 dB, 4.5 dB and 4.0 dB, respectively [Hellstrom et al, 1998]. Recently, Bhagat & Davis (2008) measured hearing thresholds, DPOAEs and synchronized SOAEs (SSOAEs) in 20 subjects after listening to music during 30 minutes at a preset listening level. There were no significant differences in hearing thresholds before and after music exposure. There were, however, significant reductions in DPOAE half-octave band levels centered from 1.4 to 6.0 kHz, but variable shifts in frequency and level of SSOAEs [Bhagat & Davis, 2008].

From these TTS studies, we may be conclude that there are only slight, if any, reductions in hearing thresholds after listening to PMPs, but changes in OAEs might be early warning signs of the harmful effects of high levels of music exposure. There are however some shortcomings, as well as considerable variability in literature regarding temporary hearing damage after listening to PMPs. First, there is only one study [Pugsley et al, 1993] which included a control group to evaluate the threshold changes in a experimental group based on the test-retest reliability of hearing thresholds in a control group. Second, Lee et al (1985) considered thresholds shifts of at least 10 dB to be significant while others only reported the mean or median TTS [Hellstrom, 1991; Turunen-Rise et al, 1991; Hellstrom et al, 1998]. Third, there are methodological differences in music exposure, as well as in the determination of output levels. The music exposure ranged from one hour to three hours with different genres of music: with rock/fusion music [Lee et al, 1985], pop music [Turunen-Rise et al, 1991], contemporary music [Pugsley et al, 1993] or the favorite music cassette of the subjects [Hellstrom, 1991; Hellstrom et al, 1998]. Mainly, user-preferred listening levels were used with either standard headphones [Hellstrom, 1991; Turunen-Rise et al, 1991; Hellstrom et al, 1998] or user-preferred headphones [Lee et al, 1985]. However, one study [Pugsley et al, 1993] did not perform output measures to correlate with the results from the hearing test. The output levels were measured on an artificial ear with coupler [Lee et al, 1985], on KEMAR [Turunen-Rise et al, 1991], or via a miniature microphone in the external ear canal [Hellstrom, 1991; Hellstrom et al, 1998].

There are also several studies investigating the permanent auditory effects caused by long-term listening to PMPs. Wong et al (1990) found no differences in mean hearing thresholds between 78 young PCP users and 25 non-users [Wong et al, 1990]. However, the half-octave frequencies 3.0 and 6.0 kHz were not tested. Meyer-Bisch (1996) compared high definition audiometry in three groups. There were significant poorer hearing thresholds in the most exposed PCP group (n=54, > 7hrs/wk) compared to the controls (n=358). No significant differences were seen between the less exposed PCP group (n=195, 2-7 hrs/wk) and the control group. There was also twice more subjective auditory suffering - presence of tinnitus and/or hearing fatigue - in the total PCP group than in the controls [Meyer-Bisch, 1996]. LePage & Murray (1998) noticed a decline in click-evoked OAEs significantly proportional with increasing PCP listening time from less than one hour to more than six hours per week [LePage & Murray, 1998]. Mostafapour et al (1998) evaluated hearing thresholds, speech reception threshold and speech discrimination in 50 subjects with estimated lifetime exposure of PMPs low, medium or high. No significant differences between the three groups were found [Mostafapour et al, 1998]. Peng et al (2007) found significant differences in hearing thresholds at conventional and extended high-frequencies between 120 PMP users and 30 controls, but no significant differences between the three subgroups of PMP use (one to three years, three to five years, longer than five years) were seen. Moreover, the hearing thresholds at extended high-frequencies of normal-hearing subjects at conventional frequencies were significantly higher than those of the control group. Therefore, the authors concluded that long-term use of PMPs could induce NIHL, and extended high-frequency audiometry is more sensitive than audiometry at conventional frequencies [Peng et al, 2007]. Montoya et al (2008) found a reduction of TEOAE and DPOAE incidence and amplitudes, as well as an increase in DPOAE thresholds with longer duration of listening to PMPs in years, and for more hours per week [Montoya et al, 2008].

The results of the aforementioned studies might indicate that with more extensive use of PMPs, hearing deteriorates. However, several shortcomings in these studies can be pointed out. First, in some studies [LePage & Murray, 1998; Peng et al, 2007], there was no consideration of other sources of leisure noise. So, it is impossible to distinguish hearing damage caused by PMPs from deterioration caused by several confounding sources of leisure noise. Second, mostly either the duration of use in years [Peng et al, 2007], or the use per week [Meyer-Bisch, 1996; LePage & Murray, 1998] of PMPs was investigated. In our opinion, the lifetime noise exposure from PMPs must be evaluated encompassing both parameters. Third, subjects were not always representative for the population [Wong et al, 1990; Mostafapour et al, 1998]. It is possible that with a more representative group, more extreme listening habits appear. Finally, the mentioned listening habits are based on a retrospective estimation by the subjects which could lead to errors in the quantification of PMP usage.

Previously, risk assessments were established, and ranged from 0.065 to 30% [Catalano & Levin, 1985; MRC Institute of Hearing Research, 1986; Rice et al, 1987a; Clark, 1991; Ising et al, 1994; Ising et al, 1995; Passchier-Vermeer, 1999; Williams, 2005]. Moreover, PMPs are supplementary sound sources and might accumulate with other noise exposure [Meyer-Bisch, 1996]. The variability in risk assessment could be explained by the definition for NIHL and the damage-risk criteria for hearing loss, which are directly adopted from occupational settings. According to some authors, extrapolation of occupational risk criteria to leisure noise exposures is not justified because of the differences in spectral and temporal pattern between industrial noise and music [Turunen-Rise et al 1991; Mostafapour et al 1998; Metternich & Brusis, 1999; Smith et al 2000; Fligor and Cox 2004]. Amplified music emphasizes low-frequencies, and is characterized with transients superimposed on a relatively steady-state signal [Peng et al, 2007]. As such, it can be assumed that A-weighted sound levels underestimate the low-frequency contribution, and C-weighted sound levels could be proposed. However, industrial criteria are usually expressed in dBA. Moreover, it was also found that aversive sounds – noise or disliked music - induced larger TTSs than enjoyable sounds [Lindgren & Axelsson, 1983; Swanson et al, 1987]. Nevertheless, the regulation for occupational noise exposure is based on the exposure level and duration of noise exposure which also determines leisure noise exposure and there are currently no criteria available for this latter source. Thus, the criteria adopted from occupational noise exposure can be applied to evaluate the impact of leisure noise, although this must be done with caution. Therefore, users should be warned for the gradual and insidious development of hearing loss associated with long-term listening to PMPs at high intensity levels [Smith et al, 2000].

## 2. Attendance of Discotheques, Nightclubs or Live Concerts

### 2.1. Attendance habits

Generally, it is assumed that discotheques or nightclubs have a larger impact on young people's hearing than concerts. The noise exposure in the latter can be louder, but are attended less frequently and lead to less overall noise immission [Smith et al, 2000; Serra et al, 2005]. In 700 adolescents ranging in age from 16 to 25 years, attending discotheques regularly was found to be 79%, whereas attendance at pop and rock concerts and techno parties was 53% and 36% respectively [Mercier & Hohmann, 2002]. The average hours per week in 1323 adolescents (age range 28-58 years) was 4.4 for nightclubs/ pubs and 2.4 for concerts [Jokitulppo et al, 2006]. An average of 6.2 hours per week was determined for discotheque attendance [Zenner et al, 1999; Maassen et al, 2001].

Some tendencies regarding gender and age differences can be found in discotheque, nightclubs or concert attendance. First, more males (91%) attended nightclubs than females (84%) which was investigated in 494 university students [Meecham & Hume, 2001]. Meyer-Bisch (1996) also found more occasionally discotheque attendance in females, and more frequent attendance (at least twice a month) by males. Further, a higher proportion of males regularly (once a month) or intensively (twice a month) attended concerts. Second, attending discotheques and concerts was reported more often in older exposed (19-23 years) than younger exposed (15-16 years) adolescents [West & Evans, 1990]. Moreover, the highest proportion of attendance was at 21-22 years, and rare after 28 years [Meyer-Bisch, 1996]. It was reported that the highest median visits per month was at the age of 17-18 years, with a decreasing trend from 22 years [Zenner et al, 1999; Maassen et al, 2001]. However, the more extreme noise exposure habits indicate that visits of more than twice a month was exceeded at the age of 13 years, with the highest 10% value of approximately seven visits a month at 19 years.

The mean of sound levels, measured in discotheques and rock concerts was 103.4 dBA [Clark, 1991]. Smith et al (2000) reported sound levels in nightclubs and discotheques ranging from 85 to 105 dBA with a mean of 101 dBA. Another study found sound levels in nightclubs in the range of 97 to 106 dBA [Meecham & Hume, 2001]. Factors influencing these sound levels are: measurement position, time in the evening, variations between clubs, as well as between evenings in the same club [Ising, 1994; Smith et al, 2000; Meecham &

Hume, 2001]. Recently, average sound levels for concerts ranged from 95 to 102 dBA for pop concerts, 97 to 103 dBA for heavy metal concerts, and 96 to 107 dBA for rock concerts with maximum sound levels 126, 113 and 118 dBA, respectively [Opperman et al, 2006]. So, it is clearly a misconception that some music genres, especially rock and heavy metal concerts, are louder than pop concerts.

As in listening habits of PMPs, it is difficult to establish general attendance habits in a representative sample of adolescents. Moreover, there are only few studies addressing the sound levels with respect of the influencing parameters.

### 2.2. Short- and long term effects

Clark (1991) reported that research in the seventies and eighties regarding temporary auditory effects indicate moderate TTS up to 30 dB recovering within hours to days after noise exposure [Clark, 1991]. For example, Axelsson & Lindgren (1978) found mean TTSs at 4 kHz of approximately 12 dB in listeners, and 10 dB in pop musicians. TTSs amounted up to 45 dB HL [Axelsson & Lindgren, 1978]. More recently, in a small population (n=22) TTSs after rock concerts were found to be 10.9, 9.8 and 20.9 dB depending on the position in the arena with respective $L_{Aeq}$ of 89.29, 99.6 and 101.3 dBA [Yassi et al, 1993]. Peak levels were almost 140 dBA which is assumed to cause irreversible acoustic trauma due to impulse noise. Sixty percent of the subjects assessed the sound levels as too loud or intolerable. However, only slightly more than half the subjects were aware of their TTSs which is a cause for concern and emphasizes the insidious nature of NIHL. The average TTS after attending discotheques increased from 6.2 dB to 10.01 dB with increasing attendance from one to two hours [Liebel et al, 1996]. Significant effects on TEOAE reproducibility and amplitudes were also found, but not on DPOAEs. Therefore, OAEs were regarded as not ideal measures of hearing shifts after noise exposure. Opperman et al (2006) found that largest mean hearing shifts were located at 3 and 4 kHz. Significant hearing shifts, according to OSHA and ASHA criteria, were present in 64% of the subjects wearing no earplugs, whereas in 27% wearing earplugs. This might be explained by the fact that the real-world attenuation of hearing protection devices is less than theoretically established mainly by the fitting of the earplugs into ear canal. Therefore, it is important to instruct adolescents correctly wearing earplugs.

The permanent auditory effects of concert and discotheque attendance in adolescents can be considered more dangerous than the use of PMPs [Meyer-Bisch, 1996; Mercier & Hohmann, 2002; Biassoni et al, 2005]. However, only few studies evaluated the long-term auditory effects of attending discotheques, nightclubs or concerts. Meyer-Bisch (1996) noticed a significant reduction in hearing thresholds, especially at 4 kHz, in the concert group as compared to the control group which never or only occasionally used a PMP and went only rarely to concerts or discotheques. No significant differences in hearing thresholds between the discotheque attendees and control group could be established. However, there was three times more auditory suffering in the discotheque group than the controls, whereas in the concert group this was four times higher than in the control group. Meecham and Hume (2001) reported no significant association between attendance of nightclubs and occurrence of post exposure tinnitus, but they indicate that attendance increased the risk of and reduced recovery from tinnitus after noise exposure.

## 3. Conclusion

It can be concluded that there is a large variation in listening and attendance habits of the most popular music-related leisure noise activities. Gender and age differences are two major sociodemographic factors partially explaining the variation in habits. More research is needed to extensively evaluate the type of leisure noise activities, as well as listening or attendance habits in a representative sample of adolescents.

TTS studies indicate that there are only slight reductions in hearing thresholds after listening to PMPs, but more damage seem to be present after attending discotheques, nightclubs or live concerts. However, more sensitive methods to evaluate minimal cochlear changes should be incorporated in future TTS studies with consideration of the mentioned shortcomings of the existing studies.

Furthermore, PTS studies indicate that visiting discotheques, nightclubs or concerts poses more risk to hearing than listening to PMPs. The measured sound pressures levels indicate theoretically that frequently attending these activities might cause hearing loss. As previously mentioned however, a clear association between hearing loss and attendance of these activities has not been proven yet, and more research is needed addressing hearing loss in young people with more extensive listening habits for multiple sources of leisure noise.

## PREVENTION OF NOISE-INDUCED HEARING LOSS CAUSED BY LEISURE NOISE

It is currently inconceivable that several parties would take place without music exposure. However, it is remarkable that young people tend to listen to music in almost every environment, individually using their PMPs, as in groups in discotheques, nightclubs, concerts festivals etc. Plath (1998) describes this phenomenon as the fear of silence, as well as the reduction of unwanted background noise by listening to music [Plath, 1998a; Plath, 1998b]. However, adolescents extent this behavior to excessive music-listening in which music has to be felt, consistent with exuberant behavior [Clark, 1991]. Zenner et al (1999) and Maassen et al (2001) mentioned that such behavior compensates for the frustration and problems experienced by adolescents. Florentine et al (1998) stated that music-listening behavior is sometimes associated with dependency-like disorders [Florentine et al, 1998], and recently, it was found that there was a correlation between general risk behavior such as smoking, drinking and leaving school on the one hand, and risk behavior regarding loud music on the other hand [Bohlin & Erlandsson, 2007].

Hetu & Fortin (1995) analyzed the temporal and spectral features of discotheque music, especially house music. It was postulated that the pulsating character of house music influences cardiac activity, and thus the general level of arousal. Moreover, low-frequency emphasizing maximizes beat perception, mid-frequency reduction prevents annoyance by permitting communication, and high-frequency enhancement allows perception of high-pitched sounds to stress the beat. Furthermore, these authors described the phenomenology of music-listening explaining the possessing of music. First, penetration of the music environment is limited due to the high sound pressure levels, as well as uninterrupted nature of discotheque or nightclub music (confinement). Second, listeners are enclosed in a musical field shared by other listeners (immersion). Third, music is heard without any focus of attention needed; communication is hardly impossible (passive hearing). Finally, the music and the light show are responsible for auditory, vestibular and proprioceptive sensations (excitement) [Hetu & Fortin, 1995].

The opposite of such excessive social lifestyle is presented when adolescents experience a hearing loss which affects their quality of life [Arlinger, 2003]. The handicap of NIHL in adolescents has an impact on the individual in interactions, but also in their broader communications with family and friends, as well as on the society. Their educational achievement is hampered, and eventually also their employability. In Argentina, pre-employment medical examination is failed in a high percentage of young people because of hearing loss [Serra et al, 2005]. Therefore, it is important to prevent NIHL, in occupational settings, but also during leisure activities.

Preventive strategies should incorporate a two-layered approach. First, by educating the adolescents and second, by protective measures such as legislation. It was reported that not only adolescents, but several other parties are involved in the prevention of NIHL. To prevent NIHL caused by discotheque attendance, the authorities, discotheque owners and decorators, as well as disc-jockeys are possible responsible [Vogel et al, 2009a]. Preventing NIHL due to PMP-listening, manufacturers of earphones and MP3 players, authorities, music industry, parents, media and community centers are potentially involved [Vogel et al, 2009b].

Improving the awareness and knowledge regarding the problems associated with excessive loud music-listening, consequences and preventive measures should be aimed for. Chung et al (2005) conducted a web-based survey, and found that only 8% of the 3310 respondents indicate hearing loss as a 'very big problem' [Chung et al, 2005]. Among the seven health concerns – hearing loss, sexually transmitted diseases, alcohol or drug abuse, depression, smoking, nutrition and weight issues and acne – hearing loss was perceived as the least 'very big problem'. Further, others reported that knowledge regarding the irreversibility of NIHL was limited [Weichbold & Zorowka, 2002; Shah et al, 2009]. Others have found a greater awareness of the risks in their population [Crandell et al, 2004; Rawool & Colligon-Wayne, 2008]. However, since there is still a great deal of unawareness, or al lot of misconceptions regarding to NIHL caused by leisure noise, information is necessary. Hearing education campaigns improve the knowledge and awareness of NIHL, and improve motivation to protect the hearing [Becher et al, 1996]. However, it was found that the behavior of adolescents did not change: the frequency of discotheque attendance after a hearing education campaign even increased, the average duration of discotheque attendance, the use of hearing protection and their listening behavior using headphones was not influenced by the campaign [Weichbold & Zorowka, 2002; Weichbold & Zorowka, 2003; Weichbold & Zorowka, 2007]. Only the use of regeneration breaks at discotheques during which the ears can rest in a silent environment was increased. However, after the campaign, sound levels were more often judged as too loud, and the authors hypothesize that there might be less resistance for political action at that point.

It is possible that behavioural changes in adolescents are not achieved because the consequences of their behavior, hearing loss, is not immediately perceived or not experienced as serious enough. Widen & Erlandsson (2004) found that subjects reporting tinnitus and noise sensitivity are more worried regarding hearing loss than those without symptoms, and were more likely to report the use of hearing protectors [Widen et al, 2006]. Moreover, subjects with permanent tinnitus assessed loud music-listening as more risky, and subjects with only occasional tinnitus listened more often to loud music [Bohlin & Erlandsson, 2007]. It was found that, even after perceiving hearing loss and/or tinnitus, only 14% was willing to avoid noisy leisure activities, 86% was prepared to reduce their attendance at such activities, and 12% did not have any intention to change their behavior regarding music exposure. So, previous hearing-related symptoms do not necessarily implicate a more responsible behavior in the future. However, they sometimes trigger behavioral changes [Bogoch et al, 2005].

The high sound levels in discotheques, concerts and other parties are quite easily ascribed to the demands of the attendees by nightclub or discotheque owners and concert organizers. However, Mercier & Hohmann (2002) report that the sound levels are judged too high by 43%, 47% and 52% of the visitors in discotheques, concerts and techno parties, respectively. It was reported that sound levels in discotheques was at least sometimes perceived as too loud by over 60% of adolescents [Weichbold & Zorowka, 2002], and it should be more quiet by more than 40% [Weichbold & Zorowka, 2005]. Also, at festivals, the sound levels were too loud for 25% of the attendees [Mercier et al, 2003]. It was even found that 85% of adolescents would not change their attendance behavior even if sound levels in discotheques were lowered, and almost 10% would visit discotheques more often when the sound levels were turned down [Weichbold & Zorowka, 2005]. Therefore, besides hearing conservation campaigns, more effort should be undertaken from politicians to regulate the sound levels in various establishments, as well as supervise the compliance of the legislation. Vogel et al (2008) also states that MP3 players should be equipped with a clear indicator of the volume, as well as with a warning signal when a hazardous doses is reached [Vogel et al, 2008].

# CASE STUDIES

## 1. Short-term Auditory Effects

### 1.1. Case one

Case one represents a 26-year old male which participated at our current study on leisure noise exposure. He mentioned a five-hour attendance in a nightclub about nine hours before his visit. There was bilateral a normal otoscopy, type A tympanogram and present middle ear muscle reflexes at 1.0 kHz. Pure-tone audiometry and DPOAEs were performed, and are reflected in Figure 1 and 2, respectively. Pure-tone audiometry revealed normal hearing at the right ear, and a audiometric notch of 30 dBHL at 4 kHz at the left ear. DPOAEs evoked with L1/L2=65/55 dBSPL showed reduced emission amplitudes at the right ear and significantly deteriorated amplitudes at the left ear.

### 1.2. Case two

Case two is a 24-year old male participating at the study regarding the short-term auditory effects of listening to an MP3 player during one hour. He listened to poprock music at a loud, but comfortable listening level. Pure-tone audiometry and DPOAEs (L1/L2=65/55 dBSPL) were measured before and after exposure. Normal otoscopy, type A tympanogram and normal middle ear muscle reflexes at 1.0 kHz were obtained before music exposure. Figure 3 and 4 show the results of the right ear for audiometry and DPOAEs, respectively, before and after the listening session. Temporary thresholds shifts varied between 5 and 10 dB, which can be regarded as the test-retest reliability of hearing thresholds. The emission amplitudes decreased considerably; the largest temporary emissions shifts were 4.4, 6.1 and 4.0 dB at frequency band with centre frequencies 4.0, 6.0 and 8.0 kHz.

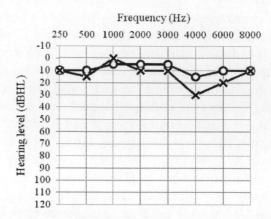

Figure 1. Hearing thresholds at octave frequencies from 250 to 8000 Hz, and half-octave frequencies 3000 and 6000 Hz for the right ear (circles) and left ear (crosses).

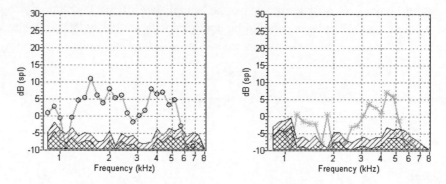

Figure 2. DPOAE amplitudes (grey lines) and noise amplitudes (shaded areas) from 841 to 8000 Hz for the right ear (right) and left ear (left).

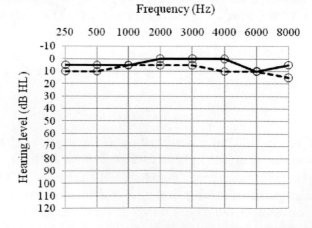

Figure 3. Pure-tone audiometry of case number two. The solid line represents the pre-exposure measurement; the dashed line the post-exposure measurement of listening to a PMP for one hour.

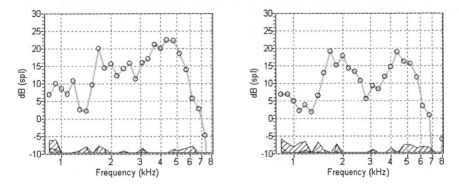

Figure 4. DPOAE amplitudes (grey lines) and noise amplitudes (shaded areas) of case number two: pre-exposure measurement (right) and post-exposure measurement (left) of listening to a PMP for one hour.

## 2. Long-term Auditory Effects

### 2.1. Case three

Case three is a 22-year old male student participating at our current study regarding leisure noise exposure. There was a bilateral normal otoscopy, type A tympanogram and normal middle ear muscle reflexes at 1.0 kHz. Pure-tone audiometry was measured (Figure 5) and shows bilateral (quasi-)normal hearing thresholds at conventional frequencies. Extended high-frequency audiometry was performed at 10.0, 12.5 and 16.0 kHz. Hearing thresholds were lowered, with the largest hearing loss of 60 dBHL at 16.0 kHz for the right ear. Figure 6 represents the DPOAEs (L1/L2=65/55 dBSPL) and reduced emission amplitudes are observed at both ears, with the left ear more deteriorated than the right ear. His noise exposure history can be described as substantially, as reflected in Table 1. He listens to his PMPs at maximum volume setting, mostly while using public transportation. After attending a discotheque, he usually experiences a post-exposure tinnitus.

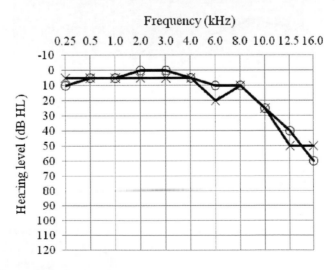

Figure 5. Reflected are the hearing thresholds at frequencies from 0.250 to 16.0 kHz of both ears (right ear: circles; left ear: crosses) of case number three.

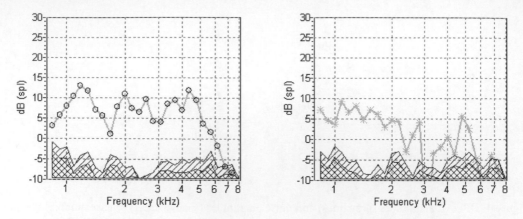

Figure 6. DPOAE amplitudes (grey lines) and noise amplitudes (shaded areas) for both ears (right ear: right figure; lef ear: left figure) of case number three.

**Table 1. Summary of the noise history of case number three.**

| Leisure activity | Weekly or monthly exposure (hours) | Duration of exposure (years) |
|---|---|---|
| Listening to a PMP | 9 hrs/wk | 7 |
| Listening to a stereo | 14 hrs/wk | 7 |
| Attendance of discotheques or parties | 15 hrs/wk | 6 |
| Attendance of live concerts | 6 hrs/month | 4 |
| Visiting a cinema or theater | 2 hrs/month | 6 |
| Attendance of sport events | 5 hrs/wk | 3 |

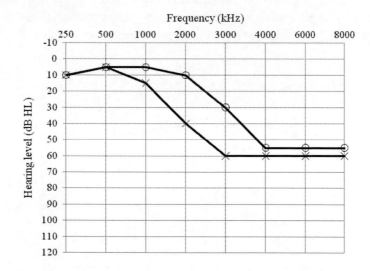

Figure 7. Pure-tone audiometry for case number four for the right ear (circles) and lef ear (crosses).

## 2.2. *Case four*

Case four is a male of 22 years old. He also voluntarily participated at a current study regarding leisure noise exposure. Since six years, he experiences a hearing loss and tinnitus at both ears. A high-frequency hearing loss, especially at 4 and 6 kHz, was confirmed by a ENT-specialist. He wears hearing protector devices rigorously, and a hearing test is performed yearly. At the time of testing, normal otoscopy, type A tympanogram and normal middle ear muscle reflexes at 1.0 kHz were obtained. Pure-tone audiometry (Figure 7) reveals bilateral high-frequency sensorineural hearing loss from 2.0 kHz at the left ear and 3.0 kHz at the right ear. DPOAEs (L1/L2=65/55 dBSPL) were measured and revealed absent emission amplitudes in the high-frequencies, and slightly more preserved emission amplitudes at the right ear (Figure 8).

## 3. Conclusion

These case studies illustrate the short- and long-term auditory effects of leisure noise exposure. In cases with hearing loss as established with pure-tone audiometry, the emission amplitudes are also reduced. Moreover, in cases with audiometric normal hearing, emission amplitudes indicate cochlear damage. Therefore, it can be concluded that OAEs complement pure-tone audiometry in the detection of cochlear hearing loss caused by noise exposure and more specifically leisure noise exposure. The clinical utility of OAEs in the diagnosis of NIHL must be further explored.

## REGULATION

There is increasing excessive noise exposure everywhere. Long-term exposure to high noise levels have caused moderate to severe hearing problems in millions of industrial workers [Dobie, 2008]. Moreover, recent studies of environmental noise have demonstrated that children compared to workers may receive more decibels from an 8-hour working day in a factory and that persons regularly attending sport events are exposed to intensity levels exceeding all federal guidelines (WHO, 1997).

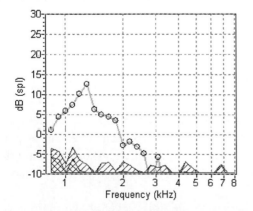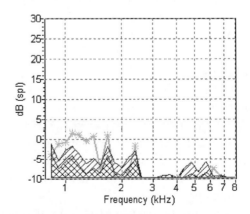

Figure 8. DPOAE amplitudes (grey lines) and noise amplitudes (shaded areas) measured in case number four for the right ear (right figure) and left ear (left figure).

**Table 2. Permissible Noise Exposure (OSHA, 1992).**

| Exposure duration per day (hours) | Exposure level (dBA) |
|---|---|
| 8 | 90 |
| 6 | 92 |
| 4 | 95 |
| 3 | 97 |
| 2 | 100 |
| 1 | 105 |
| ½ | 110 |
| ¼ | 115 |

Most of the guidelines, criteria and legislation are setup for occupational purposes. Estimations of the risk for developing a non-occupational hearing loss is nowadays compared to hearing loss caused by occupational exposure. The problem of noise and hearing conservation is regulated in specific standards, regulations and legislations for recordkeeping and the general industry. A regulation is a rule prescribed by the government and is more formal than a standard. A standard is a set of rules or guidelines, but can be developed also by consensus groups, such as the American National Standards Institute (ANSI). Legislation consists of laws prescribed by the American Congress or by local governing bodies [Sutter, 1996]. In Europe, these standards and legislations are expressed as European Community Directives. The most recent directive is Directive 2003-10-EC of the European Parliament and Council on the minimum health and safety requirements regarding the exposure of workers to the risks arising from physical agents (Directive 2003-10-EC, 2003). Other nations use a code of practice, which has less legal force than regulations and legislations. An example of this is the Australian national standard in which a 35 page code of practice provides the guidelines on how the standard, described in two short paragraphs, should be implemented. Finally, recommendations are sometimes used, which act more as guidelines rather than enforceable rules [Sutter, 1996].

Most of these standards are based on little valid, reliable, and scientific data. Political, social and economical factors have often strong influence on the final rules and regulations. As a consequence permissible safety exposure limits (PEL), rules and guidelines differ very much according to country.

An overview of all standards, rules and regulations of the different countries and states is not within the scope of this chapter. As an example the different parameters of the 1910.95 OSHA Noise Standard are provided here (OSHA, 1992).

In the 1910.95 OSHA Noise Standard, PELs for noise are described as the maximum duration of exposure per working day, permitted for various noise intensity levels (in dBA). The exposure-duration table of the OSHA standard is described in Table 2.

The PELs depend on two parameters, a criterion level and an exchange rate. The criterion level is the steady noise intensity level, which is allowed for a full eight-hour working day. This is 90 dBA in most jurisdictions, but in Europe and other nations these values may be much lower.

Applying the equal-energy rule of sound, increasing the noise level above the criterion level, must result in a decrease of the allowed exposure time. This level-duration relation depends on the exchange rate. The exchange rate is the amount by which the permissible exposure level can be increased when the exposure duration is divided by two. There are worldwide two types of exchange rates in use: 3 dBA and 5 dBA exchange rates. These two exchange rates produce different guidelines worldwide. The 3 dBA exchange rate is more stringent. The maximum permitted duration for a 105 dBA noise exposure using the 3 dBA exchange rate is 15 minutes, whereas it is one hour with the 5 dBA exchange rate. Most international experts evaluate the 3 dBA rule as more logical for occupational noise exposure. As can be seen in Table 2, the OSHA advices a PEL of 90 dBA and an exchange rate of 5 dBA. The US Army and Air Force now use 3 dB exchange rates.

Since most of the regulations and standards across the world are made for occupational purposes, one should be cautious to extrapolate these criteria and permissible exposure levels to the situations of leisure noise exposure.

There is an increasing need for an international debate on legislation and regulation of noise exposure outside occupational activities. Legislation on output levels of personal music players and sound levels in discotheques, nightclubs, live concerts or at festivals is urgently needed and should not be based on occupational regulations and legislations.

## CONCLUSION

NIHL is the result of long-term noise exposure in occupational setting, as well as during non-occupational, leisure activities. These leisure activities include participation in non-musical activities, as well as music-related exposure. The most common sources of music exposure during leisure activities are listening to PMPs, and attending discotheques, nightclubs, or live concerts.

An increased prevalence of NIHL in youth caused by these leisure noise exposures is assumed in the mainstream media. However, scientific results concerning this issue are equivocal. There is a definite amount of high-frequency hearing loss in young people, but there are only small associations observed between leisure noise exposure and hearing loss as determined by pure-tone audiometry and clear, firm evidence of an increased prevalence of NIHL is not yet noticed.

Several explanations are possible. First, it could be that leisure noise exposure is insufficient to cause widespread hearing loss. Second, recent technological improvements in PMPs, and subsequently improved listening comfort and habits do not cause hearing loss yet. Finally, it is suggested that pure-tone audiometry is not sensitive enough to detect minimal cochlear damage.

Nevertheless, the aforementioned sources of leisure noise can be hazardous for hearing in some highly susceptible, or even in many young people with extreme listening or attendance habits. Therefore, further research on several domains is essentially to prevent NIHL in young people.

First, a careful inventory of leisure activities and listening habits in a representative sample of adolescents is needed, as well as a well-grounded understanding of music-listening habits. As mentioned above, there are gender differences in listening habits, and these habits also tend to change during life. Therefore, factors determining risk behavior regarding noise exposure must be further explored. We prefer a multidisciplinary context with at least a hearing specialist and psychologist to gain insight in risk behavior excessive music listening by adolescents.

Second, the long-term risks of cumulative noise exposures of adolescents must be evaluated. We recommend using OAEs and/or extended high-frequency audiometry complementary with pure-tone audiometry. The usefulness of OAEs in the diagnosis of NIHL must be further explored, but are promising as indicated by our case studies.

Finally, hearing education campaigns should educate adolescents, and other parties involved in the prevention of NIHL. As education is not enough to induce behavioral changes in adolescents, we insist in a strict legislation to limit sound levels in several establishments with high intensity levels, as well as a limitation of the output levels of PMPs.

# REFERENCES

Airo, E., Pekkarinen, J. & Olkinuora, P. S. (1996). Listening to music with earphones: an assessment of noise exposure. *Acta Acustica*, *82*, 885-94.

Alberti, P. (1998). Traumatic sensorineural hearing loss. In H. Ludman & A. Wright (Eds.), *Diseases of the ear* (6th, pp. 483-494). London: Arnold/Hodder Headline.

American College of Occupational and Environmental Medicine. Position Statement on noise-induced hearing loss. 2002. Available at: http://www.acoem.org/guidelines. aspx?id=846. Accessed on June 16, 2009.

Arlinger, S. (2003). Negative consequences of uncorrected hearing loss--a review. *Int J Audiol*, *42 Suppl 2*, 2S17-20.

Attias, J., Horovitz, G., El-Hatib, N. & Nageris, B. (2001). Detection and Clinical Diagnosis of Noise-Induced Hearing Loss by Otoacoustic Emissions. *Noise Health*, *3*, 19-31.

Augustsson, I. & Engstrand, I. (2006). Hearing ability according to screening at conscription; comparison with earlier reports and with previous screening results for individuals without known ear disease. *Int J Pediatr Otorhinolaryngol*, *70*, 909-13.

Axelsson, A. & Lindgren, F. (1978). Temporary threshold shift after exposure to pop music. *Scand Audiol*, *7*, 127-35.

Axelsson, A. & Prasher, D. (1999). Tinnitus: A warning signal to teenagers attending discotheques? *Noise Health*, *1*, 1-2.

Axelsson, A. & Prasher, D. (2000). Tinnitus induced by occupational and leisure noise. *Noise Health*, *2*, 47-54.

Axelsson, A., Jerson, T. & Lindgren, F. (1981b). Noisy leisure time activities in teenage boys. *Am Ind Hyg Assoc J*, *42*, 229-33.

Axelsson, A., Jerson, T., Lindberg, U. & Lindgren, F. (1981a). Early noise-induced hearing loss in teenage boys. *Scand Audiol*, *10*, 91-6.

Axelsson, A., Rosenhall, U. & Zachau, G. (1994). Hearing in 18-year-old Swedish males. *Scand Audiol*, *23*, 129-34.

Becher, S., Struwe, F., Schwenzer, C. & Weber, K. (1996). [Risk of hearing loss caused by high volume music--presenting an educational concept for preventing hearing loss in adolescents]. *Gesundheitswesen*, *58*, 91-5.

Bhagat, S. P. & Davis, A. M. (2008). Modification of otoacoustic emissions following ear-level exposure to MP3 player music. *Int J Audiol*, *47*, 751-60.

Biassoni, E. C. et al (2005). Recreational noise exposure and its effects on the hearing of adolescents. Part II: development of hearing disorders. *Int J Audiol, 44*, 74-85.

Bogoch, I. I., House, R. A. & Kudla, I. (2005). Perceptions about hearing protection and noise-induced hearing loss of attendees of rock concerts. *Can J Public Health, 96*, 69-72.

Bohlin, M. C. & Erlandsson, S. I. (2007). Risk behaviour and noise exposure among adolescents. *Noise Health, 9*, 55-63.

Bonfils, P., Bertrand, Y. & Uziel, A. (1988). Evoked otoacoustic emissions: normative data and presbycusis. *Audiology, 27*, 27-35.

Bradley, R., Fortnum, H. & Coles, R. (1987). Patterns of exposure of schoolchildren to amplified music. *Br J Audiol, 21*, 119-25.

Brownell, W. E. (1990). Outer hair cell electromotility and otoacoustic emissions. *Ear Hear, 11*, 82-92.

Carter, N. L., Murray, N., Khan, A. & Waugh, D. (1984). A longitudinal study of recreational noise and young people's hearing. *Australian Journal of Audiology, 6*, 45-53.

Carter, N. L., Waugh, R. L., Keen, K., Murray, N. & Bulteau, V. G. (1982). Amplified music and young people's hearing. Review and report of Australian findings. *Med J Aust, 2*, 125-8.

Catalano, P. J. & Levin, S. M. (1985). Noise-induced hearing loss and portable radios with headphones. *Int J Pediatr Otorhinolaryngol, 9*, 59-67.

Céranic, B. (2007). The value of otoacoustic emissions in the investigation of noise damage. *Audiological Medicine, 5*, 10-24.

Chung, J. H., Des Roches, C. M., Meunier, J. & Eavey, R. D. (2005). Evaluation of noise-induced hearing loss in young people using a web-based survey technique. *Pediatrics, 115*, 861-7.

Clark, W. W. (1991). Noise exposure from leisure activities: a review. *J Acoust Soc Am, 90*, 175-81.

Crandell, C., Mills, T. L. & Gauthier, R. (2004). Knowledge, behaviors, and attitudes about hearing loss and hearing protection among racial/ethnically diverse young adults. *J Natl Med Assoc, 96*, 176-86.

Daniel, E. (2007). Noise and hearing loss: a review. *J Sch Health, 77*, 225-31.

Davis, A. C., Lovell, E. A., Smith, P. A. & Ferguson, M. A. (1998). The contribution of social noise to tinnitus in young people - a preliminary report. *Noise Health, 1*, 40-6.

Desai, A., Reed, D., Cheyne, A., Richards, S. & Prasher, D. (1999). Absence of otoacoustic emissions in subjects with normal audiometric thresholds implies exposure to noise. *Noise Health, 1*, 58-65.

Dobie, R. A. (2008). The burdens of age-related and occupational noise-induced hearing loss in the United States. *Ear Hear, 29*, 565-77.

European Parliament and Council. (2003). Directive 2003-10-EC on the minimum health and safety requirements regarding the exposure of workers to the risks arising from physical agents (noise), 2003-10-EC.

Fearn, R. W. & Hanson, D. R. (1984). Hearing damage in young people using headphone to listen to pop music. *Journal of sound and vibration, 96*, 147-9.

Fligor, B. J. & Cox, L. C. (2004). Output levels of commercially available portable compact disc players and the potential risk to hearing. *Ear Hear, 25*, 513-27.

Florentine, M., Hunter, W., Robinson, M., Ballou, M. & Buus, S. (1998). On the behavioral characteristics of loud-music listening. *Ear Hear, 19*, 420-8.

Gissel, S., Mortensen, J. T. & Juul, S. (2002). Evaluation of hearing ability in Danish children at the time of school start and at the end of school. *Int J Adolesc Med Health*, *14*, 43-9.

Gorga, M. P., et al. (1997). From laboratory to clinic: a large scale study of distortion product otoacoustic emissions in ears with normal hearing and ears with hearing loss. *Ear Hear*, *18*, 440-55.

Hall, A. J. & Lutman, M. E. (1999). Methods for early identification of noise-induced hearing loss. *Audiology*, *38*, 277-80.

Hanson, D. R. & Fearn, R. W. (1975). Hearing acuity in young people exposed to pop music and other noise. *Lancet*, *2*, 203-5.

Hausler, R. (2004). [The effects of acoustic overstimulation]. *Ther Umsch*, *61*, 21-9.

Heinrich, U. & Feltens, R. (2006). Mechanisms underlying noise-induced hearing loss. *Drug Discovery Today: Disease Mechanisms*, *3*, 131-5.

Hellstrom, P. A. (1991). The effects on hearing from portable cassette players: a follow-up study. *Journal of sound and vibration*, *151*, 461-9.

Hellstrom, P. A., Axelsson, A. & Costa, O. (1998). Temporary threshold shift induced by music. *Scand Audiol Suppl*, *48*, 87-94.

Henderson, D., Bielefeld, E. C., Harris, K. C. & Hu, B. H. (2006). The role of oxidative stress in noise-induced hearing loss. *Ear Hear*, *27*, 1-19.

Henderson, D., Subramaniam, M. & Boettcher, F. A. (1993). Individual susceptibility to noise-induced hearing loss: an old topic revisited. *Ear Hear*, *14*, 152-68.

Hetu, R. & Fortin, M. (1995). Potential risk of hearing damage associated with exposure to highly amplified music. *J Am Acad Audiol*, *6*, 378-86.

Hodgetts, W. E., Rieger, J. M. & Szarko, R. A. (2007). The effects of listening environment and earphone style on preferred listening levels of normal hearing adults using an MP3 player. *Ear Hear*, *28*, 290-7.

Holmes, A. E., Niskar, A. S., Kieszak, S. M., Rubin, C. & Brody, D. J. (2004). Mean and median hearing thresholds among children 6 to 19 years of age: the Third National Health And Nutrition Examination Survey, 1988 to 1994, United States. *Ear Hear*, *25*, 397-402.

Hotz, M. A., Probst, R., Harris, F. P. & Hauser, R. (1993). Monitoring the effects of noise exposure using transiently evoked otoacoustic emissions. *Acta Otolaryngol*, *113*, 478-82.

Hu, B. H., Henderson, D. & Nicotera, T. M. (2002). Involvement of apoptosis in progression of cochlear lesion following exposure to intense noise. *Hear Res*, *166*, 62-71.

Ising, H. (1994). [Potential hearing loss caused by loud music. Current status of knowledge and need for management]. *HNO*, *42*, 465-6.

Ising, H., Babisch, W., Hanel, J., Kruppa, B. & Pilgramm, M. (1995). [Empirical studies of music listening habits of adolescents. Optimizing sound threshold limits for cassette players and discoteques]. *HNO*, *43*, 244-9.

Ising, H., Hanel, J., Pilgramm, M., Babisch, W. & Lindthammer, A. (1994). [Risk of hearing loss caused by listening to music with head phones]. *HNO*, *42*, 764-8.

Jokitulppo, J. & Bjork, E. (2002). Estimated leisure-time noise exposure and hearing symptoms in a finnish urban adult population. *Noise Health*, *5*, 53-62.

Jokitulppo, J. S., Bjork, E. A. & kaan-Penttila, E. (1997). Estimated leisure noise exposure and hearing symptoms in Finnish teenagers. *Scand Audiol*, *26*, 257-62.

Jokitulppo, J., Toivonen, M. & Bjork, E. (2006). Estimated leisure-time noise exposure, hearing thresholds, and hearing symptoms of Finnish conscripts. *Mil Med*, *171*, 112-6.

Keith, S. E., Michaud, D. S. & Chiu, V. (2008). Evaluating the maximum playback sound levels from portable digital audio players. *J Acoust Soc Am*, *123*, 4227-37.

Kemp, D. T. (1978). Stimulated acoustic emissions from within the human auditory system. *J Acoust Soc Am*, *64*, 1386-91.

Konopka, W., Zalewski, P. & Pietkiewicz, P. (2001). Evaluation of Transient and Distortion Product Otoacoustic Emissions before and after shooting practice. *Noise Health*, *3*, 29-37.

Kowalska, S. & Sulkowski, W. (1997). Measurements of click-evoked otoacoustic emission in industrial workers with noise-induced hearing loss. *Int J Occup Med Environ Health*, *10*, 441-59.

Lapsley-Miller, J.A., Marshall, L. & Heller, L.M. (2004). A longitudinal study of changes in evoked otoacoustic emissions and pure-tone thresholds as measured in a hearing conservation program. *Int J Audiol*, *43*, 307-22.

Le Prell, C. G., Yamashita, D., Minami, S. B., Yamasoba, T. & Miller, J. M. (2007). Mechanisms of noise-induced hearing loss indicate multiple methods of prevention. *Hear Res*, *226*, 22-43.

Lee, P. C., Senders, C. W., Gantz, B. J. & Otto, S. R. (1985). Transient sensorineural hearing loss after overuse of portable headphone cassette radios. *Otolaryngol Head Neck Surg*, *93*, 622-5.

Lees, R. E., Roberts, J. H. & Wald, Z. (1985). Noise induced hearing loss and leisure activities of young people: a pilot study. *Can J Public Health*, *76*, 171-3.

LePage, E. L. & Murray, N. M. (1998). Latent cochlear damage in personal stereo users: a study based on click-evoked otoacoustic emissions. *Med J Aust*, *169*, 588-92.

LePage, E. L. (1998). Occupational noise-induced hearing loss: origin, characterisation and prevention. *Acoustics Australia*, *26*, 57-61.

Liebel, J., Delb, W., Andes, C. & Koch, A. (1996). [Detection of hearing loss in patrons of a discoteque using TEOAE and DPOAE]. *Laryngorhinootologie*, *75*, 259-64.

Lindeman, H. E., van der Klaauw, M. M. & Platenburg-Gits, F. A. (1987). Hearing acuity in male adolescents (young adults) at the age of 17 to 23 years. *Audiology*, *26*, 65-78.

Lindgren, F. & Axelsson, A. (1983). Temporary threshold shift after exposure to noise and music of equal energy. *Ear Hear*, *4*, 197-201.

Lipscomb, D. M. (1972). The increase in prevalence of high frequency hearing impairment among college students. *Audiology*, *11*, 231-7.

Litke, R. E. (1971). Elevated high-frequency hearing in school children. *Arch Otolaryngol*, *94*, 255-7.

Loth, D., Avan, P., Menguy, C. & Teyssou, M. (1992). [Secondary auditory risks from listening to portable digital compact disc players]. *Bull Acad Natl Med*, *176*, 1245-52.

Lucertini, M., Moleti, A. & Sisto, R. (2002). On the detection of early cochlear damage by otoacoustic emission analysis. *J Acoust Soc Am*, *111*, 972-8.

Maassen, M., et al. (2001). Ear damage caused by leisure noise. *Noise Health*, *4*, 1-16.

MacLean, G. L., Stuart, A. & Stenstrom, R. (1992). Real ears sound pressure levels developed by three portable stereo system earphones. *Am J Audiol* 52-5.

Mansfield, J. D., Baghurst, P. A. & Newton, V. E. (1999). Otoacoustic emissions in 28 young adults exposed to amplified music. *Br J Audiol*, *33*, 211-22.

Meecham, E. A. & Hume, K. I. (2001). Tinnitus, attendance at night-clubs and social drug taking in students. *Noise Health*, *3*, 53-62.

Melnick, W. (1991). Human temporary threshold shift (TTS) and damage risk. *J Acoust Soc Am*, *90*, 147-54.

Mercier, V. & Hohmann, B. W. (2002). Is Electronically Amplified Music too Loud? What do Young People Think? *Noise Health*, *4*, 47-55.

Mercier, V., Luy, D. & Hohmann, B. W. (2003). The sound exposure of the audience at a music festival. *Noise Health*, *5*, 51-8.

Metternich, F. U. & Brusis, T. (1999). [Acute hearing loss and tinnitus caused by amplified recreational music]. *Laryngorhinootologie*, *78*, 614-9.

Meyer-Bisch, C. (1996). Epidemiological evaluation of hearing damage related to strongly amplified music (personal cassette players, discotheques, rock concerts)--high-definition audiometric survey on 1364 subjects. *Audiology*, *35*, 121-42.

Mills, J. H. & Going, J. A. (1982). Review of environmental factors affecting hearing. *Environ Health Perspect*, *44*, 119-27.

Montgomery, J. K. & Fujikawa, S. (1992). Hearing thresholds of students in the second, eighth, and twelfth grades. *Language, Speech, and Hearing Services in School*, *23*, 61-3.

Montoya, F. S., Ibarguen, A. M., Vences, A. R., del Rey, A. S. & Fernandez, J. M. (2008). Evaluation of cochlear function in normal-hearing young adults exposed to MP3 player noise by analyzing transient evoked otoacoustic emissions and distortion products. *J Otolaryngol Head Neck Surg*, *37*, 718-24.

Morata, T. C. (2007). Young people: their noise and music exposures and the risk of hearing loss. *Int J Audiol*, *46*, 111-2.

Mostafapour, S. P., Lahargoue, K. & Gates, G. A. (1998). Noise-induced hearing loss in young adults: the role of personal listening devices and other sources of leisure noise. *Laryngoscope*, *108*, 1832-9.

MRC Institute of Hearing Research (1986). Damage to hearing arising from leisure noise. *Br J Audiol*, *20*, 157-64.

Niskar, A. S., et al. (1998). Prevalence of hearing loss among children 6 to 19 years of age: the Third National Health and Nutrition Examination Survey. *JAMA*, *279*, 1071-5.

Niskar, A. S., et al. (2001). Estimated prevalence of noise-induced hearing threshold shifts among children 6 to 19 years of age: the Third National Health and Nutrition Examination Survey, 1988-1994, United States. *Pediatrics*, *108*, 40-3.

Nordmann, A. S., Bohne, B. A. & Harding, G. W. (2000). Histopathological differences between temporary and permanent threshold shift. *Hear Res*, *139*, 13-30.

Norton, S. J. (1992). Cochlear function and otoacoustic emissions. *Seminars in Hearing*, *13*, 1-14.

Occupational Safety and Health Administration. 1992. Occupational Noise Exposure, 1910-95.

Opperman, D. A., Reifman, W., Schlauch, R. & Levine, S. (2006). Incidence of spontaneous hearing threshold shifts during modern concert performances. *Otolaryngol Head Neck Surg*, *134*, 667-73.

Passchier-Vermeer, W. (1999). Pop music trough headphones and hearing loss. *Noise Control Eng J*, *47*, 182-6.

Peng, J. H., Tao, Z. Z. & Huang, Z. W. (2007). Risk of damage to hearing from personal listening devices in young adults. *J Otolaryngol*, *36*, 181-5.

Persson, B. O., Svedberg, A. & Gothe, C. J. (1993). Longitudinal changes in hearing ability among Swedish conscripts. *Scand Audiol*, *22*, 141-3.

Plath, P. (1998a). [Socio-acousis. Non-occupationally-induced hearing loss due to noise, 1]. *HNO, 46*, 887-92.

Plath, P. (1998b). [Sociacusis. Non-occupationally induced hearing damage by noise, 2]. *HNO, 46*, 947-52.

Plinkert, P. K., Hemmert, W. & Zenner, H. P. (1995). [Comparison of methods for early detection of noise vulnerability of the inner ear. Amplitude reduction of otoacoustic emissions are most sensitive at submaximal noise impulse exposure]. *HNO, 43*, 89-97.

Probst, R., Harris, F. P. & Hauser, R. (1993). Clinical monitoring using otoacoustic emissions. *Br J Audiol, 27*, 85-90.

Probst, R., Lonsbury-Martin, B. L. & Martin, G. K. (1991). A review of otoacoustic emissions. *J Acoust Soc Am, 89*, 2027-67.

Pugsley, S., Stuart, A., Kalinowski, J. & Armson, J. (1993). Changes in hearing sensitivity following portable stereo system use. *Am J Audiol, 2*, 64-7.

Rabinowitz, P. M., Slade, M. D., Galusha, D., xon-Ernst, C. & Cullen, M. R. (2006). Trends in the prevalence of hearing loss among young adults entering an industrial workforce 1985 to 2004. *Ear Hear, 27*, 369-75.

Rawool, V. W. & Colligon-Wayne, L. A. (2008). Auditory lifestyles and beliefs related to hearing loss among college students in the USA. *Noise Health, 10*, 1-10.

Rice, C. G., Rossi, G. & Olina, M. (1987a). Damage risk from personal cassette players. *Br J Audiol, 21*, 279-88.

Rice, C.G., Breslin, M. & Roper, R.G. (1987b). Sound levels from personal cassette players. *Br J Audiol, 21*, 273-278.

Schmuziger, N., Fostiropoulos, K. & Probst, R. (2006). Long-term assessment of auditory changes resulting from a single noise exposure associated with non-occupational activities. *Int J Audiol, 45*, 46-54.

Serra, M. R. et al (2005). Recreational noise exposure and its effects on the hearing of adolescents. Part I: an interdisciplinary long-term study. *Int J Audiol, 44*, 65-73.

Shah, S., Gopal, B., Reis, J. & Novak, M. (2009). Hear today, gone tomorrow: an assessment of portable entertainment player use and hearing acuity in a community sample. *J Am Board Fam Med, 22*, 17-23.

Sliwinska-Kowalska, M. & Jedlinska, U. (1998). Prolonged exposure to industrial noise: cochlear pathology does not correlate with the degree of permanent threshold shift, but is related to duration of exposure. *J Occup Health, 40*, 123-31.

Sliwinska-Kowalska, M. & Kotylo, P. (2008). Evaluation of individuals with known or suspected noise damage to hearing. *Audiological Medicine, 5*, 54.

Smith, P. A., Davis, A., Ferguson, M. & Lutman, M. E. (2000). The prevalence and type of social noise exposure in young adults in England. *Noise Health, 2*, 41-56.

Spaeth, J., Klimek, L., Doring, W. H., Rosendahl, A. & Mosges, R. (1993). [How badly does the "normal-hearing" young man of 1992 hear in the high frequency range?]. *HNO, 41*, 385-8.

Strauss, P., Quante, M., Strahl, M., Averhage, H. & Bitzer, M. (1977). [Is hearing of the students damaged by environmental noise in their leisure time?]. *Laryngol Rhinol Otol (Stuttg), 56*, 868-71.

Sutter, A. H. (1996). Current Standards for Occupational Exposure to Noise. In A. Axelsson et al. (Eds.), *Scientific Basis of Noise-Induced Hearing Loss* New York: Thieme Medical Publishers.

Swanson, S. J., Dengerink, H. A., Kondrick, P. & Miller, C. L. (1987). The influence of subjective factors on temporary threshold shifts after exposure to music and noise of equal energy. *Ear Hear, 8*, 288-91.

Talaska, A. E. & Schacht, J. (2007). Mechanisms of noise damage to the cochlea. *Audiological Medicine, 5*, 3-9.

Torre, P., III (2008). Young adults' use and output level settings of personal music systems. *Ear Hear, 29*, 791-9.

Turunen-Rise, I., Flottorp, G. & Tvete, O. (1991). Personal cassette players ('Walkman'). Do they cause noise-induced hearing loss? *Scand Audiol, 20*, 239-44.

Vogel, I., Brug, J., Hosli, E. J., van der Ploeg, C. P. & Raat, H. (2008). MP3 players and hearing loss: adolescents' perceptions of loud music and hearing conservation. *J Pediatr, 152*, 400-4.

Vogel, I., Brug, J., van der Ploeg, C. P. & Raat, H. (2007). Young people's exposure to loud music: a summary of the literature. *Am J Prev Med, 33*, 124-33.

Vogel, I., Brug, J., van der Ploeg, C. P. & Raat, H. (2009a). Prevention of adolescents' music-induced hearing loss due to discotheque attendance: a Delphi study. *Health Educ Res.*

Vogel, I., Brug, J., van der Ploeg, C. P. & Raat, H. (2009b). Strategies for the prevention of MP3-induced hearing loss among adolescents: expert opinions from a Delphi study. *Pediatrics, 123*, 1257-62.

Weichbold, V. & Zorowka, P. (2002). [Effect of information about hearing damage caused by loud music. For adolescents the music in discoteques is too loud despite loudness limits]. *HNO, 50*, 560-4.

Weichbold, V. & Zorowka, P. (2003). Effects of a hearing protection campaign on the discotheque attendance habits of high-school students. *Int J Audiol, 42*, 489-93.

Weichbold, V. & Zorowka, P. (2005). [Will adolescents visit discotheque less often if sound levels of music are decreased?]. *HNO, 53*, 845-1.

Weichbold, V. & Zorowka, P. (2007). Can a hearing education campaign for adolescents change their music listening behavior? *Int J Audiol, 46*, 128-33.

West, P. D. & Evans, E. F. (1990). Early detection of hearing damage in young listeners resulting from exposure to amplified music. *Br J Audiol, 24*, 89-103.

Widen, S. E. & Erlandsson, S. I. (2004). Self-reported tinnitus and noise sensitivity among adolescents in Sweden. *Noise Health, 7*, 29-40.

Widen, S. E., Holmes, A. E. & Erlandsson, S. I. (2006). Reported hearing protection use in young adults from Sweden and the USA: effects of attitude and gender. *Int J Audiol, 45*, 273-80.

Williams, W. (2005). Noise exposure levels from personal stereo use. *Int J Audiol, 44*, 231-6.

Wong, T. W., Van Hasselt, C. A., Tang, L. S. & Yiu, P. C. (1990). The use of personal cassette players among youths and its effects on hearing. *Public Health, 104*, 327-30.

World Health Organization. 1997. Prevention of noise-induced hearing loss: report of an informal consultation held at the World Health Organization, Geneva, on 28-30 October 1997.

Yassi, A., Pollock, N., Tran, N. & Cheang, M. (1993). Risks to hearing from a rock concert. *Can Fam Physician, 39*, 1045-50.

Zenner, H. P., et al. (1999). [Hearing loss caused by leisure noise]. *HNO, 47*, 236-48.

Zogby, J. (2006). Survey of teens and adults about the use of personal elctronic devices and head phones. *Am Speech Lang Hear Assoc.*

In: Deafness, Hearing Loss and the Auditory System
Editors: D. Fiedler and R. Krause, pp.111-135

ISBN: 978-1-60741-259-5
©2010 Nova Science Publishers, Inc.

*Chapter 3*

# CURRENT CONCEPTS IN RADIATION-INDUCED SENSORI-NEURAL HEARING LOSS

## *Wong-Kein Low*

Department of Otolaryngology, Singapore General Hospital, Singapore 169608

## ABSTRACT

Sensori-neural hearing loss is a frequent complication of radiotherapy of head and neck tumours, when the auditory pathways have been included in the radiation field. This chapter focuses on the review of three aspects of radiation-induced SNHL that have a significant impact on modern day medicine: 1) effect of radiation on retro-cochlear nervous pathways, 2) cellular and molecular processes involved in radiation-induced ototoxicity, 3) combined ototoxic effects of radiation and cisplatin. A model of radiation-induced damage of the sensor-neural auditory system has been proposed, which is based on the concept of dose-dependent, reactive oxygen species related cochlear cell apoptosis without significant damage to the retro-cochlear pathway. This model supports the feasibility of cochlear implantation, should one be clinically indicated in such patients. It can explain clinical observations such as radiation-induced sensori-neural hearing loss being dose-dependent and affects the high frequencies more than the lower frequencies. It also opens up the possibility of preventive strategies targeted at different stages of the apoptotic process. The use of anti-oxidants which target upstream pathways, appear promising. In particular, it may have a major role in chemo-radiation where combined ototoxic effects lead to significant sensori-neural hearing loss.

## I. INTRODUCTION

Radiation-induced sensori-neural hearing loss (SNHL) has long been recognized as a complication of radiotherapy (RT) for head and neck tumours, when the auditory pathways had been included in the radiation fields. It is believed that radiation therapy has been a much larger etiologic factor of hearing loss than suspected and should clearly be recognized as a major factor in the etiology of adult hearing disorders [1,2,3]. In recent years, improved radiotherapy techniques can potentially reduce unnecessary radiation exposure to ear structures. Nevertheless, radiation-induced SNHL remains an important cause of hearing loss clinically, especially in chemo-radiation [4].

In the past, SNHL resulting from radiotherapy which involved inner ear structures was deemed inevitable and conventional hearing aids were prescribed to improve hearing when necesary. With recent advancements in medical science and technology, modern hearing devices and preventive measures based on molecular and cellular processes have become available. Nowadays, there is a need to better understand the effects of radiation on the auditory system in order to effectively manage radiation-induced SNHL. Seemingly irrelevant questions in the past have become important today. This chapter focuses on the review of three aspects of radiation-induced SNHL which have a significant impact on modern day medicine:

1. Effect of radiation on retro-cochlear nervous pathways. Cochlear implants are widely used nowadays and are indicated for patients with severe to profound hearing loss due to cochlear damage. In cochlear implantation, a pre-requisite for a successful outcome is intactness of the retro-cochlear pathways. It is, therefore, important to ascertain if radiotherapy damages the retro-cochlear pathways.
2. The cellular and molecular processes involved in radiation-induced ototoxicity. It becomes necessary to understand these processes as they can potentially be targeted by medical intervention strategies that are available today.
3. The combined ototoxic effects of radiation and cisplatin (CDDP). Chemo-radiotherapy using CDDP is increasingly being used to treat advanced head and neck cancers, and the extent of inner ear damage by combined therapy should be appreciated [5].

## II. CHARACTERISTICS OF RADIATION-INDUCED SNHL

### Existence of Radiation-Induced SNHL

*Animal studies*

The effects of radiation on the inner ear was documented as early as 1905, when Ewald placed radium beads in the middle ear of pigeons and noted labyrinthine symptoms [6]. In 1933, Girden & Culler were first to report the effects of radiation on hearing [7]. Experimenting on dogs subjected to various X-ray doses, a hearing impairment averaging 5.5 dB was recorded. Novotny (1951) studied the ionizing effects of radiation in guinea pigs and found a hearing impairment of about 8.4dB at 4000 Hz [8]. Kozlov (1959) also noted a hearing imparment of 3.9–9.1dB over 500–8000 Hz in guinea pigs [9]. Gamble et al. (1968) subjected the ears of 50 guinea pigs to 500–6000 rads of radiation and found decreased sensitivity of cochlear microphonics of 20–40dB, particularly in the high frequencies [10]. This was consistent with microscopic findings which demonstrated damage to the Organ of Corti and cochlear duct in rats, after doses of 100–3000 rads [11]. Tokimoto & Kanagawa (1985) in their study on guinea pigs concluded that even in the absence of gross anatomical cochlear changes, post-irradiation functional hair cell defects could exist [12].

Histologically, Keleman (1963) studied temporal bones in rats which had received 100–3000 rads of radiation [11]. Haemorrhage was noted to be the most prominent finding with destruction of the cochlear duct, organ of corti and its surrounding elements. Early changes of the stria vascularis accompanied by significant inflammatory responses, were found in the inner ears of guinea pigs that had received 6000 rads of radiation [10].

### *Human studies*

Several clinical studies have recorded SNHL in patients who have had RT for head and neck malignancies, where inner ear structures were included in the radiation fields. Leach (1965) observed SNHL in some of the 56 patients who had received 3000–12000 rads of RT for different head and neck cancers [13]. Morretti (1976) retrospectively studied 137 post-irradiated patients with nasopharyngeal carcinoma (NPC), and found 7 to have SNHL of at least 10dB [14].

There had also been suggestions that radiation did not result in significant SNHL [15]. After a systematic review of the literature, it was concluded that the conflicting results from the various studies were attributable to variations in patient groups, size, study design, follow-up period, radiotherapy techniques and presentation of audiometric results [16]. From the pooled data generated from this systematic review, it was found that about one-third of patients who had received 70 Gy in 2 Gy per fraction near the inner ear, developed hearing loss of at least 10dB at 4 kHz.

Schnecht & Karmody (1966) reported the histological features of a deafened man who had received 5,220 rads of radiation to the region of the ears several years ago [17]. Degeneration of the Organ of Corti was noted, with atrophy of the basilar membrane, spiral ligament and stria vascularis. Progressive hearing loss across the various frequencies had been attributed to obliterating endarteritis and eventual fibrosis, leading to vascular compromise [14].

## Prevalence and Epidemiology

It had been difficult to establish the exact prevalence of radiation-induced hearing loss because statistics relating to ototoxicity were often not well kept or easily interpreted [2]. Not only was hearing not often considered important in the face of life-threatening diseases, hearing losses were frequently not recorded in those who did not survive. Clinical studies had reported varying prevalence, depending on factors such as dose, period of follow-up and definition/criteria used for hearing loss [16]. In NPC where the radiation dose received by the ear is relatively high, the incidence of post-RT SNHL had been reported to be as high as 24% [18].

In SNHL after RT in NPC patients, sex and age were found to be independent prognostic factors [18]. Males were noted to be more susceptible than females in developing SNHL after radiation. Older patients were at greater risk, as pre-existing degenerative changes could have made them more vulnerable to radiation injury [19]. Post-RT middle ear effusion was identified to be another predicting factor, as toxic materials from chronic inflammation could affect the inner ear [20]. However, it is argued that the development of post-RT middle ear effusion could have been just another manifestation of radiation damage related to individual variation in susceptibility to radiation [18].

## Effect of Radiation Dose

Gamble et al. (1968) found in guinea pigs that the extent of inner ear injury correlated with the radiation dose applied [10]. Bohne et al. (1985) confirmed in chinchillas that the higher the radiation dose received, the greater the damage to the inner ear [21]. A systematic review on human studies reported increasing loss with increasing dose, starting at about 40 Gy applied in 2 Gy per fraction [16]. Guidelines for tolerance doses in normal tissues are being used in clinical practice [22].

It is noteworthy that early human studies had reported the effects of very high doses of radiation to the ears, doses that are no longer used in clinical practice today [23,24]. Although these could have potentially provided rare opportunities to study the effect of excessively high doses of radiation on the inner ear in humans, documentation of the audiometric data was so poor that it was impossible to draw conclusions on the relationship between high radiation dose and SNHL.

## High Frequency Hearing Loss

High frequency hearing levels were affected more than those in the lower frequencies after irradiation [16,25]. This corresponded to histological observations made in animals that the basal part of the cochlea (which respond to higher frequency sounds) was usually more damaged by radiation than the apical part. Keleman (1963) demonstrated in rats that the apical turn of the cochlea was least affected by radiation doses of 100-3000 rads [11]. Winther (1970) similarly reported in guinea pigs that post-irradiated apical hair cells remained intact while the outer hair cells of the 2 basal turns were affected [26]. Early threshold shifts at high stimulus frequencies are indicators of probable subsequent shifts to low frequencies [27].

## Early vs. Late Onset

Traditionally, radiation-induced SNHL is regarded to have either early or late onsets [25]. In early-onset SNHL, hair cell damage in guinea pigs occurred as early as 6 hrs. following radiation of 4,000–7,000 rads [26]. Tokimoto & Kanagawa (1985) demonstrated in guinea pigs that sensori-neural loss appeared 3–10 hrs depending on dose administered, and outer hair cells in the basal turn of the cochlea were destroyed about 6 hrs after radiation [12]. In humans, SNHL often occurred near the end or shortly after the completion of fractionated RT [28]. Early-onset SNHL due to inflammatory causes or transient functional disturbances in the stria vascularis, may recover with time (18,28].

In late-onset hearing loss, Schuknecht & Karmordy (1966) observed marked atrophy of the cochlear stria vascularis in a patient who had developed hearing loss 8 years after radiotherapy (5200 rads) for carcinoma of the ear [17]. Grau et al. (1991) studied 22 NPC patients with well-documented pre- and post-RT hearing levels over 7-84 months, and found SNHL (especially the higher frequencies) developing 12 months post-RT [29]. Merchant et al. (2004) were of the opinion that radiation-induced SNHL could only occur 4 years after irradiation [30]. Delayed-onset hearing loss was found to correlate with age, pre-existing

SNHL and radiation dosage [31]. Late-onset radiation-induced SNHL had generally been attributed to progressive vascular compromise from radiation-induced vasculitis obliterans [14].

However, after a review of the relevant literature, Sataloff et al. (1994) were not convinced that late-onset hearing loss existed at all [32]. They argued that although significant hearing losses over the whole spectrum of the speech range were often seen several years after radiation, there was little or no convincing evidence to support the notion that hearing loss developing several years following radiation was causally related to radiation therapy itself. Nevertheless, the existence of early-onset radiation-induced SNHL and its progressive course had been well documented [19,33]. SNHL observed in patients years after radiotherapy may well be a result of the progressive nature of radiation-induced inner ear damage, rather than from an event which only begins after a long post-irradiation period.

## III. EFFECT OF RADIATION ON RETRO-COCHLEAR PATHWAYS

Modern RT for head and neck tumours can potentially induce SNHL, as the cochlea and parts of the auditory neural pathways are often included in the radiation fields. Kwong et al. (1996) reported sensori-neural hearing loss in NPC patients after RT, but did not differentiate between sensory or neural deafness [18]. Radiation-induced SNHL is generally believed to be a result of cochlear damage [32]. However, it cannot be assumed that retro-cochlear deafness does not occur, whether alone or in combination with cochlear deafness. The intactness of retro-cochlear auditory pathways is essential, if cochlear implantation were to be considered for restoration and rehabilitation of hearing loss in such patients.

### The Sensori-Neural Auditory Pathways

According to Hackney (1987), the hair cells of the Organ of Corti transduce vibrations within the cochlea into neural signals [34]. Outer hair cells are contractile and may contribute to mechanical feedback processes, whilst the inner hair cells are apparently the primary sensory cells being innervated by the majority of the afferent fibres. These run in the cochlear nerve to the brain stem where they bifurcate, projecting cochleotopically to the dorsal and ventral cochlear nuclei. A divergence continued in the main routes taken by the ascending pathways; one runs bilaterally from the ventral cochlear nucleus to the superior olivary complex and then to the inferior colliculi, the other runs from the dorsal cochlear nucleus to the contralateral inferior colliculus. Fibres from the brainstem nuclei travelling to each inferior colliculus form a tract, the lateral lemniscus, and may make contact with one of the nuclei within it. The pathway continues to the medial geniculate bodies and on to the auditory cortex, preserving its cochleotopicity at all levels. A descending system parallels the ascending system throughout. The presence of commissural and decussating connections from the level of the brainstem onwards, provides the anatomical basis for the analysis of binaural information. The division of the pathway forms the anatomical substrate for the parallel processing of different features of the auditory environment.

## Mechanisms of Damage to the Nervous System

Awwad (1990) gave an account on radiation damage to the 3 main cell categories found in the central nervous system namely neurons, vascular endothelial cells and glial cells [35]. Glial cells have a slow turn-over rate with a small precursor (stem-cell) compartment (1%). Endothelial cells also have a slow turn-over rate but proliferate rapidly after injury. Neurons are non-proliferating end-cells in the adult organism. Myelination of the nerve axons is accomplished by the oligodendrocytes in the central nervous system and by Schwann cells in the peripheral nerves. The following 4 types of damage can be demonstrated in the rat spinal cord:

(a) Transient demyelination is mediated by damage to the oligodendrocytes. In man, transient myelopathy has a relatively short latent period of 3 months and is reversible within 3 months. The main manifestations are paraesthesia and an electric shock-like pain, which are common after irradiation to cervical spine

(b) White matter necrosis has a latency period of about 3-6 months and requires doses >20Gy. It is mediated by oligodendrocyte damage interacting with vascular injury. This probably is responsible for early myelopathy found in humans

(c) Vascular damage has a latency period of >7 months and requires relatively lower doses (<20Gy). This type of injury probably causes progressive myelopathy in man

(d) Spinal nerve root necrosis is caused by damage to the Schwann cells and results in radiculopathy. For example, irradiation to the cauda equina results in flaccid paralysis and muscle atrophy. However, there are no sensory manifestations indicating that in man, the ventral roots are selectively damage

## Cerebral and Brainstem Damage

Temporal lobe necrosis after RT for NPC occurs. It can easily be missed as only one third of these patients present with classical epilepsy and the latent period could range from 1.5 to 13 years (median five years) [36]. Temporal lobe necrosis can result in cognitive dysfunction, epilepsy and theoretically, central hearing dysfunction. However, because of bilateral innervation to the auditory cortex, unilateral cortical damage does not normally cause significant hearing problems.

Brainstem necrosis after RT for NPC is notorious because damage to the cochlear ganglia and other neuronal cells can result in neural deafness and other even more serious neurological complications [37,38]. Grau et al. (1991) concluded that the deleterious effects of irradiation on hearing should be kept in mind in both treatment planning and post-RT follow-up, based on their prospective study of 22 patients evaluated prior to and 7-84 months after radiotherapy for NPC [29]. They found that auditory brainstem evoked responses in 4 patients were severely abnormal and 2 had clinical signs of brainstem dysfunction. Grau et al. (1992) had shown by dose response analysis, a correlation between total radiation doses received by the brainstem and the incidence of pathologic brainstem evoked response audiometry (BERA) [38]. Patients who had received RT doses of 59Gy or less to the brainstem had normal BERA, whereas 4 of 6 patients who had received a dose of 68 Gy manifested brainstem dysfunction. Fortunately, the risk of this major complication has been minimized by the routine use of effective shielding techniques in modern radiotherapy regimes [39].

## Spiral Ganglia and Cochlear Nerve Damage

There have only been limited studies on the spiral ganglia and auditory nerve after radiation. Although the brainstem is well shielded during RT, the retro-cochlear auditory pathways at the level of the spiral ganglia and cochlear nerve remain at risk as these structures are not effectively shielded during treatment. In addition to the direct damage of these structuies, secondary changes could also result from hair cell loss.

Namura et al. (1997) demonstrated in rabbits, loss of ganglion cell bodies and cochlear ganglia after more than 40 Gy of gamma radiation [40]. On the other hand, Keleman (1963) did not observe any effect on the cochlear nerve fibres after single doses of photon radiation less than 20 Gy [11]. As the effects of radiation on nervous tissues could be related to dose, Bohne et al. (1985) studied the effects of ionising radiation on the ear by exposing chincillas to 40 to 90 Gy of radiation, fractionated at 2 Gy per day [21]. The animals were sacrificed two years after completion of treatment and the temporal bones were studied microscopically. Dose dependent degeneration of sensory and supporting cells as well as loss of 8th nerve fibres in the Organ of Corti, were observed. In ears exposed to 40-50Gy of radiation, the incidence of nerve fibre damage was 31%; whereas in ears exposed to 60-90Gy, the incidence was 62%. The strength of this paper laid in the use of fractionated doses (which resembled clinical practice) and the relatively long post-treatment follow-up. However, because hearing tests were not performed in the study, it could not be ascertained if hearing ability correlated with the degree of 8th nerve fibre damage. It is pointed out that in an experiment on guinea pigs using auditory brainstem responses to measure hearing thresholds before and after applying radiation ranging from 57.5 to 70Gy, no threshold changes were observed even up to 12 months post-RT [41].

## Necropsy Studies

In a necropsy study on a patient who had hearing loss and previous radiotherapy for NPC, preservation of Organ of Corti and degeneration of auditory nerve were observed [42]. However, because tumour invasion and infection of the auditory nerve were also present, it was not possible to substantiate the cause of auditory nerve degeneration. Leach (1965) reported a patient with NPC who had received 40Gy of radiation [13]. He became progressively deaf and died 1 year later. The pathology report noted spiral ganglion and nerve atrophy.

## Clinical Studies

Anteunis et al. (1994) studied 18 patients who had received RT for parotid tumours at daily doses of 2.0 to 2.5 Gy, to a total dose of 50 Gy [43]. For malignancies, an additional booster dose to a total of 60-70 Gy was given. Although post-RT BERA at 2 years showed significant inter-aural I-V latency difference in 3 patients (2 of whom were sub-clinical), pre-RT data was not available.

There had been 2 clinical studies on the effect of RT on retro-cochlear pathways in NPC patients, but each had a follow-up period of only up to 1 year. Lau et al. (1992) prospectively studied 49 patients, and found a statistical difference between pre- and post-RT I-III intervals which suggested retro-cochlear auditory damage [37]. However, retro-cochlear damage was not observed in a similar study conducted by Leighton et al. (1997) [39]. The conflicting result was attributed to the difference in techniques used during RT as in the later, special efforts were made to confine radiation to anterior surface of the pons and medulla. The ability of the retro-cochlear pathways to remain intact after irradiation is supported by case reports. Coplan et al. (1981) described a 12 year-old girl who had received 5,000 rads of radiation for optic glioma [44]. She developed SNHL 2 years after radiotherapy and no audiologic signs of retro-cochlear damage were observed. Talmi et al. (1988) reported SNHL in a 35 year-old woman who had received a high total radiation dose of 23,900 rads for facial hemangioma [24]. Again, there was no evidence of retro-cochlear damage with 90% speech discrimination, normal BERA and stapedial reflex.

## Gamma Radiosurgery for Acoustic Neuroma

Gamma knife stereotactic radiosurgery has become a popular modality of treatment for acoustic neuroma [45]. As hearing preservation is often an important consideration in the management of acoustic neuroma, what is known about the effects of radiation on the cochlear nerve is of great clinical relevance to such patients [46,47]. Hirsch & Noren (1988) reported 64 patients with acoustic neuroma which were treated with stereotactic radiosurgery with doses ranging from 1,800 to 5,000 rads [48]. In these patients, 54% had pronounced deterioration of thresholds and/or speech discrimination; BERA was abnormal in all but one ear. In a more recent report by Bush et al. (2008), patients who received gamma knife treatment with dose ranging from 12.5-16 Gy (mean 13.8 Gy) were studied [49]. Of those patients with useful audition pre-treatment, 42% maintained useful hearing post-treatment after a mean follow-up of 33.6 months. However, because the post-irradiation hearing results are often confounded by the tumour effect on the cochlear nerve, acoustic neuroma is not a suitable clinical model to study the effects of radiation on the retro-cochlear auditory pathways [50].

## Long-term Effects of Radiotherapy on Retro-Cochlear Pathways in NPC Patients

It can be seen that earlier literature gave conflicting views on the effect of radiotherapy on the retro-cochlear pathways. It is pointed out that many of the clinical studies were retrospective and were based on small numbers of patients with short periods of follow-up. A longer period of follow-up is necessary as any hearing loss associated with irradiation may be gradual in development and slow in onset and irradiation damage to the nervous tissue is delayed in manifestation [2,18]. We therefore, embarked on a prospective study on the long-term effects beyond 1 year after irradiation in NPC patients [51]. NPC has provided a good clinical model to study the effects of radiation on the auditory pathways. In NPC, relatively high doses of radiation are used in standard treatment regimes where significant doses in relatively narrow dose ranges are delivered to specific ear structures. Although this could limit the ability to study the effect of dose on hearing, useful correlations could be made between specific dose ranges and any observed changes in hearing.

In this study, 27 newly diagnosed NPC patients who were treated by RT alone were prospectively studied. Evoked response audiometry was carried out prior, during and at 3, 18 and 48 months after RT. Waves 1-5, 1-3 and 3-5 latencies were measured. The study showed no statistically significant difference in 1-5, 1-3 and 3-5 inter-wave latencies recorded during RT and post-RT, as compared to those recorded before RT (p >0.05). Similarly, a subset of 16 ears which recorded post-RT hearing deterioration, also did not have statistically significant difference (p=0.366) between the pre- and post-RT wave 1-5 latencies. This suggested that although the radiation delivered to the auditory system had damaged the cochlea, the retro-cochlear pathway was spared. The study suggested that in patients who have had radiotherapy for nasopharyngeal carcinoma, the retro-cochlear auditory pathways are functionally intact even in the longer term.

In the same study, the mean radiation doses delivered to the cochlea and internal auditory meatus ranged from 24.1-62.2 Gy and 14.4 – 43.4 Gy respectively. Based on the actual doses applied to the auditory pathways, more meaningful correlations between radiation dose and retro-cochlear damage in humans could be derived. Most clinical studies on radiation-induced SNHL reported only the total dosage received by the patients for tumours in the head and neck region, and assumed that the ear structures received the full dosage prescribed. This is not necessarily the case because specific ear structures may not have received the full radiation dose but a gradation in dosage.

## Feasiblity of Cochlear Implantation in Irradiated Ears

The finding that retro-cochlear pathways remained functionally intact after irradiation suggested that cochlear implantation could be a viable option for hearing restoration should one be clinically indicated in these patients.

To further substantiate that the retro-cochlear auditory pathways remained functionally intact after RT, a case-control study of cochlear implant recipients who had prior irradiation for NPC was conducted in our clinic [52]. They received their RT 11-28 years prior to cochlear implantation and the post-implant follow-up period ranged from 9 to 46 months. The implanted ear of each patient had favourable pre-operative promontory stimulation results. Post-implant, all patients were satisfied with their hearing outcomes and the improvement in speech discrimination scores was comparable to the controls.

## IV. CELLULAR AND MOLECULAR BASIS OF OTOTOXICITY

The above review therefore suggests that radiation-induced SNHL in doses used clinically, is mainly an intra-cochlear event. The cellular and molecular processes involved in ototoxicity from non-radiation causes such as from CDDP, aminoglycoside and acoustic trauma had been well described. Protecting hair cells from irreversible degradation has been a primary objective because of the finite number of hair cells in the inner ear. Hair cells stop differentiating during development and are post-mitotic in nature so that the number of cells one is born with (about 16,000) is a life-time supply [53].

## Non-Radiation Causes of Ototoxicity

Given the similarities in audiometric changes and cochlear pathology from different causes of hearing loss like noise, ototoxic drugs and aging, there may be a common factor underlying these seemingly different etiologies [54]. The cellular and molecular mechanisms leading to hearing loss appear to be similar and a final common pathway may hinge upon apoptosis [53,55].

According to Miller & Marx (1998), apoptosis is a highly regulated active form of programmed cell death which allows a cell to self-degrade in order for the body to eliminate unwanted or dysfunctional cells [56]. Apoptosis can be triggered in a cell through either the extrinsic pathway or the intrinsic pathways [57]. The extrinsic pathway is initiated through the stimulation of the transmembrane death receptors, such as the Fas receptors, located on the cell membrane. In contrast, the intrinsic pathway is initiated through the release of signal factors by mitochondria within the cell. The Bcl-2 family of proteins and the caspase cascade had been found to be important in effecting downstream pathwauys. The apoptotic processes are modulated by the p53 tumor suppressing gene.

Over the past decade, a growing body of evidence suggests the importance of ROS as a possible mechanism leading to sensori-neural hearing loss [55]. There is compelling evidence implicating reactive oxygen species (ROS) in damage associated with cochlear ischemia, noise trauma, presbycusis, meningitis-associated hearing loss and aminoglycoide and CDDP ototoxicity [58].

It is well established that ROS are generated in hair cells exposed to CDDP, aminoglycosides and noise [55]. Studies have reported that enhancing antioxidant levels through drug application or genetic manipulation, promotes hair cell survival and preserve function [59]. Hair cell death is potentiated when knockout mice lacking the enzymes responsible for maintaining antioxidant homeostasis are exposed to loud noise [60]. Although the relationship between ROS and other cell death events is not fully understood, recent studies have shown that mitochondria-associated oxidants are involved in processes which regulate cytochrome c translocation and caspase activation in the central nervous system [61].

## Radiation-Induced Ototoxicity

Although CDDP and gentamicin have been shown to induce cochlear cell apoptosis the cellular and molecular processes resulting from radiation-induced ototoxicity was still unclear. We therefore, embarked on a study aimed at investigating the biophysical changes of dose-related gamma radiation-induced cochlear cell apoptosis in the OC-k3 cochlear cell line [62]. Using flow cytometry and TUNEL assay, radiation-induced apoptosis was found to be dose-dependant with a greater degree of apoptosis resulting after 20 Gy than 5 Gy. Apoptosis occurred predominantly at 72 hrs post-irradiation and microarray analysis showed associated dose-dependant apoptotic gene regulation changes (Figure 1). Western blotting revealed phosphorylation occurring at 3, 24, 48 and 72 hrs post-irradiation and p53 up-regulation at 72 hrs. Although early activation of c-jun occurred at 3 hrs, it was not sustained with time. Associated dose-dependant intracellular generation of ROS was also demonstrated (Figure 2). The study demonstrated for the first time, a dose-dependant radiation-induced cochlear cell apoptosis which was associated with ROS generation and with p53 possibly playing an important role. A model of radiation-induced SNHL based on ROS and p53 dependant cochlear hair cell apoptosis, was therefore proposed.

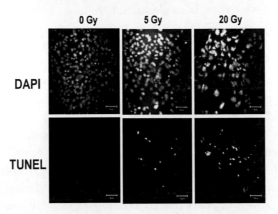

Figure 1. **TUNEL assay confirms irradiation-induced apoptosis in OC-k3 cells at 72 hrs and is dose related.** The cells were counterstained with DAPI, a nuclear-specific dye. More TUNEL positive nuclei were demonstrated at 72 hrs after 20 than 5 Gy of irradiation. The bar scale represents 50 micron. The results are representative of 3 separate experiments. Source: Low et al. [62], reproduced with kind permission of Springer and Business Media.

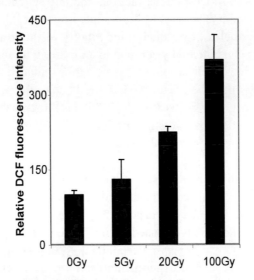

Figure 2. **Radiation-induced generation of ROS is dose related.** Intracellular generation of ROS in OC-k3 cells was detected 1 hr after treatment with different doses of radiation. The value for each dose was calculated as a relative intensity of DCF fluorescence compared to 0Gy, which was set at 100. Each value represents the mean ± SD of 3 separate experiments. Significantly more intracellular ROS were generated by higher doses of radiation (p<0.0001, one-way ANOVA). Source: Low et al. [62], reproduced with kind permission of Springer and Business Media.

## An Apoptotic Model in Radiation-Induced SNHL

It is known that many other different etiologies of SNHL (such as ageing and drug toxicity) share similar cell death mechanisms where a final common pathway is apoptosis [53]. Dose-dependant radiation-induced apoptosis has already been well described in non-cochlear cell systems and is generally accepted as an important mechanism of cell death *in vivo* [63]. Hence, by relating our findings to what is already known, it is not unreasonable to expect radiation-induced cochlear hair cell apoptosis also occurring in an *in vivo* situation.

Radiation-induced SNHL has been described to have either early or late-onset [25]. Radiation-induced early-onset SNHL occur within hours or days after completion of treatment whereas late-onset radiation-induced SNHL may manifest months or years after exposure. As radiation was demonstrated to have resulted in cochlear cell apoptosis as early as 72 hrs after exposure, it is concievable that early-onset SNHL is the result of radiation-induced cochlear cell apoptosis [62]. The possibility of the same mechanism being applied in late-onset SNHL should be further appraised.

In a review paper, Sataloff & Rosen (1994) were not convinced that radiation-induced late-onset SNHL existed at all [32]. They argued that although significant hearing losses over the whole spectrum of the speech range were often seen several years after radiation, there was little or no convincing evidence to support the notion that hearing loss developing several years following radiation was causally related to radiation therapy itself. Late-onset radiation-induced SNHL had generally been attributed to progressive vascular compromise from radiation-induced vasculitis obliterans [14]. It is interesting that radiation-induced SNHL has no correlation with vestibular dysfunction although in a minute structure like the inner ear, both hearing and vestibular functions is expected to be affected by significant radiation-induced vascular changes [64]. Despite the fact that the late sequelae of radiation have often been ascribed to vascular injury, Withers (1992) pointed out that it has not been supported by hard evidence [65]. Nevertheless, by reducing the vitality of the irradiated tissues, radiation-induced vascular changes can potentially compound an injury without being the cause.

On the other hand, it is well accepted.that radiation-induced SNHL is progressive in nature. Wang et al. (2003) observed that SNHL started soon after RT and progressed during long-term follow-up [19]. Grau & Overgaard (1996) also found that the radiation-induced SNHL occurred in the early post-radiation period and progressed [33]. The majority of patients reached a plateau in severity by 2 years but a few progressed to severe hearing loss [5].

It is well known that radiation can result in late biological effects [66]. In animal studies, it was observed that radiation-induced cell death could possibly occur 2 years after irradiation and beyond, even without vascular occlusion [21]. This may represent a late biological response to the initial cellular damage caused by irradiation. Bohne et al. (1985) were of the opinion that most of the microscopic vascular and supporting structural changes seen in the early post-radiation period in animal experiments do not exist in clinical practice. They felt that these changes were the result of radiation fields which were not uniform, used in large single doses or due to the short survival time of the animal. Indeed, by simulating radiation as used in clinical situations, they demonstrated histologically radiation-induced cochlear cell degeneration in animals in the absence of damage to the supporting structures and with the supplying blood vessels remaining patent even up to 2 years post-radiation. This implied that delayed hair cell death could have resulted from the initial direct ionic effects of radiation, causing SNHL. This is supported by the observation that delayed cochlear hair cells apoptosis could occur in noise-induced deafness [54].

Therefore, taken together, apoptotic cochlear hair cell death due to the ionic effects of radiation explains not only early-onset but possibly, also "late"-onset radiation-induced SNHL. The integrity of normal tissues or organs depends on the maintenance of a certain number of normally functioning mature cells. When the depletion of functioning cells reaches a critical level, a clinically detectable effect becomes apparent [35]. Therefore, people having limited hair-cell loss may be sub-clinical, whereas those with substantial hair cell loss experience SNHL. Pre-treatment SNHL has been found to be a risk factor for further sensori-neural hearing deterioration after chemo-radiation [67]. This could merely be a reflection of increased cochlear hair cell loss after treatment, in an organ, which consists of a finite number of post-mitotic non-regenerating hair cells. In radiation-induced SNHL, a patient experiences hearing loss when a critical mass of hair cells is lost and it may take several months or even years after radiation exposure, before this stage is finally reached. In a recent prospective study on patients who had radiotherapy for head and neck tumours, a number developed reduced DPOAE measurements 1 month after treatment [68]. These patients went on to develop SNHL 12 months post-radiation which again, may be a reflection of progressive cochlear hair cell loss. Hence, "late"-onset radiation-induced SNHL may well represent the later stages of the progression in hair cell degeneration initiated by direct cellular injury during irradiation. Alternatively, irradiated cells may have been rendered more susceptible to further ototoxic insults such as subsequent exposure to loud noise and ototoxic medications.

## The Role of p53

In CDDP-induced ototoxicity, DNA damage and ROS generation both activate p53, which plays a pivotal role in cochlear hair cell apoptosis [55]. In a study on HEI-OC1 cells derived from the cochlea, CDDP caused an increase in p53 at 3 hrs prior to the activation of Bax, cytochrome-c, caspase 8 and 9 [69]. In another CDDP-induced apoptosis experiment using cochlear organotypic cultures prepared from rats at postnatal day 3-4, significant up-regulation of phospho-p53 serine 15 expression was found and apoptosis was suppressed by the p53 inhibitor pifithrin-α [70]. Therefore, taken together, p53 is likely to play a role in radiation-induced cochlear hair-cell apoptosis.

It is well established that p53 plays a key role in the cellular response to nuclear DNA damage [71]. It regulates cell cycle arrest and dictates cell fate like senescence, apoptosis and DNA repair. It is believed that the nature of DNA damage enables p53 to selectively discriminate between promotors in the induction of target genes, thereby regulating their expression and subsequent cellular outcome [72]. Hence, radiation-induced p53 activation can cause a delay in cell cycle progression, predominantly at the G1-S transition, allowing the damaged DNA to be repaired before replication and mitosis occur [73]. However, if repair fails, p53 may trigger the destruction of cells through apoptosis. It has been been shown that p53 induces apoptosis through a transciption-dependent or independent mechanism [74,75]. It regulates proapoptotic genes functions in the nucleus whereas cytoplasmic p53 directly activates proapoptotic Bcl-2 proteins to permeabilise mitochondria and initiate apoptosis; PUMA couples this nuclear and cytoplasmic proapoptotic function of p53 [76]. The significance of p53 in radiation-induced apoptosis remains complex and depends on the existence of other pathways of cell cycle control and response to injury. Several genes that are specifically induced by p53 were discovered to play a potential role in mediating its effects on cell death including Bcl-2 family members like Bax [77].

## The Role of ROS

There has also been compelling evidence in animal models, implicating ROS in the damage associated with cochlear ischemia, noise trauma, presbycusis, meningitis-associated hearing loss and aminoglycoside and CDDP ototoxicity [58]. Although the exact relationship between ROS and other cell death events is still not fully understood, ROS is believed to play a key role in the promotion of apoptosis by affecting mitochondrial permeability, release of cytochrome c and activation of p53 and caspases [55,69]. Moreover, it is increasingly recognized that apoptosis plays an important role in radiation-induced cell death [78]. In the OC-k3 inner ear cell line, dose-dependant intracellular generation of ROS was demonstrated [62]. This suggested that ROS could be an important triggering factor in the apoptotic process

The role of ROS in radiation-induced SNHL could explain the observation that high frequency hearing is preferentially damaged by radiation [57]. In an animal study on aminoglycoside ototoxicity, outer hair- cell death in the Organ of Corti were observed to follow a base-to-apex gradient, which was eliminated by the addition of antioxidants [79]. This was attributed to the outer hair cells in the basal coil (respond to higher frequency sounds) having much lower levels of glutathione than those in the apical region (respond to lower frequency sounds) and therefore, a lower anti-oxidant capacity [57].

## Protection against Radiation-Induced Cochlear Cell Apoptosis

An apoptotic model of radiation-induced SNHL offers the potential of using agents to manipulate the apoptotic balance in cochlear cells in favour of cell survival. A prerequisite for the successful use of anti-apoptotic treatment is that is must be safe and must not interfere with the efficacy of the treatment. Treatment of the inner ear is especially feasible because the delivery of these medications to the inner ear transtympanically would decrease systemic side effects and be more target specific [58].

The use of anti-apoptotic factors is potentially an important intervention strategy for sensori-neural hearing loss, which can be directed at upstream or downstream signaling processes [57]. An upstream intervention such as the use of anti-oxidants, protect the cochlea from the processes that lead to apoptotic cell death and is likely to be more effective than downstream measures.

We investigated the protective effect of the anti-oxidant L-N-acetylcysteine (L-NAC) on radiation-induced cochlear cell death [80]. The OC-k3 cochlear cell line was studied before and after 20 Gy of γ-irradiation. Using 3-[4,5-dimethylthiazol-2-yl]-2,5-diphenyltetrazolium bromide cell viability assays, it was was shown that L-NAC increased the viability of cells after irradiation. Flow cytometry and TUNEL assay both showed cell apoptosis at 72 hrs post-irradiation, which was reduced by the addition of L-NAC. Generation of ROS was demonstrated using 2', 7'-dichlorofluorescein diacetate at 1 hr post-irradiation, which was diminished by L-NAC (Figure 3).

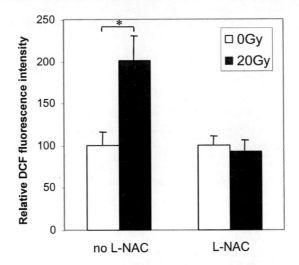

Figure 3. **L-NAC reduces intracellular ROS generated by γ-irradiation.** (A) OC-k3 cells on coverslips were irradiated (0 or 20Gy) in the presence or absence of L-NAC. Images were captured using confocal laser scanning microscopy. Cells were labeled with DCFDA, which fluoresces as green when oxidized by ROS. The nuclei were stained with DAPI (blue). (B) DCF fluorescence intensity was measured at 1h post-irradiation (0 or 20Gy) in the presence or absence of L-NAC. The results (mean ± SD) were normalized in relation to 0Gy, which was given an arbitrary value (relative DCF fluorescence intensity) of 100. The data was generated from three independent experiments. The asterisk indicates the presence of significant differences in relation to 0Gy ($p<0.0001$). Source: Low et al. [80], reproduced with kind permission of Taylor & Francis.

The finding that L-NAC reduced ROS generation and cochlear cell apoptosis after irradiation, suggests that anti-oxidants can potentially be used clinically to prevent radiation-induced SNHL. High drug concentrations can possibly be delivered topically through the middle ear while minimizing systemic side effects.

## Alternative Cell Death Mechanisms in Radiation-Induced SNHL

Based on the understanding of aminoglycoside ototoxicity, Rizzi & Hirose (2007) opined that apoptotic pathways are clearly responsible for hair cell demise [81]. Our own work has also suggested that in radiation-induced SNHL, apoptotic cell death is important with p53 possibly playing a major role [62]. However, it is pointed out that a number of different mechanisms leading to cell deaths have been desribed in the literature and may well be also involved in radiation-induced SNHL.

Firstly, necrotic cell death is expected to occur, especially in high radiation doses. Although this is a passive form of cell death which does not encompass activation of any specific cellular program, ROS can contribute to the death process by affecting lipid peroxidation of the cell membrane [54].

Secondly, p53-independent mechanisms had been described. It had been noted that apoptosis induced by high LET radiation was not affected by cellular p53 gene status [82]. Ionising radiation has been found to induce caspase-dependent but p53-independent cell death in Drosophilia [83]. This may possibly be due to ceramide formation as ceramide has been shown to trigger caspase activation during gamma-induced apoptosis of human glioma cells lacking functional p53 [84].

Thirdly, caspase-independent programmed cell death mechanisms had also been described in recent years. Non-caspase proteases such as cathepsins, calpains and granzymes are involved, resulting in intra-cellular signaling processes that lead to apoptotic- or necrotic-like morphological forms of programmed cell death [85]. Indeed, leupeptin, a calpain inhibitor, had been shown to protect inner ear cells from aminoglycoside ototoxicity [86].

It can therefore, be argued that ototoxicity based on only one stereotypical form of active cell death is likely to be an over-simplification. The coexistence of multiple cell death mechanisms in the same tissue is thought to be common and may even occur in the same cell population [87]. Multiple cellular organelles may trigger several pathways that may act independently or in concert [85]. This has implications for attempts to attenuate or prevent drug-induced hearing loss through manipulation of apoptotic pathways, in that downstream inhibition of a single pathway may not be sufficient to block all cell deaths. Nevertheless, intervention in the early upstream stages of ototoxicity when the different modes of cell deaths share common initial signaling processes, may be feasible. Such upstream intervention approaches include strategies directed at the generation of ROS [87]. In a sudy on humans, the principle of anti-oxidant protection against otoxicity was demonstrated [88]. In this double-blinded placebo-controlled study on patients receiving gentamicin treatment for acute infections, significantly more patients developed hearing loss in the placebo group compared to the group protected by aspirin, an anti-oxidant. Hence, anti-oxidants appear promising in protecting against radiation-induced SNHL in a clinical setting.

# V. COMBINED EFFECTS OF RADIATION AND CDDP ON SNHL

## Combined Chemo-Radiotherapy for Head and Neck Tumours

Combined chemo-radiotherapy is increasingly being used clinically to treat advanced head and neck cancers. In RT of tumours in the head and neck region, the auditory pathways are often included in the radiation fields and radiation-induced SNHL may result. CDDP, widely used as an effective anti-neoplastic drug for these cancers, is also well known to cause ototoxicity. Therefore, in combined therapy, the synergistic ototoxic effects of CDDP and radiation could theoretically be catastrophic for the patient and is a clinical issue that deserves attention.

## Properties of CDDP

CDDP is widely used in the treatment of epithelial malignancies such as lung, head and neck, ovarian, bladder and testicular cancers. However, its clinical use is limited by its severe adverse reactions which include not only ototoxicity but also renal toxicity from renal tubular necrosis and interstitial nephritis, gastrointestinal toxicity and peripheral neuropathy [89].

There are various speculations why CDDP is ototoxic whereas most anti-neoplastics are not [90]. Firstly, it may be related to the small size of the molecule enabling it to cross the blood-labyrinth barrier. Secondly, CDDP is not cell cycle specific and therefore, can affect the non-dividing hair cells of the cochlea. Thirdly, mitochondria which are common in the outer hair cells and the metabolically active stria vascularis, are known to be important cellular targets for CDDP.

The mode of action of CDDP is still not completely understood but is thought to depend on hydrolysis reactions where the –Cl group is replaced by a water molecule adding a positive charge on the molecule [89]. The hydrolysis product is believed to be the active species reacting mainly with glutathione in the cytoplasm and the DNA in the nucleus, thus inhibiting replication, transcription and other nuclear functions. A number of additional properties of CDDP are now emerging, including activation of signal transduction pathways leading to apoptosis. Firing of such pathways may originate at the level of the cell membrane after damage of receptor or lipid molecules by CDDP, in the cytoplasm by modulation of proteins via interaction of their thiol groups with CDDP and finally from DNA damage via activation of the DNA repair pathways.

CDDP-induced hearing loss, first reported by Hill et al. (1972), has a prevalence ranging from as high as 91% to as low as 9 % [91,92]. Van der Hulst et al. (1988) explained that variability was a function of the terminology utilized to define ototoxic change [93]. In a review of 8 studies, most of which were in adults, the overall incidence of hearing loss was 69%. [94].

There is considerable inter-patient variability and this could possibly be contributed by variation in CDDP distribution to the inner ear or to genetic predisposition [94,95]. According to Mencher et al. (1995), pre-existing hearing loss, age and kidney function are confounding variables in the determination of CDDP ototoxicity [2]. They found that patients in poor general health were at greater risk for developing CDDP-induced hearing loss. This included the plasma albumin level, in that lower plasma albumin levels resulted in higher levels of active CDDP in the plasma. Red blood cell count, haemoglobin and hematocrit levels also resulted in higher susceptibility because of poorer oxygen transport capabilities. Intervention by blood transfusion, general nutritional support, and administration of supplemental oxygen could therefore, potentially reduce the risk of CDDP-induced hearing loss.

Morphological CDDP-induced changes in the Organ of Corti had been observed, including damage to outer hair cells (especially in the basal turn of the cochlea), inner hair cells, supporting cells, stria vascularis and spiral ganglion [96].

## Combined Ototoxicity of Radiation and CDDP

Since radiation and cisplatin are both ototoxic, their combined use may possibly result in greater SNHL than using RT alone. In fact, Skinner (1990) suggested that previous or concurrent use of other ototoxic agents with CDDP, may increase toxicity by more than simple algebric summation [94]. Indeed, there have been a number of reports which described enhanced radiatiation-induced ototoxicity when used with CDDP. In a study by Schell et al. (1989) it was found that children and young adults treated with CDDP suffered an additional 20-30dB SNHL if they had received prior cranial RT [27]. In a study on children and adolescents who had received CDDP for the treatment of solid tumours, Skinner et al. (1990) reported more severe CDDP ototoxicity in patients who had previously received RT encompassing the ear [94]. Similarly, Merchant et at (2004) observed enhanced ototoxicity in a study on children with brain tumours who were treated by pre-RT ototoxic chemotherapy [30]. Miettinen et al. (1997) also found that radiotherapy enhanced the ototoxicity of CDDP in the higher speech frequencies [95]. The results of these studies were consistent with those from case reports, which supported the argument that RTshould be considered cautiously in children treated with CDDP for intracranial malignancies [92,97].

On the other hand, there have also been reports which suggested that SNHL after combined therapy was not significantly worse than after RT alone [18,19,20,98]. In a prospective study on 32 patients with NPC who were treated by chemo-radiotherapy, Oh et al. (2004) found the incidence and features of SNHL after combined therapy for NPC to be similar to historical data from RT alone [20]. Two other studies on patients with NPC treated by chemo-radiotherapy also showed that CDDP did not have an additional adverse effect on sensor-neural hearing [18,19]. However, the dose of CDDP used in both of these later studies were relatively low (<240 mg/ sq m)

As some of the studies which showed enhanced ototoxicity were done in patients where chemotherapy was given after RT (rather than prior to RT), it had been suggested that the order in which RT and chemotherapy was administered mattered. It was proposed that in tissues that have been irradiated, post-irradiation hypereamia could cause increased sensitivity of the cochlea to CDDP damage, although enhanced toxicity could occur even up to 10 months after completion of radiation [97]. Alternatively, synergistic ototoxicity could also have resulted if radiation had provided a "predisposition" to damage or had caused changes in permeability of the inner ear and/or central nervous system barriers to CDDP [2,95].

It can be seen that that existing reports on the enhanced ototoxicity of CDDP and radiation yielded conflicting results. However, most of these reports were based on studies that were either retrospective or involved a limited number of subjects. As data emanating from randomised trials were lacking, we conducted a single-blinded randomized trial to investigate if the use of concurrent and post-radiotherapy cisplatin in patients with nasopharyngeal carcinoma resulted in a difference in post-radiotherapy sensori-neural hearing, when compared to using radiotherapy alone [99].

In the study, newly diagnosed NPC patients were randomised into the radiotherapy or chemo-radiotherapy groups. Bone conduction hearing thresholds were performed before treatment and at 1 week, 6 months, 1 year and 2 years after completion of radiotherapy. Hearing thresholds averaged over 0.5, 1 and 2kHz were found to be poorer in the chemo-radiotherapy group compared to the radiotherapy group, at 1 year (p=0.001) and 2 years (p=0.03) post-radiotherapy. Hearing thresholds at 4kHz were significantly worse for patients in the chemo-radiotherapy arm at all the post-radiotherapy time-points studied and were more severely affected than those at the lower speech frequencies. Therefore, combined chemo-radiation therapy resulted in an exaggerated form of SNHL, in particular in the higher speech frequencies.

Although high frequency hearing is generally more severely affected by radiation, threshold shifts seen early at high stimulus frequencies are indicators of probable subsequent shifts to low frequencies [27]. It has even been suggested that the audiometric criteria for monitoring ototoxicity should involve multiple-frequency averaging above 8 kHz. [2]. Frequencies that are functionally important for the intelligibility of speech are 0.5, 1, 2kHz , while the ability to perceive high frequencies are essential for speech discrimination (4kHz) [19]. By affecting speech discrimination, high frequency hearing loss can have a significant impact on the quality of life, [18].

As combined chemo-radiation increases in use in advanced head and neck cancers, normal tissue tolerance once defined for radiation alone should be redefined when used together with chemotherapy. According to Emami et al. (1991), tolerance doses (TD) 5/5 (probability of 5% complication within five years from treatment) and TD 50/5 (the probability of 50% complication within five years) of the inner ear are 60Gy and 70Gy respectively [22]. Doses below 30 Gy are said to have little effect on hearing [28,30]. In the light of the results of the present study, these may not apply in patients who had received radiotherapy combined with concurrent/adjuvant chemotherapy. In a recent sudy by Hitchcock et al. (2008), it was suggested that the threshold cochlear dose for hearing loss with CDDP-based chemotherapy and RT was as low as 10 Gy [100]. It is especially relevant to know the normal ear tissue tolerance doses today, as precise doses can nowadays be more accurately delivered by 3-dimensional techniques such as conformal or intensity modulated radiation therapy [20].

It can therefore be concluded that NPC patients who had received combined RT and concurrent/adjuvant chemotherapy using CDDP experienced greater SNHL compared to those treated by RT alone, especially to high frequency sounds in the speech range. Combined therapy appeared to have allowed the plateau representing ototoxic destruction of outer hair cells to be reached at much lower levels of CDDP, than with chemotherapy alone. Further research on the cellular and molecular processes involved in the combined ototoxicity of CDDP and radiation is warranted.

## CONCLUSION

Radiation-induced SNHL is recognized as an important side effect of radiotherapy if the auditory pathways had been included in the radiation fields. A model of radiation-induced damage of the sensor-neural auditory system is proposed, which is based on dose-dependent, ROS-related radiation-induced cochlear cell apoptosis without significant damage to the retro-cochlear pathway. This model supports the feasibility of cochlear implantation, should one be clinically indicated in such patients. It can explain clinical observations, such as radiation-induced SNHL being dose-dependent, and affects the high frequencies more than the lower frequencies. It also opens up the possibility of preventive strategies targeted at different stages of the apoptotic process. The use of anti-oxidants which target upstream pathways, appear promising. In particular, it may have a major role in chemo-radiation, where combined ototoxic effects lead to significant SNHL.

## REFERENCES

[1]  Low, WK; Fong, KW. Long-term hearing status after radiotherapy for nasopharyngeal carcinoma. *Auris Nasus Larynx*, 1998, 25, 21-4.

[2]  Mencher, GT; Novotny, G; Mencher, L; Gulliver, M. Ototoxicity and irradiation: additional etiologies of hearing loss in adults. *J Am Acad Audiol*, 1995, 6, 351-357.

[3]   Van der Putten, L; de Bree, R; Plukker, JT; Langendijk, JA; Smits, C; Burlage, FR; Leemans, CR. Permanent unilateral hearing loss after radiotherapy for parotid gland tumors. *Head Neck*, 2006, 28, 902-8.

[4]   Louis, CU; Paulino, AC; Gottschalk, S; Bertuch, AA; Chintagumpala, M; Heslop, HE; Russell, HV. A single institution experience with pediatric nasopharyngeal carcinoma: high incidence of toxicity associated with platinum-based chemotherapy plus IMRT. *J Pediatr Hematol Oncol.*, 2007, 29, 500-5.

[5]   Plowman, PN. Post-radiation sensori-neural hearing loss. *Int J Rad Oncol Biol Phys*, 2002, 589-91.

[6]   Ewald, CA. Die Wirkung des Radium auf das Labyrinth. *Zentralbl Physiol*, 1905, 10, 298-9.

[7]   Girden, E; Culler, E. Auditory effects of roentgen rays in dogs. *Am J Roentg*, 1933, 30, 215-20.

[8]   Novotny, O. Sull'azione dei raggi x sulla chiocciola della cavia. *Arch Ital Otol Rhinol Lar*, 1951, 62, 15-9.

[9]   Kozlov, MJ. Changes in the peripheric section of the auditory analyzer in acute radiation sickness. *ORL J Otorhinolaryngol Relat Spec*, 1959, 21, 29-35.

[10]  Gamble, JE; Peterson, EA; Chandler, JR. Radiation effects on the inner ear. *Arch Otolaryngol*, 1968, 88, 64-9.

[11]  Keleman, G. Radiation and ear. *Acta Otolaryngol Suppl (Stock)*, 1963, 184.

[12]  Tokimoto, T; Kanagawa, K. Effects of x-ray irradiation on hearing in guinea pigs. *Acta Otolaryngol (Stockh)*, 1985, 100, 266-72.

[13]  Leach, W. Irradiation of the ear. *J Laryngol Otol*, 1965, 79, 870-80.

[14]  Moretti, JA. Sensori-neural hearing loss following radiotherapy to the nasopharynx. *Laryngoscope*, 1976, 86, 598-602.

[15]  Evans, RA; Liu, KC; Azhar, T; Symonds, RP. Assessment of permanent hearing impairment following radical megavoltage radiotherapy. *J Laryngol Otol*, 1988, 102, 588-9.

[16]  Raajmakers, E; Engelen, AM. Is sensorineural hearing loss a possible side effect of nasopharyngeal and parotid irradiation? A systematic review of the literature. *Radiotherapy Oncol*, 2002, 65, 1-7.

[17]  Schuknecht, HF; Karmody, CS. Radionecrosis of the temporal bone. *Laryngoscope*, 1966, 76, 1416-28.

[18]  Kwong, DLW; Wei, WI; Sham, JST; Ho, WK; Yuen, PW; Chua, DTT; Au, DKK; Wu, PM; Choy, DTK. Sensorineural hearing loss in patients treated for nasopharyngeal carcinoma: A prospective study of the effect of radiation and cisplatin treatment. *Int J Rad Oncol Biol Phys*, 1996, 36, 281-9.

[19]  Wang, LF; Kuo, WR; Ho, KY; Lee, KW; Lin, CS. Hearing loss in patients with nasopharyngeal carcinoma after chemotherapy and radiation. *Kaoshsiung J Med Sci*, 2003, 19, 163-169.

[20]  Oh, YT; Kim, CH; Choi, JH; Kang, JH; Chun, M. Sensory neural hearing loss after concurrent cisplatin and radiation therapy for nasopharyngeal carcinoma. *Radiother Oncol*, 2004, 72, 79-82.

[21]  Bohne, BA; Marks, JE; Glasgow, GP. Delayed effects of ionizing radiation on the ear. *Laryngoscope*, 1985, 95, 818-28.

[22] Emami, B; Lyman, J; Brown, A; Coia, L; Goitein, M; Munzenrider, JE; Shank, B; Solin, LJ; Wesson, M. Tolerance of normal tissue to therapeutic irradiation. *Int J Radiat Oncol Biol Phys*, 1991, 21, 109-22.

[23] Thibadoux, GM; Pereira, WV; Hodges, JM; Aur, RJ. Effects of cranial radiation on hearing in children with acute lymphocytic leukemia. *J Pediatr*, 1980, 96, 403-6.

[24] Talmi, Y; Kalmanovitch, M; Zohar, Y. Thyroid carcinoma, cataract, and hearing loss in a patient afer irradiation for facial hemangioma. *J Laryngol Otol*, 1988, 102, 91-2.

[25] Talmi, YP; Finkelstein, Y; Zohar, Y. Postirradiation hearing loss. *Audiology*, 1989, 28, 121-6.

[26] Winther, FO. X-ray irradiation of the inner ear of the guinea pig – an electron microscopic study of degenerating outer hair cells of the Organ of Corti. *Acta Otolaryngol*, 1970, 69, 61-6.

[27] Schell, M; McHaney, VA; Green, AA; Kun, LE; Hayes, FA; Horowitz, M; Meyer, WH. Hearing loss in children and young adults receiving cisplatin with and without prior cranial irradiation. *J Clin Oncol*, 1989, 7, 754-760.

[28] Linskey, ME; Johnstone, PA. Radiation tolerance of normal temporal bone structures: implications for gamma knife stereotactic radiosurgery. *Int J Radiat Oncol Biol Phys*, 2003, 57, 196-200.

[29] Grau, C; Moller, K; Overgaard, M; Overgaard, J; Elbrond, O. Sensori-neural hearing loss in patients treated with irradiation for nasopharyngeal carcinoma. *Int J Radiat Oncol Biol Phys*, 1991, 21, 723-8.

[30] Merchant, TE; Gould, CJ; Xiong, X; Robbins, N; Zhu, J; Pritchard, DL; Khan, R; Heideman, RL; Krasin, MJ; Kun, LE. Early neuro-otologic effects of three-dimensional irradiation in children with primary brain tumors. *Int J Radiat Oncol Biol Phys*, 2004, 15, 1194-207.

[31] Honore, HB; Bentzen, SM; Moller, K; Grau, C. Sensori-neural hearing loss after radiotherapy for nasopharyngeal carcinoma: individualized risk estimation. *Radiother Oncol*, 2002, 65, 9-16.

[32] Sataloff, RT; Rosen, DC. Effects of cranial irradiation on hearing acuity: a review of the literature. *Am J Otol*, 1994, 15, 772-80.

[33] Grau, C; Overgaard, J. Postirradiation sensorineural hearing loss: a common but ignored late radiation complication. *Int J Radiat Oncol Biol Phys*, 1996, 36, 515-7.

[34] Hackney, CM. Anatomical features of the auditory pathway from cochlea to cortex. *British Medical Bulletin*, 1987, 43, 780-801.

[35] Awwad, HK. Radiation Oncology: Radiobiological and Physiological Perspectives. In: *Late reacting tissues: radiation damage to central nervous system*. The Netherlands: Kluger Academic Publishers, 1990, 429-47.

[36] Lee, AWN; Yau, TK. Complications of radiotherapy. In: V. C. F. Chong, & S. Y. Tsao (Eds.), *Nasopharyngeal Carcinoma*. Singapore, PA: Armour Publishing Pte Ltd, 1997, 114-127.

[37] Lau, SK; Wei, WI; Sham, JST; Choy, DTK; Hui, Y. Early changes of auditory brain stem evoked response after radiotherapy for nasopharyngeal carcinoma – A prospective study. *J Laryngol Otol*, 1992, 106, 887-892.

[38] Grau, C; Moller, K; Overgaard, M; Overgaard, J; Elbrond, O. Auditory brainstem responses in patients after radiation therapy for nasopharyngeal carcinoma. *Cancer*, 1992, 70, 2396-401.

[39] Leighton, SE; Kay, R; Leung, SF; Woo, JK; van Hasselt, CA. Auditory brainstem responses after radiotherapy for nasopharyngeal carcinoma. *Clin Otolaryngol*, 1997, 22, 350-4.

[40] Nomura, R; Hattori, T; Yanagita, N. Radiation tolerance of the cochlear nerve at the gamma-knife in rabbits. *Auris Nasus Larynx*, 1997, 24, 341-9.

[41] Greene, JS; Giddings, NA; Jacobson, JT. Effect of irradiation on guinea pig ABR thresholds. *Otolaryngol Head Neck Surg*, 1992, 107, 763-8.

[42] Gibb, AG; Loh, KS. The role of radiation in delayed hearing loss in nasopharyngeal carcinoma. *J Laryngol Otol*, 2000, 14, 139-44.

[43] Antenius, LJ; Wanders, SL; Hendriks, JJ; Langendijk, JA; Manni, JJ; de Jong, JM. A prospective longitudinal study on radiation-induced hearing loss. *Am J Surg*, 1994, 168, 408-11.

[44] Coplan, J; Post, EM; Richman, RA; Grimes, CT. Hearing loss after therapy with radiation. *Am J Dis Child*, 1981, 135, 1066-7.

[45] Chung, HT; Ma, R; Toyota, B; Clark, B; Robar, J; McKenzie, M. Audiologic and treatment outcomes after linear accelerator-based stereotactic irradiation for acoustic neuroma. *Int J Radiat Oncol Biol Phys*, 2004, 59, 1116-21.

[46] Van Eck, AT; Horstmann, GA. Increased preservation of functional hearing after gamma knife surgery for vestibular schwannoma. *J Neurosurg*, 2005, 102 Suppl, 204-6.

[47] Massager, N; Nissim, O; Delbrouck, C; Devriendt, D; David, P; Desmedt, F; Wikler, D; Hassid, S; Brotchi, J; Levivier, M. Role of intracanalicular volumetric and dosimetric parameters on hearing preservation after vestibular schwannoma radiosurgery. *Int J Radiat Oncol Biol Phys*, 2006, 64, 1331-40.

[48] Hirsch, A; Noren, G. Audiological findings after stereotactic radiosurgery in acoustic neurinomas. *Acta Otolaryngol (Stockh)*, 1988, 106, 244-51.

[49] Bush, ML; Shinn, JB; Young, AB; Jones, RO. Long-term hearing results in gamma knife radiosurgery for acoustic neuromas. *Laryngoscope*, 2008, 118, 1019-22.

[50] Kaplan, DM; Hehar, SS; Tator, C; Guha, A; Laperriere, N; Bance, M; Rutka, JA. Hearing loss in acoustic neuromas following stereotactic radiotherapy. *J Otolaryngol*, 2003, 32, 23-32.

[51] Low, WK; Burgess, R; Fong, KW; Wang, DY. Effect of radiotherapy on retro-cochlear auditory pathways. *Laryngoscope*, 2005, 15, 1823-6.

[52] Low, WK; Gopal, K; Goh, LK; Fong, KW. Cochlear implantation in postirradiated ears: outcomes and challenges. *Laryngoscope*, 2006, 116, 1258-62.

[53] Atar, O; Avraham, KB. Therapeutics of hearing loss: expectations vs reality. *Drug Discov Today*, 2005, 10, 1323-30.

[54] Henderson, D; Bielefeld, EC; Harris, KC; Hu, BH. The role of oxidative stress in noise-induced hearing loss. *Ear Hear*, 2006, 27, 1-19.

[55] Cheng, AG; Cunningham, LL; Rubel, EW. Mechanisms of hair cell death and protection. *Curr Opin Otolaryngol Head Neck Surg*, 2005, 13, 343-8.

[56] Miller, LJ; Marx, J. Apoptosis. *Science*, 1998, 281, 1301.

[57] Rybak, LP; Whitworth, CA. Ototoxicity: therapeutic opportunities. *Drug Discov Today*, 2005, 10, 1313-21.

[58] Seidman, MD; Vivek, P. Intratympanic treatment of hearing loss with novel and traditional agents. *Otolaryngol Clin North Am*, 2004, 37, 973-90.

[59]   Kawamoto, K; Ishimoto, S; Minoda, R; Brough, DE; Raphael, Y. Math1 gene transfer generates new cochlear hair cells in mature guinea pigs in vivo. *J Neurosci*, 2003, 23, 4395-400.

[60]   Ohlemiller, KK; McFadden, SL; Ding, DL; Lear, PM; Ho, YS. Targeted mutation of the gene for cellular glutathione peroxidase (Gpx1) increases noise-induced hearing loss in mice. *Assoc Res Otolaryngol*, 2000, 1, 243-54.

[61]   Chan, PH. Mitochondrial dysfunction and oxidative stress as determinants of cell death/survival in stroke. *Ann N Y Acad Sci*, 2005, 1042, 203-9.

[62]   Low, WK; Tan, MGK; Li, S; Chua, AWC; Goh, LK; Wang, DY. Dose-dependant radiation-induced apoptosis in a cochlear cell-line. *Apoptosis*, 2006, 11, 2127-36.

[63]   Verheij, M; Bartelink, H. Radiation-induced apoptosis. *Cell Tissue Res*, 2000, 301, 133-42.

[64]   Johannesen, TB; Rasmussen, K; Winther, FO; Halvorsen, U; Lote, K. Late radiation effects on hearing, vestibular function, and taste in brain tumor patients. *Int J Radiat Oncol Biol Phys*, 2002, 53, 86-90.

[65]   Withers, HR. Biologic basis of radiation therapy. In: C. A. Peretz, & L. W. Brady (Eds.), *Principles and Practice of Radiation Oncology* (2nd edition). Philadelphia: JB Lippincott Co; 1992, 64-96.

[66]   Hall, EJ. The physics and chemistry of radiation absorption. In: *Radiobiology for the Radiologist* (4th edition). Philadelphia: JB Lippincott Co; 1994, 1-13.

[67]   Zuur, CL; Simis, YJ; Lansdaal, PE; Hart, AA; Rasch, CR; Schornagel, JH; Dreschler, WA; Balm, AJ. Risk factors of ototoxicity after cisplatin-based chemo-irradiation in patients with locally advanced head-and-neck cancer: a multivariate analysis. *Int J Radiat Oncol Biol Phys.*, 2007, 68, 1320-5.

[68]   Yilmaz, YF; Aytas, FI; Akdogan, O; Sari, K; Savas, ZG; Titiz, A; Tumoz, M; Unal, A. Sensorineural hearing loss after radiotherapy for head and neck tumors: a prospective study of the effect of radiation. *Otol Neurotol.*, 2008, 29, 461-3.

[69]   Devarajan, P; Savoca, M; Castaneda, MP; Park, MS; Esteban-Cruciani, N; Kalinec, G; Kalinec, F. Cisplatin-induced apoptosis in auditory cells: role of death receptor and mitochondrial pathways. *Hear Res*, 2002, 174, 45-54.

[70]   Zhang, M; Liu, W; Ding, D; Salvi, R. Pifithrin-alpha suppresses p53 and protects cochlear and vestibular hair cells from cisplatin-induced apoptosis. *Neuroscience*, 2003, 120, 191-205.

[71]   Bristow, RG; Benchimol, S; Hill, RP. The p53 gene as a modifier of intrinsic radiosensitivity: implications for radiotherapy. *Radiother Oncol*, 1996, 40, 197-223.

[72]   Hill, R; Bodzak, E; Blough, MD; Lee, PW. p53 Binding to the p21 promoter is dependent on the nature of DNA damage. *Cell Cycle*, 2008, 7, 2535-43.

[73]   Kastan, MB; Onyekwere, O; Sidransky, D; Vogelstein, B; Craig, RW. Participation of p53 protein in the cellular response to DNA damage. *Cancer Res*, 1991, 51, 6304-11.

[74]   Caelles, C; Helmberg, A; Karin, M. p53-dependent apoptosis in the absence of transcriptional activation of p53-target genes. *Nature*, 1994, 370, 220-3.

[75]   Chao, C; Saito, S; Anderson, CW; Appella, E; Xu, Y. Phosphorylation of murine p53 at ser-18 regulates the p53 responses to DNA damage. *Proc Natl Acad Sci*, 2000, 97, 11936-41.

[76] Chipuk, JE; Bouchier-Hayes, L; Kuwana, T; Newmeyer, DD; Green, DR. PUMA couples the nuclear and cytoplasmic proapoptotic function of p53. *Science*, 2005, 309, 1732-5.

[77] El-Assaad, W; Kozhaya, L; Araysi, S; Panjarian, S; Bitar, FF; Baz E, El-Sabban, ME; Dbaibo, S. Ceramide and glutathione define two independently regulated pathways of cell death initiated by p53 in Molt-4 leukaemia cells. *Biochem J*, 2003, 376, 725-32.

[78] Shinomiya, N. New concepts in radiation-induced apoptosis: 'premitotic apoptosis' and 'postmitotic apoptosis'. *J Cell Mol Med*, 2001, 5, 240-53.

[79] Sha, SH; Taylor, R; Forge, A; Schacht, J. Differential vulnerability of basal and apical hair cells is based on intrinsic susceptibility to free radicals. *Hear Res*, 2001, 155, 1-8.

[80] Low, WK; Sun, L; Tan, MG; Chua, AW; Wang, DY. L-N-Acetylcysteine protects against radiation-induced apoptosis in a cochlear cell line. *Acta Otolaryngol*, 2008, 128, 440-5.

[81] Rizzi, MD; Hirose, K. Aminoglycoside ototoxicity. *Curr Opin Otolaryngol Head Neck Surg.*, 2007, 15, 352-7.

[82] Takahashi, A; Matsumoto, H; Yuki, K; Yasumoto, J; Kajiwara, A; Aoki, M; Furusawa, Y; Ohnishi, K; Ohnishi, T. High-LET radiation enhanced apoptosis but not necrosis regardless of p53 status. *Int J Radiat Oncol Biol Phys*, 2004, 60, 591-7.

[83] Wichmann, A; Jaklevic, B; Su, TT. Ionizing radiation induces caspase-dependent but Chk2- and p53-independent cell death in Drosophila melanogaster. *Proc Natl Acad Sci*, 2006, 103, 9952-7.

[84] Hara, S; Nakashima, S; Kiyono, T; Sawada, M; Yoshimura, S; Iwama, T; Sakai, N. Ceramide triggers caspase activation during gamma-radiation-induced apoptosis of human glioma cells lacking functional p53. *Oncol Rep*, 2004, 12, 119-23.

[85] Leist, M; Jaattela, M. Caspase-independent cell death. In: S. Grimm (Editor), *Genetics of apoptosis*. Trowbridge, UK; BIOS Scientific Publishers Ltd; 2003, 203-222.

[86] Momiyama, J; Hashimoto, T; Matsubara, A; Futai, K; Namba, A; Shinkawa, H. Leupeptin, a calpain inhibitor, protects inner ear hair cells from aminoglycoside ototoxicity. *Tohoku J Exp Med*, 2006, 209, 89-97.

[87] Jiang, H; Sha, SH; Forge, A; Schacht, J. Caspase-independent pathways of hair cell death induced by kanamycin in vivo. *Cell death and Differentiation*, 2006, 13, 20-30.

[88] Sha, SH; Qiu, JH; Schacht, J. Aspirin to prevent gentamicin-induced hearing loss. *N Engl J Med.*, 2006, 354, 1856-7.

[89] Boulikas, T. Vougiouka. Cisplatin and platinum drugs at the molecular level (Review). *Oncology Reports*, 2003, 10, 1663-82.

[90] Ekborn, A; Lindberg, A; Laurell, G; Wallin, I; Eksborg, S; Ehrsson, H. Ototoxicity, nephrotoxicity and pharmacokinetics of cisplatin and its monohydrated complex in the guinea pig. *Cancer Chemother Pharmacol*, 2003, 51, 36-42.

[91] Hill, JM; Speer, RJ; Loeb, E; MacLellan, A; Hill, NO; Khan, A. Clinical experience with cisplatinous diaminedichloride (PDD). In: M. Semosky, M. Hejzlar, & S. Masal, (Eds.), *Advances in antimicrobial and antineoplastic chemotherapy (vol 2)*. Baltimore: University Park Press, 1972, 255.

[92] Sweetow, RW; Will, TI. Progression of hearing loss following the completion of chemotherapy and radiation therapy: case report. *J Am Acad Audiol*, 1993, 4, 360-363

[93]  Van der Hulst, RJAM; Dreschlear, WA; Urbanus, NAM. High frequency audiometry in prospective clinical research of ototoxicity due to platinum derivatives. *Ann Otol Rhinol Laryngol*, 1988, 97, 133-7.

[94]  Skinner, R; Pearson, AD; Amineddine, HA; Mathias, DB; Craft, AW. Ototoxicity of cisplatinum in children and adolescent. *Br J Cancer*, 1990, 61, 927-931.

[95]  Miettinen, S; Laurikainen, E; Johansson, R; Minn, H; Laurell, G; Salmi, TT. Radiotherapy enhanced ototoxicity of cisplatin in children. *Acta Otolaryngol Suppl*, 1997, 529, 90-94.

[96]  Previati, M; Lanzoni, I; Corbacella, E; Magosso, S; Giuffre, S; Francioso, F; Arcelli, D; Volinia, S; Barbieri, A; Hatzopoulos, S; Capitani, S. Martini. RNA expression induced by cisplatin in an organ of Corti-derived immortalized cell line. *Hear Res*, 2004, 196, 8-18.

[97]  Walker, DA; Pillow, J; Waters, KD; Keir, E. Enhanced Cis-platinum ototoxicity in children with brain tumours who have received simultaneous or prior cranial irradiation. *Med Pedia Oncol*, 1989, 17, 48-52.

[98]  Kretschmar, CS; Warren, MP; Lavally, BL; Dyer, S; Tarbell, NJ. Ototoxicity of preradiation cisplatin for children with central nervous system tumors. *J Clin Oncol*, 1990, 8, 1191-8.

[99]  Low, WK; Toh, ST; Wee, J; Fook-Chong, SM; Wang, DY. Sensorineural hearing loss after radiotherapy and chemoradiotherapy: a single, blinded, randomized study. *J Clin Oncol.*, 2006, 24, 1904-9.

[100] Hitchcock, YJ; Tward, JD; Szabo, A; Bentz, BG; Shrieve, DC. Relative Contributions of Radiation and Cisplatin-Based Chemotherapy to Sensorineural Hearing Loss in Head-and-Neck Cancer Patients. *Int J Radiat Oncol Biol Phys*, 2008 Aug 14 [Epub ahead of print].

In: Deafness, Hearing Loss and the Auditory System
Editors: D. Fiedler and R. Krause, pp.137-157

ISBN: 978-1-60741-259-5
©2010 Nova Science Publishers, Inc.

*Chapter 4*

# TARGET ANTIGENS IN IMMUNE-MEDIATED HEARING LOSS: FROM RECOGNITION TO DIAGNOSTIC TOOL

## *Boulassel Mohamed-Rachid*[*]

Department of Medicine, Division of Hematology, McGill University Health Centre

## ABSTRACT

As early as 1931, immune dysfunction was hypothesized as the impairment of the inner ear's function. Since then, a variety of antigens have been described and implicated in immune-mediated hearing loss. Among these are collagen, heat shock protein-70, myelin protein P0, glycolipids, $\beta$-tubulin protein, calcium binding protein S-100$\beta$, Raf-1 protein and more recently $\beta$-actin, cochlin, $\beta$-tectorin and choline transporter-like protein 2. Of these target autoantigens, cochlin and $\beta$-tectorin seem to be specifically expressed in the inner ear. The validity of these proteins as autoantigens and their utility as clinical marker - or more importantly as predictors of hearing loss - is yet to be determined. Central to their utility is their ability to distinguish between individuals with or without immune-mediated hearing loss. Identifying one or more proteins as autoantigens predictive of hearing loss, would provide an opportunity to diagnose, treat and possibly monitor immune-mediated inner ear hearing loss.

## INTRODUCTION

The early report suggesting the implication of immune system on hearing loss dates back to 1931, when Masugi and Tomizuka reported that some idiopathic sensorineural lesions may be immune in origin [1]. Two decades later, Lehnhardt reported cases of progressive bilateral sensorineural hearing loss (SNHL) that may be resulting from antibodies directed against inner ear antigens [2]. Following that, Kikuchi in 1959 described "sympathetic otitis" by analogy to "sympathetic ophthalmia" where hearing loss occurs in the opposite ear within

---

[*] Corresponding author: McGill University Health Centre, Department of Medicine, Division of Hematology, 3650, Saint Urban Street, MCI, Room 817, Montreal, Canada, H2X 2P4, Tel: (514) 934-1934 ext. 32132 or 32625, Fax: (514) 843-2092, E-mail: rachid.boulass@muhc.mcgill.ca

weeks following surgery in the other ear [3]. Thus, he proposed an autoimmune etiology as the likely cause of the inner ear damage. In 1961, Beickert, and three years later Sasaki and Terrayama presented experimental data obtained by immunization of guinea pigs with cochlear extracts, confirming the possibility of autoimmune etiology [4, 5]. These findings were then ignored until Schiff and Brown in 1974 and Clemis in 1975, described the use of corticosteroids, antihistamines and heparin for the treatment of certain sudden deafness and progressive sensorineural hearing losses, reinforcing the hypothesis of an immune-mediated cause [6, 7]. In 1979, McCabe introduced the concept of autoimmune SNHL by describing a pattern of bilateral SNHL characterized by rapid progression over weeks to months and sometimes associated with vertigo and rarely with facial paralysis. Clinical diagnosis was established by means of a positive immune laboratory test and a positive therapeutic response to corticosteroids and immunosuppressive agents [8]. In 1983, Harris showed that the inner ear is not an immunoprivileged site as was previously theorized [9]. Since then, several studies have highlighted the importance of inner ear immune responses to protect both the auditory and balance systems from pathogens and also to cause in some instance damage to audiovestibular tissues that might lead to immune-mediated hearing loss (IMHL). This chapter describes the possible target antigens in IMHL with special regard to their usefulness in diagnosing and possibly therapeutic monitoring of patients with IMHL.

## IDENTIFICATION OF CANDIDATE ANTIGENS IN IMMUNE-MEDIATED HEARING LOSS

Development of specific "biological marker" as serological or cellular diagnostic tool for IMHL has been significantly impeded by our lack of knowledge concerning the nature of stimulants and/or antigens that initially precipitate this disease. What causes the initial activation of autoreactive lymphocytes, which are maintained in a non-pathogenic state via regulatory mechanisms, and/or their conversion to pathogenicity, is still under intensive investigations in IMHL. One generally accepted explanation is that continued stimulation of autoreactive lymphocytes is related to constant exposure to specific or non-specific antigen (s). Over the past two decades, numerous approaches have led to the identification of several candidate antigens. Such identification has at least two clear benefits. First, it allows the development of specific assay that may help diagnose, monitor and possibly predict the onside of IMHL. Second, it helps understand the immunopathological process of the disease in appropriate experimental animal model. Such understanding permits ultimately to the development of antigen-specific immunotherapy. A list of potential antigens targeted in IMHL and some of their shared features are provided in **Table 1**. The link of these antigens to IMHL has in some cases been established but their utility as a diagnostic tool including their specificity, sensitivity and practical application are yet to be determined.

## COLLAGEN

Collagen type II was the first antigen involved in the pathogenesis of IMHL [10]. This ubiquitous protein is composed of a triple helix and is involved in various functions in the body. At least twenty seven collagen types have been identified in vertebrates [11]. Collagen types I, II, III, IV, V, IX, and XI have been found in the inner ear of various animal species including humans [12-14]. Among these, collagen II has been detected in the mammalian tectorial membrane, spiral limbus, spiral ligament, and as a component of the basilar membrane [12, 15, 16]. Type IV collagen, which is believed to be involved in the pathogenesis of Alport's syndrome that results in progressive renal insufficiency and sensorineural hearing loss, was densely localized around the nerve cells and the capillary blood vessels of the stria vascularis, and beneath the epithelial cells in human and guinea pig inner ear [17,18]. Type V collagen was identified in the capillary basement membrane associated with collagen IV. Type IX collagen is less abundant and is located within the labyrinthine membranes, and within the dense fibers of the tectorial membrane [19]. Early studies by Yoo et al. have shown high levels of serum antibodies to bovine type II collagen in five out of 12 (42%) patients with otosclerosis and Ménière's disease compared to those of control subjects [10]. This data has led to the assumption that type II collagen might be involved in the pathogenesis of Ménière's disease and otosclerosis and that antibodies directed against this antigen could serve as a "biological marker" of these disorders. Subsequently, several studies have confirmed these results and have further shown the presence antibodies against type II collagen in the sera of some patients with SNHL and sudden deafness [20-22]. From experimental point of view, it was demonstrated that immunization of animals with type II collagen induced inner ear lesions characterized by spiral ganglion cell degeneration, atrophy of Corti's organ, cochlear nerve and stria vascularis, and endolymphatic hydrops. In addition, some animals develop hearing loss and vestibular dysfunction [23-28]. However, conflicting results with previous descriptions have been reported by several groups. In three unrelated studies, levels of circulating antibodies against type II collagen were not significantly higher in patients with IMHL than those in control subjects [29-31]. In another experimental study aiming at investigating the immunological, electrophysiological and morphological abnormalities following type II collagen injections, no hearing loss or inflammatory lesions in the inner ear were identified in immunized animals, despite that all animals showed very significant serum and perilymph antibody titers to type II collagen [32]. Other studies have also shown that antibodies to type II collagen are not specific for IMHL as they are found in autoimmune diseases such as rheumatoid arthritis and atrophic chronic polychondritis [33, 34]. Thus, the specificity of antibodies to type II collagen in monitoring patients with IMHL is still to be clarified.

# HEAT SHOCK PROTEIN 70 KDA

Several studies have attempted to identify disease specific circulating antibodies that bind to inner ear antigens. In 1990, Harris and Sharp used bovine inner ear antigens to study sera from fifty-four patients with bilateral SNHL and fourteen normal healthy controls. Nineteen of the patients (35%), compared to 7% in the control group, showed a single or double band corresponding to a 68 kDa antigen in the immunoblot [35]. In subsequent publications, similar results were reported by other groups and further showed that patients with rapidly progressive SNHL, Ménière's disease or sudden deafness also develop antibodies directed against the 68 kDa protein extracted from the inner ear of pig, bovine or guinea pig [36-39].

In addition, a correlation between 68 kDa protein positivity and steroid responsiveness was reported [40]. These observations have led to the hypothesis that antibodies to 68 kDa antigen might be involved in the pathogenesis of IMHL and therefore constitute an important input in the diagnosis and therapeutic monitoring of these diseases. Later on the molecular characterization of the 68 kDa protein revealed that it is identical to heat shock protein 70 kDa (HSP-70) or stress protein, which is detected in all prokaryotic and eukaryotic cells [41,42]. Increased levels of this ubiquitous protein occur after environmental stress and infections, but also in normal physiological processes [43]. In an experimental model, mice inoculated with HSP-70 produced high levels of antibodies against this protein but did not induce hearing dysfunction or cause cochlear damage in these immunized animals [44].

**Table 1. Potential target antigens in immune mediated hearing loss.**

| Candidate Antigens | Source of antigen | Inner ear tissue used | Molecular weight (kDa) | Detection technique | Distribution and body expression | Passive transfer of disease to animals | Association of antigen with human hearing loss | Ref. |
|---|---|---|---|---|---|---|---|---|
| Collagen II | Bovine Human | -- | 95 | ELISA | Ubiquitous | ± | – | [10] |
| HSP-70 | Bovine | Total | 68-70 | IF, IB ELISA | Ubiquitous | ± | – | [41,42] |
| P0 | Guinea pig | Total | 30 | IB | Ubiquitous | ± | – | [59] |
| Glycolipids | Bovine Human | Total | -- | ELISA | Ubiquitous | – | – | [64,65] |
| β-tubulin | Guinea pig | Total | 30 | IB, cDNA library screening | Ubiquitous | ± | – | [67] |
| Calcium binding protein S-100β | Rat | Total | 100 | Cell Proliferation | Ubiquitous | ± | – | [75] |
| Raf-1 protein | Guinea pig | Total | 28 | IB, ELISA | Ubiquitous | ± | – | [84] |
| β-actin | Guinea pig | Total | 42-43 | IB | Ubiquitous | ± | – | [89] |
| Cochlin | Guinea pig | Total | 58 | IB, ELISA, Cell proliferation | Specific to inner ear | + | + | [94] |
| β-tectorin | Mouse | Peptide | 36-43 | ELISA, Cell proliferation | Specific to inner ear | + | – | [101] |
| choline transporter-like protein 2 | Guinea pig | Supporting cells | 68-72 | IB | Ubiquitous | + | – | [116] |

Abbreviations: HSP-70: heat shock protein-70; P0: myelin protein P0; IF: Immunoflorescence; IB: Immunoblot; ELISA: Enzyme-linked immunosorbent assay; +: Positive evidence; ±: Conflicting results; -: lack of evidence or still unknown.

Moreover, unpublished sequencing data indicating that the 68 kDa protein is novel and distinct from HSP-70 [39]. In addition, several recent studies have shown that HSP-70 antibodies are less prevalent in patients with idiopathic progressive SNHL, Ménière's disease or sudden deafness [45-49]. Furthermore, HSP70 antibodies have been reported in the sera of normal individuals as well as in many inflammatory diseases and autoimmune and non-autoimmune conditions such as insulin-dependent diabetes mellitus, systemic lupus erythematosus (SLE), multiple sclerosis, primary biliary cirrhosis, autoimmune toxin induced interstitial nephritis, autoimmune hepatitis, peripheral and renal vascular disease and atherosclerosis, arguing against the significance of HSP-70 antibodies in the serological diagnosis of IMHL [50-55]. Therefore, whether antibodies against HSP-70 play a primary etiologic role in IMHL or occur as a secondary epiphenomenon is not yet clear. The exact relationship between HSP-70 and IMHL remains to be clarified.

## MYELIN PROTEIN P0

Using immunoblot technique, antibody activity against a 30 kDa protein extracted from human inner ear was first reported by Joliat *et al* in some patients with Ménière's disease [21]. However, the authors did not draw any conclusions regarding the character of this protein or its role in Ménière's disease at that time. Subsequently, the 30 kDa protein was localized in the modiolus and in the organ of Corti of guinea pig inner ear and antibody activity to this antigen was also described in patients with progressive SNHL and sudden deafness [39, 56-58]. Thereafter, the 30 kDa protein was identified as the protein P zero or myelin protein P0 [59]. These findings have let to the conclusions that protein P0 may play important role in the pathogenesis of IMHL and detection of anti-P0 antibodies in the sera of patients with IMHL may be valuable for early diagnosis and treatment of these conditions. However, myelin protein P0 is not specific to the inner ear since it is expressed in Schwann cells of the peripheral nervous system, where it accounts for about 50-60%, and plays an important role in the compaction of myelin by means of homophilic interaction [59]. From an experimental point of view, Matsuoka *et al* reported that injection of bovine protein P0 causes in some mice lesions of cochlear nerve and an increase in hearing thresholds of these animals [60]. However, these results were not confirmed by other recent work [61]. In addition, in a recent multicentric prospective study including 129 patients, the prevalence of anti-P0 antibodies in patients with rapidly progressive SNHL or Ménière's disease was not statistically different from that of the control subjects. Interestingly, the prevalence of anti-P0 antibodies in Ménière's disease was lower than in the control group [62]. Furthermore, anti-P0 antibodies were described in various inflammatory neuropathies including Guillain-Barré syndrome and systemic diseases [55, 63]. Thus, as for collagen and HSP-70, more clinical and experimental data are required to confirm the implication of myelin P0 protein in IMHL as well as to use anti-P0 antibodies as a serological marker of these conditions.

## SULFOGLUCURONOSYL GLYCOLIPIDS

The association between the presence of antibodies against glycolipids and IMHL was reported by Lack *et al.* and Yawamaki *et al.* who demonstrated high levels of anti-glycolipids in the sera of some patients with progressive SNHL and Ménière's disease compared to those of control subjects [64, 65]. It has thus been suggested that anti-glycolipid antibodies could be a useful marker to support the diagnosis of IMHL. In the inner ear several types of glycolipids have been described including sulphate cerebrosides and gangliosides [64, 65]. However, as the antigens cited above, glycolipids are not specific to inner ear since they were found in all neural cell membranes and involved in various cellular functions such as receptors for hormones and adhesion molecules [65]. In addition, antibodies against glycolipids are known to be present in a large variety of neurological diseases such as Guillain-Barré syndrome and peripheral demyelinating syndrome [66]. Therefore, anti-glycolipid antibodies are not specific for IMHL and need to be tested in large number of cases and non-affected controls.

## β-Tubulin

Using sera from patients with Ménière's disease to screen cochlear cDNA sequences of guinea pig, Yoo *et al.* identified β-tubulin as a potential antigen for IMHL. The nature of the 52 kDa protein extracted from the guinea pig inner ear membranous and neural fractions was then confirmed by micro sequencing to be the β-tubulin [67]. Subsequently, using enzyme-linked immunosorbent assay (ELISA) high levels of serum antibodies to β-tubulin were reported in 67 of 113 (59%) patients with Ménière's disease [68]. It was thus proposed that β-tubulin could be used as a "biological marker" for IMHL. Tubulin is the main component of microtubules, which are formed by two similar polypeptides known as α and β. This structural ubiquitous protein performs many functions in cells, including determination of cell polarity and shape, organelle transport and chromosome separation during cell division [69]. In mammals, at least seven and eight different isotypes of α and β tubulin, respectively, have been identified. In the inner ear, microtubules are prominent features of the sub-cellular anatomy of hair cells and supporting cells. Tubulin is also present in both inner hair cells and outer hair cells as loosely gathered filaments [70]. In a recent study, oral administration of β tubulin at low dose was able to induce peripheral tolerance by suppressing the experimental IMHL in mice. In addition, in antigen-specific fashion, β tubulin was able to induce changes in cytokine milieu by increasing Th2 and Th3 CD4 cell cytokines such as interleukin-4 (IL-4), IL-5, IL-13 and tumor growth factor-β (TGF-β) while suppressing Th1 CD4 cell cytokine such as interferon-γ (IFN-γ), favoring thus the potentially protective immune responses [71]. Although these findings are of importance, several studies have previously shown that antibodies to tubulin are elevated in the sera of patients with chronic inflammatory demyelinating polyneuropathy and Guillain-Barré syndrome [72, 73] thereby their usefulness as a support tool for IMHL waits confirmation.

## Calcium Binding Protein S-100β

By heterologous immunization of inbred Lewis rats with inner ear tissue, Gloddek *et al.* first established an inner-ear-specific T helper cell line that passively transferred to recipient animals induced labyrinthitis, hearing impairments and production of antibodies against inner ear components [74]. In subsequent studies, Gloddek *et al.* established that inner-ear-specific T helper cell line recognizes specifically the calcium binding protein S-100β and that this protein could serve as a potential target antigen in IMHL [75]. As for other antigens, the calcium-binding protein S-100β is not specific for the inner ear as it is expressed in the peripheral nervous system and in many other cells and tissues, including retina, skeletal muscle, adipose tissue, salivary gland and immune cells [76]. In the inner ear, calcium-binding protein S-100β is found in the stria vascularis, spiral ganglion cells, crista ampullaris and organ of Corti [75, 77]. Previous studies have identified calcium binding protein S-100β as a target antigen in experimental autoimmune encephalomyelitis, a disease mediated by specific CD4+ T cells [78]. High levels of antibodies against calcium binding protein S-100β have also been reported in patients with glioblastoma, neuroblastoma and other central nervous system-specific tumors as well as in multiple sclerosis [79-82]. Thus, the functional significance and clinical value of antibodies against calcium binding protein S-100β in IMHL remain to be established.

## RAF-1 PROTEIN

Antibody activity against a 28 kDa protein extracted from guinea pigs inner ear was first described by Suzuki *et al.* in sera of patients with Ménière's disease. The authors reported that 28% of Ménière's disease patients' sera showed a positive reaction at the 28 kDa band, corresponding to a protein specifically localized in the membranous fraction that contains the basement membrane, organ of Corti, stria vascularis, spiral ligament and vestibular epithelium of the inner ear [83]. In a subsequent study, the 28 kDa protein was identified as the proto-oncogene Raf-1 protein by microsequencing [84]. Using recombinant GST Raf-1 protein as a substrate for testing sera from patients with IMHL, 16 of 27 (59%) and 2 of 26 (8%) of patients with Ménière's disease and progressive SNHL, receptively, showed a positive reactivity, suggesting that Raf-1 antibodies are less prevalent in progressive SNHL than in Ménière's disease [84]. These findings have led to the hypothesis that Raf-1 protein could serve as a target antigen in IMHL and detection of anti-Raf-1 antibodies in the sera of patients with IMHL may be a useful tool to support the diagnostic of these conditions. The Raf-1 protein belongs to the Raf family that comprises three members, A-Raf, B-Raf and Raf-1 (also known as C-Raf), the latter being the best-studied isoform [85]. Raf family members are intermediate molecules in the mitogen-activated protein (MAP) kinase pathway and involved in a signal transduction cascade relaying extracellular signals from cell membrane to nucleus via an ordered series of consecutive phosphorylation events. Alterations activating members of the pathway have been implicated in development of carcinomas of the skin, ovary, thyroid, colon and pancreas [86]. Raf-1 protein is a serine/threonine specific MAP kinase expressed in most cells of the body including neurons [85, 86]. This non-tissue-specific protein is involved in regulation of cell proliferation and differentiation. Currently, it is not known whether the 28 kDa protein is a degradation product of the Raf-1 protein whose molecular weight is 74 kDa, or rather it is a novel protein that is very similar to the Raf-1 protein. From experimental point of view, some mice inoculated with Raf-1 protein developed a hunched posture, loss of body weight, severe skin lesions, splenomegaly, lymphadenopathy and hyperimmunoglobulinemia but did not show hearing dysfunction or cochlear damage [87]. Thus, there is a conspicuous lack of direct evidence that anti-Raf-1 antibodies are autonomously pathogenic in IMHL. Further studies have also indicted that elevated anti-Raf-1 antibodies are found in the sera of patients with SLE and Alzheimer's disease [87, 88]. Thus, the role of Raf-1 protein as a valid marker for IMHL is still to be demonstrated.

# Β-ACTIN

Using immunoblot technique, many studies have shown that sera from patients with progressives SNHL or Ménière's disease contained antibodies which reacted with multiple inner ear proteins with various molecular weights [39, 89]. Of the 120 patient suspected of having IMHL, 23 patients (19%) had antibody reacting with the 42-43 kDa protein, while in the control group only 4% had this antibody. None of the 23 patients sera showed autoantibodies to nuclear factors, which are frequently observed in patients with SLE or related disorders [89]. Efforts to identify this 42-43 kDa protein revealed that it corresponds to β-actin, a molecule which composes the cytoskeleton of most non-muscle cells [89]. β-actin is involved in many forms of cell motility and function. Within the inner ear, β-actin was found in the supporting cells, stria vascularis, spiral ganglion, sensory cells and stereocilia [90, 91]. Abnormal expression of β-actin has been found to be associated with hearing loss and vestibular disorders in animal models [92, 93], providing evidence that pathological development of actin filaments disrupts the integrity of hair cells, rendering them unable to convert mechanical stimuli into electrochemical signals and in turn leading to hearing loss. Thus, β-actin has been proposed as a potential target antigen in IMHL. However, its ubiquitous expression precludes targeting of inner ear-specific immunity. Therefore, further clinical and experimental studies are needed to confirm the interest of β-actin and corresponding antibodies in IMHL diagnosis.

# COCHLIN

When investigating sera from patients with idiopathic progressive SNHL or Ménière's disease using immunoblot against guinea pig inner ear proteins, Boulassel *et al*. found that some sera strongly react with a 58 kDa protein [94]. This 58 kDa protein was then purified and identified as cochlin, formerly known as Coch-5B2, a protein highly expressed in inner ear tissues [94]. These findings have led to the assumption that cochlin is a potential antigen in IMHL and that antibodies directed against this protein could serve as "biological marker" to help diagnose these disorders. In contrast to the above described antigens, cochlin expression is substantially confined to the inner ear in humans, whereas in mouse or guinea pig, cochlin is also expressed in the spleen, cerebrum, cerebellum/medulla, thymus and retina [56, 57, 95]. Although its function is still unknown, cochlin constitutes a major component of the extracellular matrix of the inner ear. Cochlin is found in the spiral limbus, spiral ligaments and the basilar membrane of the cochlea and throughout the vestibular end organs and it consists of three domains with an amino-terminal LCCL-domain and two von Willebrand type A domains [95 96]. In a recent study, the C-terminal but not the LCCL-domain, of the second von Willebrand type A domain of cochlin was found to have high affinity for type II collagen as well as for type I and type IV collagens [97], suggesting that cochlin interact with these collagen types, which have previously been involved in the pathogenesis of IMHL.

Along with its specific expression in the inner ear, cochlin is an interesting candidate antigen in IMHL as mutations affecting *COCH* gene, which is mapped in humans to chromosome 14q12-q13, are known to be responsible for the autosomal dominant human deafness disorder DFNA9, a non-syndromic progressive SNHL associated with vestibular dysfunction [98-100]. From experimental point of view, using epitope mapping peptide series derived from cochlin, Solares *et al* demonstrated that five weeks following immunization of SWXJ mice with peptide 131-150, auditory brainstem responses showed significantly hearing loss at all frequencies tested. The authors also found that the peptide selectively activated CD4$^+$ T cells with a pro-inflammatory Th-1 like phenotype with elevated production of IFN-γ using flow cytometry analysis. In addition, the adoptive transfer of the peptide-activated CD4$^+$ T cells into naïve mice induced hearing losses, providing confirmation that IMHL may be a T cell-mediated organ-specific immune disorder. Besides, inner ear inflammation accompanied the appearance of hearing loss after five weeks immunization with Coch peptide131-150, was most notable in the region of the spiral ligament and scala tympani where cochlin is highly expressed in the inner ear [101]. Interestingly, the same inflammation regions after Coch immunization are evident in the inner ear of humans with *COCH* gene mutations [103]. In recent study, using ELISPOT analysis Baek *et al*. reported that patients with IMHL have significantly increased frequencies of circulating cochlin-specific IFN-γ- or IL-5-producing CD4$^+$ and/or CD8$^+$ T cells. The higher frequencies of cochlin-specific T cells were accompanied by significantly higher cochlin-specific serum antibody titers in IMHL patients compared to normal hearing age- and sex-matched control subjects or patients with noise-and/or age-related hearing loss [103]. This data provides further evidence that IMHL may be a T cell-mediated organ-specific condition rather than humoral specific-immune disease although the role of antibodies can not preclude in some IMHL cases. Similarly, Tebo *et al*. reported that 9 out of 58 (14%) of patients with SNHL showed significantly elevated cochlin-specific serum antibody titers compared to zero out of 28 (0%) of healthy controls [104]. More recently, cochlin was identified to be a potential marker for the diagnostic of perilymphatic fistula, which is an abnormal connection between the middle and inner ear and associated with hearing loss and vestibular disorders [105]. Collectively, these findings implicate cochlin as a prominent target antigen for IMHL and detection of cochlin-specific immune activity may ultimately prove to be diagnostically supportive for these disorders.

## Β-TECTORIN

The pivotal role of β-tectorin in the pathogenesis of IMHL was reported by Solares *et al*. in an experimental study using β-tectorin-derived peptides to immunize SWXJ mice [101]. They showed that β-tectorin-derived peptide 71-90 was capable of inducing hearing loss within five weeks as evidenced by a significant increase in auditory brain stem response at all frequencies tested from 4 to 60 kHz compared to untreated age- and sex-matched control mice. In addition, purified CD4$^+$ T cells specific for 71-90 peptide were also capable of inducing hearing loss when transferred to γ-irradiated naïve mice, arguing in favor of a T-cell mediated hearing loss. In addition, immuno-cytochemical analysis showed that inflammation of inner ear tissues coincided with onset of hearing loss [101]. Thus, β-tectorin was proposed as a potential target antigen in IMHL. In the inner ear two tectorins have been described including α-tectorin and β-tectorin and are substantially inner ear-specific proteins in humans. Both tectorins are abundantly expressed in the tectorial membrane in the cochlea, in which the sound-induced movement of the basilar membrane is transmitted to the sensory hair bundles by the tectorial membrane [106,107]. β-tectorin holds motifs involved in sperm-egg adhesions, which appear to function in the formation of filament-based matrices [106]. So far, α-tectorin is the most studied molecules in relation to auditory function as mutations of its gene lead to autosomal dominant non-syndromic hearing impairment in both humans and mice [108-110]. Recently, β-tectorin was also involved in auditory impairments in mice as well as in humans as its expression is decreased upon thyroid hormone deficiency, which associated with hearing loss [111,112]. Using recombinant β-tectorin as a substrate for testing sera from patients with IMHL, one of 58 (2%) of patients with SNHL compared to zero of 28 (%) of healthy controls receptively, showed a positive reactivity, suggesting that β-tectorin antibodies are less prevalent in IMHL [104]. As for cochlin, β-tectorin is an interesting candidate but its clinical value to support IMHL diagnosis remains to be established and needs to be tested in a larger number of IMHL cases as well as non-affected controls.

## CHOLINE TRANSPORTER-LIKE PROTEIN 2

While developing monoclonal antibodies (mAbs) to cells isolated from the guinea pig organ of Corti, Nair *et al.* observed that mice carrying the Kresge Hearing Research Institute-3 (KHRI-3) hybridoma develop high-frequency hearing loss compared to those carrying the KHRI-5 or KHRI-6 hybridomas. Subsequently, KHRI-5 and KHRI-6 mAbs were identified to stain stereocilia while KHRI-3 mAb binds to inner ear supporting cells with a distinctive "wine-glass" pattern. In addition, KHRI-3 mAb induced loss of outer hair cells and hearing loss when infused directly into the guinea pig cochlea [Nair et al 113,114]. Collectively, these experimental studies support the view that IMHL may be an antibody-mediated disease and that antibodies to inner ear antigens in sera of patients suspected of having IMHL strongly sustain this possibility. In further investigations, using inner ear extracts Disher *et al* showed that KHRI-3 mAb and sera from IMHL patients recognize the same 68 kDa band, a protein previously identified as HSP-70 [115]. However, when protein precipitated from inner ear extracts by KHRI-3 mAb and immunoblotted, nothing in the immunoprecipitate reacted with anti-HSP-70 mAb, suggesting that KHRI-3 mAb recognized a protein distinct of HSP-70 [115]. These results confirm unpublished sequencing data indicating that the 68 kDa protein is novel [39]. Using antibody immunoaffinity purification isolate from the guinea pig inner ear supporting cell antigen with mass spectroscopy, Nair *et al* demonstrated that choline transporter-like protein 2 (CTL2) is the antigen defined by KHRI-3 mAb [116]. CTL2 is a glycoprotein with 10-11 transmembrane domains and belongs to choline transporter-like protein family that includes CTL1, CTL2, CTL3, CTL4 and CTL5. CTL2 is also known as solute carrier protein 44A2 [116,117]. The precise function of the CTL proteins, including CTL2, remains unknown but may serve as choline transporter and may also be involved in lipid metabolism and transport such as phosphatidylcholine or sphingophosphatidylcholine [117]. Choline is required for biosynthesis of acetylcholine, a primary neurotransmitter in cholinergic nerve terminals, and also an important neurotransmitter in the inner ear. In such function, CTL2 may be involved in recycling choline by supporting cells [116]. Currently, it is still unknown why the molecular weight of the 68-72 kDa protein identified by KHIR-3 mAb differs from that of the CLT2 predicted to be 80 kDa, although some plausible explanations were suggested, including post-translational modifications. In a recent study, using cochlear cross-sections, Kommareddi *et al* showed that CTL2 is more widely distributed than previously described as it is expressed in cells facing the scala media suggesting a possible role in homeostasis. Moreover, the authors showed that CTL2 and cochlin are expressed in close proximity in the inner sulcus, the spiral prominence, vessels, limbus, and spiral ligament, indicating plausible interactions [118]. In a more study, antibody activity against recombinant human CTL2 was detected in six out of 12 (50%) patients with IMHL compared to three out of 15 (20%) healthy controls. In addition, four patients with antibodies to recombinant human CTL2 responded to corticosteroids suggesting that CTL2 could serve monitoring patients with IMHL [119]. Certainly, CTL2 like cochlin and β-tectorin, is an interesting candidate antigen in IMHL but its serological usefulness to diagnose and possibly monitor IMHL patients need to be confirmed in larger clinical studies.

## OTHER CANDIDATE ANTIGENS

Multiple other candidate antigens currently under investigation in IMHL have been reported including cell-density enhanced protein tyrosine phosphatase-1, connexin 26 anti-endothelial cell antibodies and laminin as well as several inner ear antigens of various molecular weights [68,120,121]. Some of these candidate antigens were found to be partially specific to inner ear while others were not and their possible use to diagnose patients with IMHL is still to be established.

## UNIFYING FEATURES OF CANDIDATE ANTIGENS IN IMMUNE-MEDIATED HEARING LOSS

As discussed above, a plethora of candidate antigens that specifically interact with autoantibodies or autoreactive T cells has been associated with IMHL. The link between these potential candidate antigens and disease has in some cases been established by showing the ability of their derived peptides or corresponding antibodies/autoreactive lymphocytes to transfer the disease in animal models. This does show the pivotal role of autoantibodies or autoreactive T cells in mediating immune hearing loss. However, the potential contribution of each antigen to IMHL pathogenicity is still debated. What determines which antigens are selected and why are ubiquitously expressed proteins targeted in an organ-specific way? In this regard, defining shared features of antigens involved in IMHL is of paramount importance to diagnose and possibly monitor patients with suspected IMHL. Therefore, the identification of the real IMHL autoantigen (s) may clarify whether IMHL autoantibodies or autoreactive T cells are related to the etiology or rather a harmless consequence of the disease. In either case, it will allow the development of serological or cellular test, based on the immunopathogenesis of the disease that can be used to distinguish between individuals with or without IMHL. At present a variety of technologies including immunoflorescence, immunoblot, ELISA and more recently flow cytometry and ELISPOT assays are used to reveal the presence of autoantibodies or autoreactive T cells to inner ear antigens in patients with suspected IMHL. Immunoflorescence (IF), one of the oldest techniques, is not very sensitive and is based on subjective and weakly quantitative interpretation of the results as it does not require knowledge of the precise antigen (s). Because of these limitations, IF technique, may not be appropriate as a confirmatory assay to screen sera from patients with suspected IMHL. In contrast, IF technique is a useful tool when a new antigen is being characterized since it provides valuable information on possible cellular localization of the target antigen. Immunoblot is another common method used to detect anti-inner ear autoantibodies in sera of patients suspected of having IMHL. With this technique, inner ear extracts or purified inner ear antigens are first separated into discrete bands based on their molecular weights and then transferred to a nitocellulose membrane, which is incubated with varying dilutions of patient sera. The interpretation of immunoblot relies on the intensity of protein bands visualized. Immunoblot seems to be the appropriate confirmatory assay to screen sera from patients with suspected IMHL. However, like for IF technique, immunoblot is unable to quantify specific antigen-antibody interactions. The principle of ELISA is very similar to that of immunoblot. Small wells are coated with specific inner ear antigens and then various dilutions of patient sera are added. Using a spectrophotometer, the colorimetric reaction is measured to assess the amount of secondary antibody binding. Because it allows quantification of antigen-antibody reactions, ELISA seems to be the best confirmatory assay to screen sera from patients with suspected IMHL. Both flow cytometry and ELIPSOT assays are 10 to 100-fold increased sensitivity over conventional proliferation methods, to detect cytokine-producing T cell immunoreactivity in peripheral blood mononuclear cells (PBMC) using specific antigens or their corresponding derived peptides. These assays are performed using fresh or cryopreserved PBMC but are very laborious to carry out and time consuming, thereby they might not be suitable for screening patients with suspected IMHL. Regardless of the method (s) selected for detecting potential target antigens in IMHL, rigorous control measures must be observed within these assays. These should incorporate the use of negative and positive controls, and most importantly using the same source of inner ear tissues. The assays described in the literature for identifying potential target antigens in IMHL have used various sources of inner ear tissues including guinea pig, bovine, pig, rat and mice. Although antigens of these sources are likely to be homologous to human inner ear proteins, the use of human tissues in assays for specific-antigen-antibody screen is preferable. Having fresh human tissue within four to six hours after death is optimal because degradation of proteins with time could lead to erroneous results of the assay. However, for several reasons that include difficulty to obtain freshly human inner ear tissues and potential variations in the quality of the tissue between different donors, it will be preferable to use inbred and genetically homogenous rodents as source of inner ear antigens in all assays. The use of human recombinant antigens or their immunogenic derived-peptides when available is of course most suitable. By harmonizing antigen source and its preparation as well as the immunoassay, the use of inner ear autoantibodies or autoreactive T cell testing will have a great diagnostic value and may also be used in the therapeutic monitoring of patients with IMHL. Besides it may help development of antigen-specific immunotherapy. Various therapies including corticosteroids, immunosuppressant, intravenous immunoglobulin and plasmapheresis have been reported to stabilize or improve hearing loss in patients with IMHL [122-124]. Although hearing outcomes are the most important endpoint to be monitored in the therapeutic management of IMHL, a "biological marker" of disease activity such specific-inner ear autoantibodies or autoreactive T cells frequency, could be clinically relevant in monitoring these patients. Anti-inner ear autoantibody titers against HSP-70 or CTL2 have been shown to decline in response to therapeutic interventions in some cases [40, 119]. However, because of small number of patients, variations in antigens source and their specificity as well as the immunoassays used, it is difficult to interpret these results or to draw any conclusions. Long-term large studies are thus needed to assess the use of assaying anti-inner ear autoantibodies for monitoring IMHL patients. However, despite recent advances in detecting IMHL, the number of patients who fit the criteria for such a diagnosis remains very small, even at large referral centers. Therefore, without some means of pooling cases it is difficult to accumulate adequate sample size to conduct statistically meaningful studies and to investigate the usefulness of a specific inner ear autoantibody to monitor treatment response in such a population of patients. Therefore, establishment of a registry would serve as a source of well-characterized cases for both basic and translational research studies, thus fostering innovation in the field. Currently, the diagnosis of IMHL is based on clinical manifestation, auditory test results and responses to immunosuppressive therapy in addition to a battery of non-specific routine immunological tests [121,125] as the use of tissue-specific test is still lacking. Recently, two immunoblot tests for clinical use are commercially available to detect antibodies activity against HSP-70 and P0 antigens (OTOblot™ and ImmuBlot™, OTOIMMUNE Diagnostics, New York, USA) in sera of patients with suspected IMHL. In an early study, the immunoblot for the 68 kDa antigen, known as HSP-70, was found to be the best test for predicting corticosteroid responsiveness in IMHL patients with a sensitivity of 42%, a specificity of 90%, and a positive predictive value of 91% [126]. More recently, an ELISA serum assay to detect antibodies activity against HSP-70 was reported with a specificity of 84%, a sensitivity of 93% and a positive predictive value of 84% [127]. However, because of assay limitations and lack of inner ear-specificity as described earlier, these results are difficult to interpret. Until a standardized test using specific-inner ear antigen(s) is achieved, the use of these available assays will have a limited clinical value because a negative test does not rule out IMHL. As no antibody assay offers 100% specificity, a positive test using specific-inner ear antigen(s) is more likely to support the diagnosis of IMHL.

# CONCLUSION

Since the first report on IMHL, a great deal of knowledge regarding this new clinical entity has accumulated. Numerous basic and clinical studies have led to an increased understanding of this entity. Several potential candidate antigens have been identified and involved in the pathogenesis of IMHL. Most of these antigens are not specific because they were also implicated in other autoimmune and non-autoimmune diseases as well as in inflammatory conditions. Thus, their possible pathogenic nature in IMHL is still controversial. Other antigens however, appear to be more specific and are, in some cases, almost exclusively found in the inner ear. These specific antigens could have the most valuable diagnostic potential in IMHL. As such, autoantibodies to these inner ear-specific antigens have the potential to become in the near future the "serological marker" for IMHL. By standardizing and validating a simple and reproducible assay to measure the presence and titers of these inner ear-specific antibodies in IMHL patient sera, it will be possible to accurately diagnose, monitor and manage patients with this curable disease.

# REFERENCES

[1]     Masugi, M; Tomazuka, T. Über die spezifisch zytotoxischen veränderungen der nieren und der leber durch des spezifische antiserum. *Trans. Jpn. Pathol. Soc.*, 1931, 21, 329-341.

[2]     Lenhardt, E. Plotzliche Horstorungen, auf beiden Seiten gleichzeitig oder nacheinander aufgetreten. *Z. Laryngol. Rhinol. Otol.*, 1958, 37, 1-16.

[3]     Kikuchi, M. On the "sympathetic otitis". *Zibi. Rinsyo. Kyoto.*, 1959, 52, 600-605.

[4]     Beickert, P. Zur frage der empfindungsschwerhörigkeit und autoallergie. *Z. Laryngol.*, 1961, 54, 837-842.

[5]     Terrayama, Y; Sasaki, Y. Studies on experimental allergic (isoimmune) labyrinthitis in guinea pigs. *Acta. Otolaryngol.*, 1964, 58, 49-64.

[6]     Schiff, M; Brown, M. Hormones and sudden deafness. *Laryngoscope*, 1974, 84, 1959-1981.

[7]     Clemis, JD. Allergy as a cause of fluctuant hearing loss. *Otolaryngol Clin North Am.*, 1975, 8, 375-383.

[8]     McCabe, BE. Autoimmune sensorineural hearing loss. *Ann. Otol. Rhinol. Laryngol.*, 1979, 88, 585-589.

[9]     Harris, JP. Immunology of the inner ear: response of the inner ear to antigen challenge. *Otolaryngol. Head. Neck. Surg.*, 1983, 91, 17-23.

[10]   Yoo, TJ; Stuart, JM; Kang, AH; Townes, AS; Tomoda, K; Dixit, S. Type II collagen autoimmunity in otosclerosis and Meniere's Disease. *Science*, 1982, 217, 1153-1155.

[11]   Myllyharju, J; Kivirikko, KI. Collagens, modifying enzymes and their mutations in humans, flies and worms. *Trends Genet.*, 2004, 20, 33-43.

[12]   Asamura, K ; Abe, S ; Imamura, Y ; et al. Type IX collagen is crucial for normal hearing. *Neuroscience*, 2005, 132, 493-500.

[13]   Cosgrove, D; Samuelson, G; Pinnt, J. Immunohistochemical localization of basement membrane collagens and associated proteins in the murine cochlea. *Hear Res*, 1996, 97, 54-65.

[14]   Tsuprun, V; Santi, P. Ultrastructural organization of proteoglycans and fibrillar matrix of the tectorial membrane. *Hear Res*, 1997, 110, 107-118.

[15]   Dreiling, FJ; Henson, MM; Henson, OW Jr. The presence and arrangement of type II collagen in the basilar membrane. *Hear Res*, 2002, 166, 166-180.

[16]   Thalmann, I. Collagen of accessory structures of organ of Corti. *Connect Tissue Res*, 1993, 29, 191-201.

[17]   Kleppel, MM; Santi, PA; Cameron, JD; Wieslander, J; Michael, AF. Human tissue distribution of novel basement membrane collagen. *Am J Pathol.*, 1989, 134, 813-25.

[18]   Takahashi, M; Hokunan, K. Localization of type IV collagen and laminin in the guinea pig inner ear. *Ann Otol Rhinol Laryngol Suppl.*, 1992, 157, 58-62.

[19]   Slepecky, NB; Savage, JE; Yoo, TJ. Localization of type II, IX and V collagen in the inner ear. *Acta Otolaryngol.*, 1992, 112, 611-617.

[20] Helfgott, SM; Mosciscki, RA; San Martin, J; et al. Correlation between antibodies to type II collagen and treatment outcome in bilateral progressive sensorineural hearing loss. *Lancet*, 1991, 337, 387-389.

[21] Joliat, T; Seyer, J; Bernstein, J; et al. Antibodies against a 30 kilodalton cochlear protein and type II and IX collagens in the serum of patients with inner ear diseases. *Ann. Otol. Rhinol. Laryngol.*, 1992, 101, 1000-1006.

[22] Tomoda, K; Suzuka, Y; Iwai, H; Yamashita, T; Kumazawa, T. Meniere's disease and autoimmunity: clinical study and survey. *Acta. Otolaryngol.*, 1993, 500, 31-34.

[23] Yoo, TJ; Yazawa, Y; Tomoda, K; Floyd, R. Type II collagen-induced autoimmune endolymphatic hydrops in guinea pig. *Science*, 1983, 222, 65-67.

[24] Soliman, AM. Type II collagen-induced inner ear disease: critical evaluation of the guinea pig model. *Am J Otol.*, 1990, 11, 27-32.

[25] Cruz, OL; Miniti, A; Cossermelli, W; Oliveira, RM. Autoimmune sensorineural hearing loss: a preliminary experimental study. *Am J Otol.*, 1990, 11, 342-346.

[26] Takeda, T; Sudo, N; Kitano, H; Yoo, TJ. Type II collagen-induced autoimmune ear disease in mice: a preliminary report on an epitope of the type II collagen molecule that induced inner ear lesions. *Am J Otol.*, 1996, 17, 69-75.

[27] Yoo, TJ; Fujiyoshi, T; Cheng, KC; et al. Molecular basis of type II collagen autoimmune ear diseases. *Ann. N. Y. Acad. Sci.*, 1997, 830, 221-235.

[28] Meyer zum Gottesberge, AM; Gross, O; Becker-Lendzian, U; Massing, T; Vogel, WF. Inner ear defects and hearing loss in mice lacking the collagen receptor DDR1. *Lab Invest.*, 2008, 88, 27-37.

[29] Herdman, RCD; Morgan, K; Holt, PJL; Ramsden, RT. Type II collagen autoimmunity and Meniere's disease. *J. Laryngol. Otol.*, 1993, 107, 994-998.

[30] Fattori, B; Ghilardi, P; Casani, A; Migliorini, P; Riente, L. Meniere's disease: role of antibodies against basement membrane antigen. *Laryngoscope*, 1994, 104, 1290-1294.

[31] Lopez-Gonzalez, MA; Lucas, M; Sanchez, B; et al. Autoimmune deafness is not related to hyperreactivity to type II collagen. *Acta Otolaryngol.*, 1999, 119, 690-694.

[32] Harris, JP; Woolf, NK; Ryan, AF. A reexamination of experimental type II collagen autoimmunity: middle and inner ear morphology and function. *Ann Otol Rhinol Laryngol.*, 1986, 95, 176-180.

[33] Terato, K; Shimozuru, Y; Katayama, K; et al. Specificity of antibodies to type II collagen in rheumatoid arthritis. *Arthritis Rheum.*, 1990, 33, 1493-1500.

[34] Rowley, MJ; Nandakumar, KS; Holmdahl, R. The role of collagen antibodies in mediating arthritis. *Mod Rheumatol.*, 2008, 18, 429-41.

[35] Harris, JP; Sharp, P. Inner ear autoantibodies in patients with rapidly progressive sensorineural hearing loss. *Laryngoscope*, 1990, 97, 63-76.

[36] Veldman, JE; Hanada, T; Meeuwsen, F. Diagnostic and therapeutic dilemmas in rapidly progressive sensorineural hearing loss and sudden deafness. A reappraisal of immuno reactivity in inner ear disorders. *Acta. Otolaryngol. Stockh.*, 1993, 113, 303-306.

[37] Harris, JP; Moscicki, RA; Hughes, GB. Immunologic disorders of the inner ear. *In clinical otology*, 2nd edition. New York: Thieme. 1997, 381-391.

[38] Atlas, MD; Chai, F; Boscato, L. Meniere's disease: evidence of an immune process. *Am. J. Otol.*, 1998, 19, 628-631.

[39] Boulassel, MR; Deggouj, N; Tomasi, JP; Gersdorff, M. Inner ear autoantibodies and their targets in patients with autoimmune inner ear diseases. *Acta. Otolaryngol. (Stockh)*, 2001, 121, 28-34.

[40] Moscicki, RA; San Martin, JE; Quintero, CH; et al. Serum antibody to inner ear proteins in patients with progressive hearing loss. Correlation with disease activity and response to corticosteroid treatment. *JAMA*, 1994, 272, 611-616.

[41] Bloch, DB; San Martin, JE; Rauch, SD; Moscicki, RA; Bloch, KJ. Serum antibodies to heat shock protein 70 in sensorineural hearing loss. *Arch. Otolaryngol. Head. Neck. Surg.*, 1995, 10, 1167-1171.

[42] Billings, PB; Keithley, EM; Harris, JP. Evidence linking the 68 kilodalton antigen identified in progressive sensorineural hearing loss patient sera with heat shock protein 70. *Ann Otol Rhinol Laryngol.*, 1995, 104, 181-188.

[43] Rawhi, O. Heat shock proteins in autoimmune disease. *J. Clin. Immunoassay.*, 1994, 17, 129-132.

[44] Trune, DR; Kempton, JB; Mitchell, CR; Hefeneider, SH. Failure of elevated heat shock protein 70 antibodies to alter cochlear function in mice. *Hear. Res.*, 1998, 116, 65-70.

[45] García Berrocal, JR; Ramírez-Camacho, R; Arellano, B; Vargas, JA. Validity of the Western blot immunoassay for heat shock protein-70 in associated and isolated immunorelated inner ear disease. *Laryngoscope*, 2002, 112, 304-309.

[46] Samuelsson, AK; Hydén, D; Roberg, M; Skogh, T. Evaluation of anti-hsp70 antibody screening in sudden deafness. *Ear Hear.*, 2003, 24, 233-235.

[47] Yeom, K; Gray, J; Nair, TS; et al. Antibodies to HSP-70 in normal donors and autoimmune hearing loss patients. *Laryngoscope*, 2003, 113, 1770-1176.

[48] Tebo, AE; Szankasi, P; Hillman, TA; Litwin, CM; Hill, HR. Antibody reactivity to heat shock protein 70 and inner ear-specific proteins in patients with idiopathic sensorineural hearing loss. *Clin Exp Immunol.*, 2006, 146, 427-432.

[49] DiBerardino, F; Cesarani, A; Hahn, A; Alpini, D. Viral infection and serum antibodies to heat shock protein 70 in the acute phase of Ménière's disease. *Int Tinnitus J.*, 2007, 13, 90-93.

[50] Pockley, AG; Shepherd, J; Corton, JM. Detection of heat shock protein 70 (Hsp70) and anti-Hsp70 antibodies in the serum of normal individuals. *Immunol Invest.*, 1998, 27, 367-77.

[51] Wright, BH; Corton, JM; El-Nahas, AM; Wood, RF; Pockley, AG. Elevated levels of circulating heat shock protein 70 (Hsp70) in peripheral and renal vascular disease. *Heart Vessels.*, 2000, 15, 18-22.

[52] Zügel, U; Kaufmann, SH. Role of heat shock proteins in protection from and pathogenesis of infectious diseases. *Clin Microbiol Rev.*, 1999, 12, 19-39.

[53] Pockley, AG. Heat shock proteins in health and disease: therapeutic targets or therapeutic agents? *Expert Rev Mol Med.*, 2001, 3, 1-21.

[54] Pockley, AG; Georgiades, A; Thulin, T; de Faire, U; Frostegård, J. Serum heat shock protein 70 levels predict the development of atherosclerosis in subjects with established hypertension. *Hypertension.*, 2003, 42, 235-238.

[55] Boulassel, MR. Clinical significance of autoantibodies to inner ear antigens in sera of patients with systemic diseases. *Clin Exp Med.*, 2008, 8, 59-60.

[56] Cao, MY; Deggouj, N; Gersdorff, M; Tomasi, JP. Guinea pig inner ear antigens: extraction and application to the study of human autoimmune inner ear disease. *Laryngoscope*, 1996, 106, 207-212.

[57] Cao, MY; Gersdorff, M; Deggouj, N; Tomasi, JP. The localization and specificity of guinea pig inner ear antigenic epitopes. *J Laryngol Otol.*, 1995, 109, 19-23.

[58] Tomasi, JP; Lona, A; Deggouj, N; Gersdorff, M. Autoimmune sensorineural hearing loss in young patients: an exploratory study. *Laryngoscope*, 2001, 111, 2050-2053.

[59] Cao, MY; Dupriez, VJ; Rider, M; et al. Myelin protein Po as a potential autoantigen in autoimmune inner ear disease. *FASEB.*, 1996, 14, 1635-1640.

[60] Matsuoka, H; Cheng, KC; Krug, MS; Yazawa, Y; Yoo, TJ. Murine model of autoimmune hearing loss induced by myelin protein P0. *Ann. Otol. Rhinol. Laryngol.*, 1999, 108, 255-264.

[61] Boulassel, MR; Guérit, JM; Denison, S; et al. No evidence of auditory dysfunction in guinea pigs immunized with myelin P0 protein. *Hear. Res.*, 2001, 152, 10-16.

[62] Pham, BN; Rudic, M; Bouccara, D; et al. Antibodies to myelin protein zero (P0) protein as markers of auto-immune inner ear diseases. *Autoimmunity*, 2007, 40, 202-207.

[63] Steck, AJ; Schaeren-Wiemers, N; Hartung, HP. Demyelinating inflammatory neuropathies, including Guillan-Barré syndrome. *Curr. Opin. Neurol.*, 1998, 11, 311-318.

[64] Lake, GM; Sismanis, A; Ariga, T; Yamawaki, M; Gao, Y; Yu, RK. Antibodies to glycosphingolipid antigens in patients with immune-mediated cochleovestibular disorders. *Am. J. Otol.*, 1997, 18, 175-178.

[65] Yamawaki, M; Ariga, T; Gao, Y; Tokuda, A; Yu, JS; Sismanis, A; Yu, RK. Sulfoglucuronosyl glycolipids as putative antigens for autoimmune inner ear disease. *J. Neuroimmunol.*, 1998, 84, 111-116.

[66] Yu, RK; Yoshino, H; Ariga, T. The role of glycosphingolipids in peripheral neuropathies and related disorders. In M. Nicolini, & P. S. Zatta (Eds.), *Glycobiology and the Brain*. New York, Plenum, Press. 1993, 155-177.

[67] Yoo, TJ; Tanaka, H; Kwon, SS; et al. β-Tubulin as an autoantigen for autoimmune inner ear disease. In: O. Sterkers, E. Ferrary, R. Dauman, J. P. Sauvage, & P. Tran Ba Huy, (Eds.), Ménière's Disease 1999—Update. *Proceedings of the 4th International Symposium on Ménière's Disease*, Paris, France. The Hague, The Netherlands: Kugler Publications, 2000, 529-35.

[68] Yoo, TJ; Du, X; Kwon, SS. Molecular mechanism of autoimmune hearing loss. *Acta Otolaryngol Suppl.*, 2002, 548, 3-9.

[69] Hallworth, R; Luduena, RF. Differential expression of beta tubulin isotypes in the adult gerbil cochlea. *Hear. Res.*, 2000, 148, 161-172.

[70] Banerjee, A; Jensen-Smith, H; Lazzell, A; et al. Localization of betav tubulin in the cochlea and cultured cells with a novel monoclonal antibody. *Cell Motil Cytoskeleton.*, 2008, 65, 505-14.

[71] Cai, Q; Du, X; Zhou, B; Cai, C; Kermany, MH; Yoo, T. Induction of Tolerance by Oral Administration of Beta-Tubulin in an Animal Model of Autoimmune Inner Ear Disease. *ORL J Otorhinolaryngol Relat Spec.*, 2009, 71, 135-141.

[72] Tagawa, Y; Yuki, N; Hirata, K. The 301 to 314 amino acid residue of beta-tubulin is not a target epitope for serum IgM antibodies in chronic inflammatory demyelinating polyneuropathy. *J Neurol Sci.*, 1999, 163, 44-46.

[73] Connolly, AM; Pestronk, A. Anti-tubulin autoantibodies in acquired demyelinating polyneuropathies. *J Infect Dis.*, 1997, 176 Suppl 2, S157-159.

[74] Gloddek, B; Gloddek, J; Arnold, W. A rat T-cell line that mediates autoimmune disease of the inner ear in the Lewis rat. *Oto. Rhino. Laryngol.*, 1999, 61, 181-187.

[75] Gloddek, B; Lassmann, S; Gloddek, J; Arnold, W. Role of S-100beta as potential autoantigen in an autoimmune disease of the inner ear. *J. Neuroimmunol.*, 1999, 101, 39-46.

[76] Zimmer, DB; Cornwall, EH; Landar, A; Song, W. The S100 protein family: history, function, and expression. *Brain Res Bull.*, 1995, 37, 417-429.

[77] Foster, JD; Drescher, MJ; Hatfield, JS; Drescher, DG. Immunohistochemical localization of S-100 protein in auditory and vestibular end organs of the mouse and hamster. *Hear Res.*, 1994, 74, 67-76.

[78] Kojima, K; Wekerle, H; Lassmann, H; Berger, T; Linington, C. Induction of experimental autoimmune encephalomyelitis by CD4+ T cells specific for an astrocyte protein, S100 beta. *J Neural Transm Suppl.*, 1997, 49, 43-51.

[79] Ishiguro, Y; Kato, K; Akatsuka, H; Iwata, H; Ito, F; Watanabe, Y; Nagaya, M. Comparison of calbindin D-28k and S-100 protein B in neuroblastoma as determined by enzyme immunoassay. *Jpn. J. Cancer. Res.*, 1996, 87, 62-67.

[80] Bertsch, T; Casarin, W; Kretschmar, M; et al. Protein S-100B: a serum marker for ischemic and infectious injury of cerebral tissue. *Clin Chem Lab Med.*, 2001, 39, 319-23.

[81] Schmidt, AP; Tort, AB; Amaral, OB; et al. Serum S100B in pregnancy-related hypertensive disorders: a case-control study. *Clin Chem.*, 2004, 50, 435-438.

[82] Sen, J; Belli, A; Petzold, A; et al. Extracellular fluid S100B in the injured brain: a future surrogate marker of acute brain injury? *Acta Neurochir.*, 2005, 147, 897-900.

[83] Suzuki, M; Krug, MS; Cheng, KC; Yazawa, Y; Bernstein, J; Yoo, TJ. Antibodies against inner-ear proteins in the sera of patients with inner-ear diseases. ORL. *J. Otorhinolaryngol. Relat. Spec.*, 1997, 59, 10-17.

[84] Cheng, KC; Matsuoka, H; Lee, KM; Kim, N; Krug, MS; Kwon, SS; Mora, M; Yoo, TJ. Proto-oncogene Raf-1 as an autoantigen in Meniere's disease. *Ann. Otol. Rhinol. Laryngol.*, 2000, 109, 1093-1098.

[85] Chong, H; Vikis, HG; Guan, KL. Mechanisms of regulating the Raf kinase family. *Cell Signal.*, 2003, 15, 463-469.

[86] Roberts, PJ; Der, CJ. Targeting the Raf-MEK-ERK mitogen-activated protein kinase cascade for the treatment of cancer. *Oncogene*, 2007, 26, 3291-3310.

[87] Yoo, TJ; Du, X; Kwon, SS. Molecular mechanism of autoimmune hearing loss. *Acta Otolaryngol Suppl.*, 2002, 548, 3-9.

[88] Mei, M; Su, B; Harrison, K; Chao, M; Siedlak, SL; Previll, LA; Jackson, L; Cai, DX; Zhu, X. Distribution, levels and phosphorylation of Raf-1 in Alzheimer's disease. *J Neurochem.*, 2006, 99, 1377-1388.

[89] Boulassel, MR; Tomasi, JP; Deggouj, N; Gersdorff, M. Identification of β-actin as a candidate autoantigen in autoimmune inner ear disease. *Clin. Otolaryngol. Allied. Sci.*, 2000, 25, 535-541.

[90] Flock, A; Bretscher, A; Weber, K. Immunohistochemical localization of several cytoskeletal proteins in inner ear sensory and supporting cells. *Hear Res.*, 1982, 7, 75-89.

[91]  Nakazawa, K; Spicer, SS; Gratton, MA; Schulte, BA. Localization of actin in basal cells of stria vascularis. *Hear Res.*, 1996, 96, 13-19.

[92]  Sobin, A; Flock, A; Bagger-Sjöbäck, D. Freeze-fracturing of vestibular sensory epithelia in a strain of the waltzing guinea pig. *Acta. Otolaryngol. Stockh.*, 1983, 4, 207-214.

[93]  Sobin, A; Anniko, M; Flock, A. Rods of actin filaments in type I hair cells of the Shaker-2 mouse. *Arch Otorhinolaryngol.*, 1982, 236, 1-6.

[94]  Boulassel, MR; Tomasi, JP; Deggouj, N; Gersdorff, M. COCH5B2 is a target antigen of anti-inner ear antibodies in autoimmune inner ear diseases. *Otol. Neurotol.*, 2001, 22, 614-618.

[95]  Robertson, NG; Morton, CC. Beginning of a molecular ear in hearing and deafness. *Clin. Genet.*, 1999, 55, 149-159.

[96]  Ikezono, T; Omori, A; Ichinose, S; Pawankar, R; Watanabe, A; Yagi, T. Identification of the protein product of the Coch gene (hereditary deafness gene) as the major component of bovine inner ear protein. *Biochim Biophys Acta.*, 2001, 1535, 258-65.

[97]  Nagy, I; Trexler, M; Patthy, L. The second von Willebrand type A domain of cochlin has high affinity for type I, type II and type IV collagens. *FEBS Lett.*, 2008, 582, 4003-4007.

[98]  Robertson, NG; Resendes, BL; Lin, JS; et al. Inner ear localization of mRNA and protein products of COCH, mutated in the sensorineural deafness and vestibular disorder, DFNA9. *Hum Mol Genet.*, 2001, 10, 2493-2500.

[99]  Fransen, E; Verstreken, M; Verhagen, WI; et al. High prevalence of symptoms of Meniere's disease in three families with a mutation in the COCH gene. *Hum. Mol. Genet.*, 1999, 8, 1425-1429.

[100] de Kok, YJ; Bom, SJ; Brunt, Tm; et al. A Pro51Ser mutation in the COCH gene is associated with late onset autosomal dominant progressive sensorineural hearing loss with vestibular defects. *Hum. Mol. Genet.*, 1999, 8, 361-366.

[101] Solares, CA; Edling, AE; Johnson, JM; et al. Murine autoimmune hearing loss mediated by CD4+ T cells specific for inner ear peptides. *J Clin Invest.*, 2004, 113, 1210-1217.

[102] Robertson, NG; Cremers, CW; Huygen, PL; et al. Cochlin immunostaining of inner ear pathologic deposits and proteomic analysis in DFNA9 deafness and vestibular dysfunction. *Hum Mol Genet.*, 2006, 15, 1071-1085.

[103] Baek, MJ; Park, HM; Johnson, JM; et al. Increased frequencies of cochlin-specific T cells in patients with autoimmune sensorineural hearing loss. *J Immunol.*, 2006, 177, 4203-4210.

[104] Tebo, AE; Szankasi, P; Hillman, TA; Litwin, CM; Hill, HR. Antibody reactivity to heat shock protein 70 and inner ear-specific proteins in patients with idiopathic sensorineural hearing loss. *Clin Exp Immunol.*, 2006, 146, 427-432.

[105] Ikezono, T; Shindo, S; Sekiguchi, S; et al. Cochlin-Tomoprotein: A Novel Perilymph-Specific Protein and a Potential Marker for the Diagnosis of Perilymphatic Fistula. *Audiol Neurootol.*, 2009, 14, 338-344.

[106] Killick, R; Legan, PK; Malenczak, C; Richardson, GP. Molecular cloning of chick beta-tectorin, an extracellular matrix molecule of the inner ear. *J Cell Biol.*, 1995, 129, 535-47.

[107] Legan, PK; Richardson, GP. Extracellular matrix and cell adhesion molecules in the developing inner ear. *Semin Cell Dev Biol.*, 1997, 8, 217-224.

[108] Verhoeven, K; Van Laer, L; Kirschhofer, K; et al. Mutations in the human a-tectorin gene cause autosomal dominant non-syndromic hearing impairment. *Nat Genet*, 1998, 19, 60-62.

[109] Mustapha, M; Weil, D; Chardenoux, S; et al. An α-tectorin gene defect causes a newly identified autosomal recessive form of sensorineural pre-lingual non-syndromic deafness, DFNB21. *Hum Mol Gen*, 1999, 8, 409-412.

[110] Legan, PK; Lukashkina, VA; Goodyear, RJ; et al. A targeted deletion in a-tectorin reveals that the tectorial membrane is required for the gain and timing of cochlear feedback. *Neuron*, 2000, 28, 273-285.

[111] Knipper, M; Richardson, G; Mack, A; et al. Thyroid hormone-deficient period prior to the onset of hearing is associated with reduced levels of b-tectorin protein in the tectorial membrane: implication for hearing loss. *J Biol Chem*, 2001, 276, 39046-39052.

[112] Zou, P; Muramatsu, H; Sone, M; Hayashi, H; Nakashima, T; Muramatsu, T. Mice doubly deficient in the midkine and pleiotrophin genes exhibit deficits in the expression of beta-tectorin gene and in auditory response. *Lab Invest.*, 2006, 86, 645-53.

[113] Nair, TS; Raphael, Y; Dolan, DF; et al. Monoclonal antibody induced hearing loss. *Hear Res.*, 1995, 83, 101-13.

[114] Nair, TS; Prieskorn, DM; Miller, JM; Mori, A; Gray, J; Carey, TE. In vivo binding and hearing loss after intracochlear infusion of KHRI-3 antibody. *Hear Res.*, 1997, 107, 93-101.

[115] Disher, MJ; Ramakrishnan, A; Nair, TS; et al. Human autoantibodies and monoclonal antibody KHRI-3 bind to a phylogenetically conserved inner-ear-supporting cell antigen. *Ann N Y Acad Sci.*, 1997, 830, 253-65.

[116] Nair, TS; Kozma, KE; Hoefling, NL; et al. Identification and characterization of choline transporter-like protein 2, an inner ear glycoprotein of 68 and 72 kDa that is the target of antibody-induced hearing loss. *J Neurosci.*, 2004, 24, 1772-1779.

[117] O'Regan, S; Traiffort, E; Ruat, M; Cha, N; Compaore, D; Meunier, FM. An electric lobe suppressor for a yeast choline transport mutation belongs to a new family of transporter-like proteins. *Proc Natl Acad Sci*, U S A., 2000, 97, 1835-1840.

[118] Kommareddi, PK; Nair, TS; Raphael, Y; et al. Cochlin isoforms and their interaction with CTL2 (SLC44A2) in the inner ear. *J Assoc Res Otolaryngol.*, 2007, 8, 435-446.

[119] Kommareddi, PK; Nair, TS; Vallurupalli, M; et al. Autoantibodies to recombinant human CTL2 in autoimmune hearing loss. *Laryngoscope*, 2009, 119, 924-32.

[120] Lunardi, C; Bason, C; Leandri, M; et al. Autoantibodies to inner ear and endothelial antigens in Cogan's syndrome. *Lancet*, 2002, 360, 915-921.

[121] Agrup, C; Luxon, LM. Immune-mediated inner-ear disorders in neuro-otology. *Curr Opin Neurol.*, 2006, 19, 26-32.

[122] Harris, JP; Weisman, MH; Derebery, JM; et al. Treatment of corticosteroid-responsive autoimmune inner ear disease with methotrexate: a randomized controlled trial. *JAMA*, 2003, 290, 1875-1883.

[123] Alexander, TH; Weisman, MH; Derebery, JM; et al. Safety of high-dose corticosteroids for the treatment of autoimmune inner ear disease. *Otol Neurotol.*, 2009, 30, 443-448.

[124] Broughton, SS; Meyerhoff, WE; Cohen, SB. Immune-mediated inner ear disease: 10-year experience. *Semin Arthritis Rheum.*, 2004, 34, 544-548.

[125] Yehudai, D; Shoenfeld, Y; Toubi, E. The autoimmune characteristics of progressive or sudden sensorineural hearing loss. *Autoimmunity*, 2006, 39, 153-8.

[126] Hirose, K; Wener, MH; Duckert, LG. Utility of laboratory testing in autoimmune inner ear disease. *Laryngoscope*, 1999, 109, 1749-1754.

[127] Munari, L; Charchat, S; Rodrigues, L; et al. An ELISA serum assay for autoantibodies to HSP70 in immune-mediated hearing loss. *J Immunol Methods*, 2003, 283155-161.

In: Deafness, Hearing Loss and the Auditory System
Editors: D. Fiedler and R. Krause, pp.159-180

ISBN: 978-1-60741-259-5
©2010 Nova Science Publishers, Inc.

*Chapter 5*

# DAMAGE OF CHRONIC SUBLETHAL HYPOXIA TO THE IMMATURE AUDITORY BRAINSTEM

## *Ze Dong Jiang*[*]

Department of Paediatrics, University of Oxford, John Radcliffe Hospital,
Oxford, United Kingdom

## ABSTRACT

Acute severe or lethal hypoxia is well known to damage the immature auditory system. However, limited information is available about whether chronic sublethal hypoxia also damages this system. Previous studies in animal experiments showed that chronic sublethal hypoxia adversely affects the immature cerebral cortex. Recent studies have revealed that chronic sublethal hypoxia damage functional integrity of the immature auditory system in both human infants and animal models of chronic sublethal hypoxia. In human infants, a typical clinical problem that is associated with chronic sublethal hypoxia is bronchopulmonary dysplasia (BPD), a major perinatal problem that often leads to neurodevelopmental deficits. In recent years, the influence of this problem on the immature brain has attracted considerable attention. The understanding of the influence of chronic sublethal hypoxia associated with BPD on the immature auditory system remains very limited. Brainstem auditory function has recently been studied in very preterm infants who suffered chronic sublethal hypoxia due to BPD. In the maximum length sequence brainstem auditory responses the components that reflect central auditory function were significantly abnormal, while the components that reflect peripheral neural function of the auditory system did not show any major abnormalities. The results suggest that chronic sublethal hypoxia damage neural conduction, reflecting impaired myelination and synaptic dysfunction, in the immature central auditory system, with no major effect on neural function of the peripheral auditory system. Newborn rats reared in chronic sublethal hypoxia showed a significant reduction in myelination in major white tracts and a patchy distribution of the residual myelination in the auditory brainstem. There was also a reduction in myelin basic protein expression. It appears that chronic sublethal hypoxia inhibits myelination and the expression of myelin basic protein in the

---

[*] Corresponding author: Telephone: ++44 1865 221364; Telefax: ++44 1865 221366. E-mail address: zedong.jiang@paediatrics.ox.ac.uk.

auditory brainstem. These recent novel findings provide new insights into our understanding of the influence of chronic sublethal hypoxia on functional integrity of the very immature auditory system.

# INTRODUCTION

Development of the brain, including the central auditory system, in the very early life is characterized by sequential periods of cellular proliferation, migration of glia and neurons into appropriate cortical positions, synaptogenesis and the emergence of cortical connectivity with other cortical and subcortical regions of the brain (Lagercrantz and Ringstedt, 2001). Oxygen deprivation or hypoxia is a well recognized cause of brain damage, with significant long-term consequences. Acute severe or lethal hypoxia occurring during the perinatal period, which is often associated with ischemia, can seriously damage the immature brain (Vannucci, 1990). Hypoxic-ischemic insult frequently results in brainstem auditory lesions (Dambska et al., 1987; Leech and Alvord, 1977; Myers, 1977; Natsume et al., 1995; Pasternak, 1993). By comparison, little is known about the effect of chronic sublethal hypoxia on the auditory system until very recently.

In animal experiments, some investigators showed evidence that chronic sublethal hypoxia adversely affects the immature brain (Curristin et al., 2002; Schwartz et al., 2004; Stewart et al., 1997; Weiss et al., 2004). A typical clinical problem that is associated with chronic sublethal hypoxia in very preterm infants is bronchopulmonary dysplasia (BPD) (Greenough and Milner, 2005). Infants who suffer BPD often experience frequent episodes of hypoxaemia or prolonged hypoxaemia. Recent studies have revealed that these infants have major impairment in the immature central auditory function (Jiang et al., 2006a,2007a,2009a,2010; Wilkinson et al., 2007). In the brainstem auditory evoked responses (BAERs), infants with BPD showed major abnormalities in the components that mainly reflect functional integrity of the central auditory brainstem. Such abnormalities suggest poor myelination and synaptic dysfunction in the auditory brainstem, which may well be related to or due to chronic sublethal hypoxia that occurs during the course of BPD. Preliminary experiments in newborn rats reared in chronic sublethal hypoxia confirm that chronic sublethal hypoxia affects myelination in the immature auditory brainstem. These studies provide clear evidence that chronic sublethal hypoxia damages the immature central auditory system.

# ABNORMALITIES IN THE IMMATURE BRAIN (- EVIDENCE FROM ANIMAL EXPERIMENTS)

Examination of the brain in newborn rats exposed to chronic sublethal hypoxia revealed a significant decrease in brain weight, cortical volume, white matter volume and progressive cerebral ventriculomegaly (Ment et al., 1998; Stewart et al., 1997). Such abnormalities mimic those seen in preterm infants in neuroimaging studies (Peterson et al., 2000; Hüppi et al., 1996,2001; Muphy et al., 2001). The rat model of chronic sublethal hypoxia also showed a significant reduction in total cortical cell number and Glia (Schwartz et al., 2004). On the other hand, neuron numbers were only slightly reduced. After returning to normoxic environment, there was some recovery of glial cell numbers, but no significant recovery of neuronal cell numbers. During the period of hypoxic exposure western blot analyses of Bcl-2 and Bax protein levels showed a ratio favorable to Bax at multiple time points (Schwartz et al., 2004). Apparently, chronic or prolonged exposure to hypoxia during the pre- and perinatal period alters the production and maintenance of glial and neuronal cells. Glia and neurons demonstrate differential patterns of vulnerability and recovery following subsequent periods of normoxic exposure.

Mice are another rodent model for the premature brain. In newborn mice subjected to chronic sublethal hypoxia, there was an accentuation in genes subserving presynaptic function and a suppression in genes involved with synaptic maturation, postsynaptic function, and neurotransmission (Curristin et al., 2002). Other significantly affected pathways included those that involved with glial maturation, vasculogenesis, and components of the cortical and microtubular cytoskeleton. It appears that there is a global dysynchrony in the maturation programs of the developing brain which undergoes sublethal postnatal hypoxia. Waves of inappropriate apoptosis, possibly as a result of impaired synaptogenesis, may lead to a permanent loss of cortical complexity and an irreversible injury after hypoxia.

Neonatal chronic sublethal hypoxia can also cause direct neuronal damage and modifies the environment for axonal re-growth in the immature brain of experimental mice. Many oligodendrocyte-specific proteins were reduced in abundance in the hypoxic neonatal brain, including the axon outgrowth-regulating surface protein, myelin associated glycoprotein (MAG). There was a dramatically decrease in the level of the axon outgrowth inhibitor Nogo-A in oligodendrocytes of CNS white matter, and a moderate decrease in another myelin protein - MAG (Weiss et al., 2004).

Regenerating CST fibers in some strains of mice lacking Nogo-A/B or treated with a NgR antagonist assumed many ectopic locations (GrandPréet al., 2002; Kim et al., 2003). Mice reared under chronic sublethal hypoxia exhibited misplaced collateral connections and corticofugal sprouting. This is unlikely to be solely caused by a loss of myelin-derived inhibition of axon sprouting. Instead, the fiber misrouting is the result of loss of myelin inhibitors in combination with the mild hypoxic insult to the neuron itself. Anterograde axonal tracing in cortex demonstrated ectopic corticofugal fibers in the corticospinal tract, corpus callosum, and caudate nucleus in animals reared in chronic sublethal hypoxia (Weiss et al., 2004). All these findings indicate that chronic sublethal hypoxia adversely affects the immature brain.

## ABNORMALITIES IN IMMATURE BRAIN CENTRAL AUDITORY FUNCTION (- EVIDENCE FROM HUMAN INFANTS WITH BPD)

### Perinatal Hypoxia and the Auditory Brainstem

Hypoxemia disturbs the metabolism of neurons, depresses the electrophysiological function of synapses, and interferes with nerve conduction (Jiang, 2008; Johnston et al., 2001). This can lead to neural impairment and dysfunction of the brain. Hypoxia occurring during early life often results in neurodevelopmental disorders, including auditory impairment (Dixon et al., 2002; Gonzales and Miller, 2006; Jiang, 2008; Johnston et al., 1995,2001; Levene, 2001; Levene and Evans, 2005; Marlow et al., 2005; Rennie et al., 2007; Volpe, 2001; Wilkinson and Jiang, 2006). This is particularly obvious in preterm infants (Jiang et al., 2005a,2009b,c; Pinto-Martin et al., 1999; Volpe, 1998,2001; Paneth, 1999). Considerable evidence suggests that neurodevelopmental disorders in infants born very prematurely often link to hypoxic events during the perinatal period.

Auditory neurons in the neonatal brainstem are vulnerable to hypoxic-ischaemic insult. Histopathological studies revealed that following perinatal hypoxia-ischemia discrete hypoxic-ischaemic lesions are very common in the auditory brainstem, including loss of neurones with gliosis or ischaemic cell changes in the cochlear nuclei, superior olive and inferior colliculus (Dambska et al., 1987; Leech and Alvord, 1977; Myers, 1977; Natsume et al., 1995; Pasternak, 1993). The inferior colliculus – a major auditory centre in rostral regions of the auditory brainstem - receives widespread auditory input from the brainstem. This nucleus has very high metabolic rates and is particularly vulnerable to hypoxia-ischaemia. Animal experiments showed that auditory neurons in the immature brainstem are sensitive to severe hypoxiemia (Jiang et al., 2005b,2006c; Inagaki et al., 1987). Electrophysiological studies in human infants after perinatal asphyxia also demonstrate that the auditory brainstem is vulnerable to severe hypoxia, particularly when associated with ischemia (Hecox, et al., 1981; Jiang, 1995,1998,2008; Jiang and Tierney, 1996, Jiang et al., 2001; Kileny et al., 1980; Wilkinson and Jiang 2006). Therefore, acute severe or lethal hypoxia, which is often associated with ischemia, can seriously damage the immature, particularly central, auditory system. However, the influence of chronic sublethal hypoxia on the immature auditory brainstem remains unclear.

In human infants, hypoxia is particularly prevalent among those who are born very prematurely (Hack et al., 1995; Vohr and Msall, 1997). Such infants often undergo chronic or prolonged periods of sublethal hypoxia (Poets et al., 1995). With the increase in survival rate for critically ill preterm infants, there is an increased concern of brain damage and neurodevelopmental disorders, including auditory problems, in the survivors. Animal experiments demonstrated that chronic sublethal hypoxia adversely affects the immature cerebral cortex (Ment et al., 1998; Stewart et al., 1997 Curristin et al., 2002 Schwartz et al., 2004Weiss et al., 2004). It is possible that the immature central auditory system is also affected by chronic sublethal hypoxia.

In very preterm infants, a typical clinical problem that is associated with chronic sublethal hypoxia is bronchopulmonary dysplasia (BPD) - a severe type of chronic lung disease. It is a major lung disease that causes hypoxaemia of pulmonary origin in infants who are born very prematurely (Greenough and Milner, 2005; Katz-Salamon et al., 2000; Murphy et al., 2001; Skidmore et al., 1990). The survivors of infants with BPD have a high incidence of neurological impairment and developmental deficits, such that BPD has increasingly become one of the highest risk factors of neurodevelopmental problems (Böhm and Katz-Salamon 2003; Gregoire et al., 1998; Katz-Salamon et al., 2000; Kurzner et a., 1988; Meisels et al., 1987; Murphy et al., 2001; Northway et al., 1990; Perlman 2001; Short et al., 2003; Singer et al., 1997; Thompson et al., 2007; Vohr et al., 2000).

Infants who suffer BPD often experience frequent episodes of hypoxaemia or prolonged hypoxaemia. Such hypoxaemia plays an important role in the development of neurological impairment and deficit in infants with BPD. An earlier study suggests that neurophysiological organization of the immature brain is altered in infants with BPD (Scher et al., 1992). Recent studies in human infants and animal models revealed that chronic sublethal hypoxia damages the immature central auditory system (Jiang et al., 2006a,2007a,2009a,2010; Wilkinson et al., 2007).

## Electrophysiological Methods to Study the Auditory Brainstem

The brainstem auditory evoked response (BAER) (also known as auditory brainstem response or ABR) reflects functional integrity of the auditory brainstem. It is the electrophysiological activity of large numbers of sequentially activated neurons at successively higher levels of the brainstem auditory pathway following acoustic stimulation (Chiappa, 1990; Henderson-Smart et al., 1991; Jiang, 2008; Wilkinson and Jiang, 2006). The maturational phases of central components of the BAER overlap or parallel the critical period of brainstem myelination, axonal sprouting, formation of central synaptic connections, improvement of synaptic efficiency, increase in axonal diameter and development of central dendritic properties (Krumholz et al., 1985; Moore et al., 1995,1997; Ponton et al. 1996; Wilkinson and Jiang, 2006). BAER changes with chemical alterations of myelination and synaptic function. The measurements of BAER variables are related to myelination and synaptic function along the brainstem auditory pathway of the developing brain.

As a non-invasive objective test, BAER is particularly suitable in very young or sick infants. It is the major tool to detect auditory impairment in high-risk infants, and an important component in universal hearing screening. It has also been widely used to examine functional integrity and development of the central auditory system in infants with perinatal problems that affect the brainstem auditory pathway (Henderson-Smart et al., 1991; Wilkinson and Jiang, 2006). In both human subjects and experimental animals the BAER is shown to be very sensitive to arterial blood oxygen levels and hypoxia or hypoxia-ischaemia (Inagaki et al., 1997; Jiang et al., 2005b,2006c; Sohmer et al., 1986a,b; Urbani and Lucertini, 1994; Volpe, 2001). The BAER plays an important role in assessment of cerebral and auditory function in infants after perinatal hypoxia or hypoxia-ischaemia (e.g. Hecox, et al., 1981; Jiang, 1995,1998,2008; Jiang and Tierney, 1996; Jiang et al., 2001; Kileny et al., 1980; Majnemer et al., 1988; Wilkinson and Jiang 2006).

In addition to conventional averaging techniques, a relatively new technique - the maximum length sequence (MLS) – has also been employed to record and process BAER (Eysholdt and Schreiner, 1982). Some previous authors used the MLS BAER to study sensorineural hearing impairment and auditory processing disorders (Eysholdt and Schreiner, 1982; Jirsa, 2001; Lina Granade et al., 1994). A major advantage of this technique is that it can present acoustic stimuli at much higher repetition rates (up to 1,000/sec or even higher) than possible using conventional averaging techniques (Bell et al., 2001,2002; Eysholdt and Schreiner, 1982; Jiang, 2008; Jirsa, 2001; Lasky, 1997; Lasky et al., 1996,1998; Lina Granade et al., 1994; Picton et al., 1992). The very high-rate stimulation provides a much stronger temporal/ physiological challenge to auditory neurons in the brainstem. Such a stimulus "stress" offers a potential to improve the detection of some neuropathology which may not be detected by presenting less stressful stimuli (i.e. low-rate stimulation) using conventional averaging techniques (Jiang, 2008; Wilkinson and Jiang, 2006).

The MLS BAER has been studied in newborn infants (Lasky et al., 1992; Weber and Roush, 1993; Jiang et al., 1999). More recently, the MLS has been employed to study BAER in infants with various perinatal problems, particularly perinatal asphyxia (Jiang 2008; Jiang et al., 2000,2003,2005a,2006b;2007b,2008,2009a,b,c,2010; Wilkinson and Jiang, 2006; Wilkinson et al., 2007; Yin et al., 2008). In both human infants and animal models, perinatal hypoxia-ischaemia has been shown to exert a major damage to the neonatal auditory brainstem (Jiang, 2008; Jiang et al., 2005b,2006c,2000,2003,2008,2009a,b,c,2010). There is a characteristically dynamic change in wave latencies and interpeak intervals during the neonatal period in infants after perinatal hypoxia-ischemia (Jiang, 2008; Jiang et al., 2003). The MLS BAER can detect some auditory abnormalities or impairment that cannot be shown by conventional BAER. Now, the MLS technique has become a valuable method to improve the diagnostic value of BAER for central auditory impairment in infants with perinatal problems that affect the brainstem auditory pathway (Jiang 2008; Jiang et al., 2000,2003,2005a,2006b;2007b, 2008,2009a,b,c,2010; Wilkinson and Jiang, 2006; Wilkinson et al., 2007). This high-rate stimulation, or 'stimulus stress', offered by the MLS technique is particularly valuable for detection of early and subtle auditory abnormalities that may not be detected by conventional BAER or other methods (Jiang, 2008; Jiang et al., 2007b; Wilkinson and Jiang, 2006).

## Impaired Central Auditory Function

More recently, the MLS BAER has been employed to study central auditory function in very preterm infants with BPD (Wilkinson et al., 2007; Jiang et al., 2009a,2010). The following results were obtained from the analysis of data that were reported in earlier studies (Jiang et al., 2009a, 2010; Wilkinson et al., 2007) plus additional data that have been accumulated after this report. The criteria of BPD included requirement for supplementary oxygen or ventilatory support beyond 36 weeks of postconceptional ages of 36 weeks to maintain $PaO_2$ >50 mmHg, clinical signs of chronic lung respiratory disease and radiographic evidence of BPD (persistent strands of density in both lungs) (Greenough and Milner, 2005; Northway et al., 1990). To minimize any possible confounding effect of major brain lesions on the MLS BAER any BPD infants who had concomitant major brain lesions (e.g. severe intraventricular haemorrhage and periventricular leucomalacia) were excluded.

The MLS BAER was recorded at term equivalent age, i.e. 37-42 weeks postconceptional age. The data obtained in very preterm infants with BPD were compared with those obtained in age-matched healthy very preterm infants, i.e. very preterm infants who had no BPD and any other major perinatal problems. Figure 1 shows a typical MLS BAER waveforms in a BPD infant recorded at term age, and MLS BAER waveforms in a normal term infants.

Compared with healthy very preterm infants, BPD infants demonstrated major abnormalities in MLS BAER central components, that is, the components that mainly reflect or are related to central neural function, including wave V latency (Figure 2) and I-V (Figure 3) and particularly III-V interpeak intervals (Figure 5). Such abnormalities were particularly significant at very higher rates (455/sec and 910/sec). In contrast, no apparent abnormalities were found in the components that are mainly related to peripheral auditory function, including wave I and III latencies. There were also no major abnormality in I-III interval, which reflects functional integrity of the more peripheral or caudal regions of the auditory brainstem, although the interval tended to be longer than that in the healthy very preterm infants at high rate-stimulation (Figure 4). These results implies that the increase in wave V latency and I-V interval in the infants with BPD was fundamentally produced by the significant increase in III-V interval, which reflects functional integrity of the more central or rostral regions of the auditory brainstem (Jiang et al., 2009e). This is supported by the increase in the III-V/I-III interval ratio at all click rates, mainly at higher rates (Figure 6).

In the BAER, each of wave components requires the integrity of an anatomically diffuse system comprising a set of neurons, their axons and the neurons on which they terminate. The latencies and, particularly, interpeak intervals in the BAER primarily reflect nerve conduction velocity associated with axonal diameter, myelination and synaptic function along the brainstem auditory pathway. Other factors, such as neural orientation and synchronization, are also involved. In the immature auditory brainstem, the BAER changes with maturation of myelination and synaptic function. The abnormalities found in infants with BPD indicate that neural conduction, mainly related to myelination, in the more central or rostral regions of the auditory brainstem is delayed or impaired during the course of BPD.

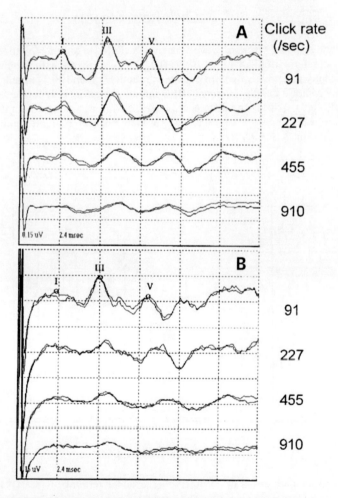

Figure 1. Sample recordings of the MLS BAER from a normal term infant (A, gestation 39 weeks) and a BPD infant (B, gestation 26 weeks) at 40 weeks postconceptional age. Compared with the term infant, the BPD infant shows an increase in wave V latency, I-V and particularly III-V interpeak intervals. The increase in III-V interval is most significant at 455/s and 910/s.

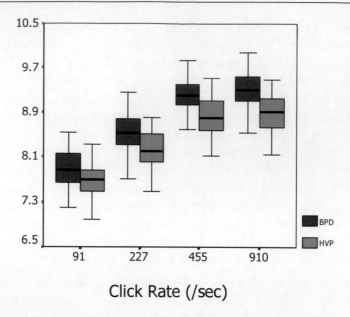

Figure 2. Means and standard errors of wave V latency recorded at term age with 91-910/sec clicks. HVP, healthy very preterm infants without BPD. The latency increases with increasing click rate, and correlates significantly and positively with click rate in both HVP and BPD infants (all P <0.01). Analysis of variance shows that the latency in BPD infants is significantly longer than in HVP infants at all click rates (P <0.01-0.001). The differences increase with increasing click rate. Regression analysis demonstrates that the slope of wave V latency-rate function is significantly steeper in BPD infants than in HVP infants (P <0.05).

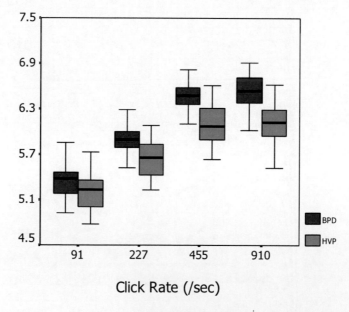

Figure 3. Means and standard errors of I-V interval recorded at term age with 91-910/sec clicks. The interval increases with increasing click rate, and correlates significantly and positively with click rate in both HVP and BPD infants (all P <0.01). The interval in BPD infants is significantly longer than in HVP infants at all click rates (P <0.01-0.0001). The differences increase with increasing click rate. The slope of I-V interval-rate function is significantly steeper in BPD infants than in HVP infants (P <0.01).

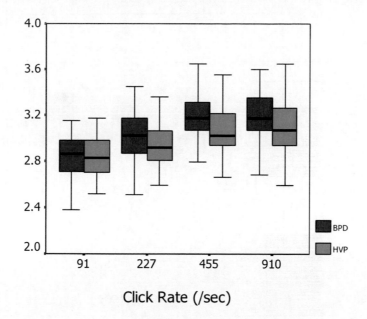

Figure 4. Means and standard errors of I-III interval recorded at term age with 91-910/sec clicks. The interval increases with increasing click rate, and correlates significantly and positively with click rate in both HVP and BPD infants (all P <0.01). The interval in BPD infants is similar to that in HVP infants at lower rates (91/sec), but longer than HVP infants at higher rates (227-910/sec, all P <0.05). The slope of I-V interval-rate function in BPD infants is similar to that in HVP infants, without any significant differences.

The change in the BAER with the increase in stimulus presentation rate, i.e. stimulus rate-dependent change, primarily reflects neural processes concerning the efficacy of central synaptic transmission, as well as neural synchronisation and metabolic status of auditory neurons in the brainstem following the presentation of a physiological challenge (Jiang, 2008; Jiang et al., 2000,2002,2003,2004; Ken-Dror et al., 1987; Lasky 1997). The abnormalities in MLS BAER central components in the infants with BPD generally increased with the increase in the rate of clicks. The slopes of wave V latency-rate function, and I-V and particularly III-V interval-rate functions tended to be increased in the infants with BPD, suggesting that there is an increased in stimulus rate-dependent changes in MLS BAER central components. Apparently, auditory neurons in the more central regions of the auditory brainstem in infants with BPD are vulnerable to physiological/temporal challenge of acoustic stimulation, resulting in a decreased efficacy of central synaptic transmission. Therefore, in addition to myelination, central synaptic efficacy in the auditory brainstem is also affected during the course of BPD.

A major clinical event in infants with BPD is frequent episodes of hypoxaemia or prolonged hypoxaemia (Greenough and Milner, 2005). Our infants with BPD showed major abnormalities in MLS BAER central components, reflecting impaired functional integrity and development of the auditory brainstem. Since none of our BPD infants had any concomitant major brain lesions that may exert confounding effect on the MLS BAER, the MLS BAER abnormalities are most likely to be attributable mainly to frequent episodes of hypoxaemia or prolonged sublethal hypoxaemia, which is associated with BPD (Jiang et al., 2009a,2010; Wilkinson et al., 2007).

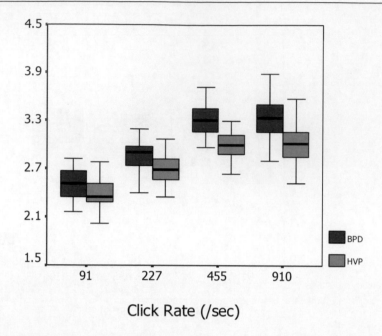

Figure 5. Means and standard errors of III-V interval recorded at term age with 91-910/sec clicks. The interval increases with increasing click rate, and correlates significantly and positively with click rate in both HVP and BPD infants (all P <0.01). The interval in BPD infants is significantly longer than in HVP infants at all click rates (P <0.01-0.0001). The differences increase with increasing click rate. The slope of III-V interval-rate function is significantly steeper in BPD infants than in HVP infants (P <0.01).

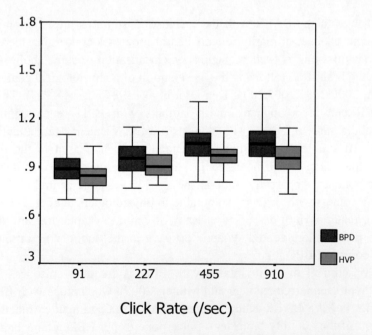

Figure 6. Means and standard errors of III-V/I-III interval ratio recorded at term age with 91-910/sec clicks. The interval increases with increasing click rate, and correlates significantly and positively with click rate in both HVP and BPD infants (all P <0.01). The interval in BPD infants is significantly longer than in HVP infants at all click rates (P <0.05-0.0001). The differences increase with increasing click rate. The slope of the interval ratio-rate function is significantly steeper in BPD infants than in HVP infants (P <0.01).

In BPD, the prolonged hypoxaemia is often associated with periods of oxygen desaturation, as well as suboptimal respiratory mechanics (Greenough and Milner, 2005). Infants with BPD are invariably associated with therapy in high oxygen concentrations for prolonged periods. The prolonged exposure to high oxygen concentrations has complex biochemical microscopic and gross anatomical effects on lung tissues, which can injure the immature lung and cause further hypoxemia. Furthermore, infants with BPD often have other associated adverse clinical conditions or complications, such as very immaturity, respiratory distress syndrome, patent ductus arteriosus, disrupted alveolar and capillary development, pulmonary interstitial emphysema, oxygen toxicity, and perinatal infection and inflammation (Greenough and Milner, 2005). These adverse conditions may exert some effects on the immature auditory system. But the major effect that contributes to the MLS BAER abnormalities seen in the infants with BPD remains chronic sublethal hypoxia.

In contrast to the major increase in the III-V interval, there were no apparent abnormalities in MLS BAER components that are mainly related to peripheral auditory function, including wave I and III latencies. There were also no appreciable abnormality in the I-III interval, which reflects functional status of the more peripheral or caudal regions of the auditory brainstem. These results suggest that functional status of the more peripheral regions of the auditory brainstem in BPD infants is relatively intact or only slightly affected. Therefore, chronic sublethal hypoxia does not have a major effect on functional integrity of the more peripheral regions of the auditory brainstem.

The major abnormalities in the MLS BAER variables that mainly reflect central neural function in infants with BPD suggest a significant delay in neural conduction, mainly reflecting impaired myelination, in the more central regions of the auditory brainstem. These infants also had a certain degree of abnormalities in click rate-dependent changes in MLS BAER central components, mainly reflecting a decreased efficacy of synaptic transmission. Therefore, chronic sublethal hypoxia associated with BPD has a detrimental effect on functional integrity of the auditory brainstem. However, peripheral neural function of the auditory pathway does not seem to be significantly affected.

## No Major Neuronal Impairment

Compared with wave latencies and interpeak intervals, the amplitudes of various wave components in the BAER have a relatively large across subject variability, which limits the usefulness of wave amplitudes (Chiappa 1990; Psatta and Matei, 1988). More recently, some BAER studies show that under well-controlled and consistent experimental conditions, the amplitudes of BAER waves, particularly wave V, are useful variables to reflect neuronal function of the auditory brainstem (Jiang, 1998,1999; Jiang and Tierney, 1996; Jiang et al., 2001,2006d,2008,2009a,b,d) A significant reduction in wave amplitudes after perinatal asphyxia is mainly related to impairment in neuronal function of the auditory brainstem (Jiang et al., 2006d,2008,2009a,b).

To examine whether there is any neuronal impairment in the auditory brainstem wave amplitudes in the MLS BAER have recently studied in infants with neonatal BPD (Jiang et al., 2009a). The amplitudes of waves I, III and V in the infants with BPD at 91-910/s clicks were all similar to those in the healthy very preterm infants, typically as shown by wave V amplitude at various click rates in Figure 7. At some rates, the amplitudes of waves III and V in the infants with BPD tended to be greater than those in the healthy very preterm infants. No significant differences were found between the two groups in any wave amplitudes at any click rates. Similarly, the V/I (Figure 8) and V/III amplitude ratios in the infants with BPD did not any significant differences from those in the healthy very preterm infants at any click rates.

As in the healthy very preterm infants, the amplitudes of waves I, III and V in the infants with BPD were all reduced with the increase in click rates, and were correlated significantly and negatively with the repetition rate of click stimuli. Regression analysis showed that both the intercepts and slopes of the amplitude-rate functions for waves I, III and V in the infants with neonatal BPD were similar to those in the healthy very preterm infants, without any significant differences. The V/I amplitude ratio did not show any significant and systematic change with varying click rate, which was similar to that in the healthy very preterm infants.

Taken together, there are no appreciable abnormalities in wave amplitudes in the MLS BAER. Such relatively normal wave amplitudes are in sharp contrast to the abnormal findings in wave latencies and intervals. It appears that neonatal BPD does not have any major effect on the neural origin of the amplitudes, which is more related to neuronal function, of MLS BAER components, although it has a significant effect on the neural origin of wave latencies and intervals, which is more related to neural conduction and myelination of the brainstem.

Acute severe or lethal hypoxia-ischemia can cause serious neuronal impairment and/or death in the neonatal brain and central auditory system. This results in fewer neurons contributing to BAER wave amplitudes and/or smaller contribution from each neuron, neural asynchrony, and a decrease in membrane potential of neurons, as reflected by a significant reduction in wave amplitudes in the MLS BAER in infants after perinatal asphyxia (Jiang et al., 2006d,2008,2009a,b). In neonatal BPD, however, the chronic sublethal hypoxia may be not severe enough to cause any major damage to neural origin of wave amplitudes in the MLS BAER, and thus there are no appreciable abnormalities in the amplitudes.

## IMPAIRED MYELINATION IN THE IMMATURE AUDITORY BRAINSTEM (- EVIDENCE FROM ANIMAL EXPERIMENTS)

During the perinatal and postnatal period the human central auditory pathway experiences considerable synaptogenesis, and after term there is a tremendous growth of dendrites (Moore et al., 1995,1997; Ponton et al., 1997; Norman 1975; Yakovlev and Lecour, 1967). Myelination occurs during the second growth spurt of the brain, which takes place in the second half of gestation and lasts well into the second postnatal year of later (Dobbing 1974). The auditory pathways in the brainstem myelinate early and rapidly before term, whereas other fibre systems at the level of the brainstem myelinate later at a slower rate (Brody et al., 1987; Yakovlev and Lecour, 1967). At term the auditory pathway is myelinated in 95% of infants. Neonatal BPD in very preterm infants occurs before term, corresponding to later phase of the second half of gestation. It is presumable that the rapid myelination of the auditory brainstem occurring during this period could be interfered by chronic sublethal hypoxia associated with neonatal BPD.

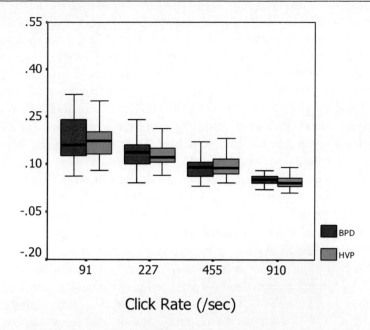

Figure 7. Means and standard errors of wave V amplitude recorded at term age with 91-910/sec clicks. The amplitude decreases with increasing click rate, and correlates significantly and negatively with click rate in both HVP and BPD infants (all P <0.01). The amplitude in BPD infants is similar to those in HVP infants at all click rates. The slope of wave V amplitude rate-function in BPD infants does not differ significantly from HVP infants.

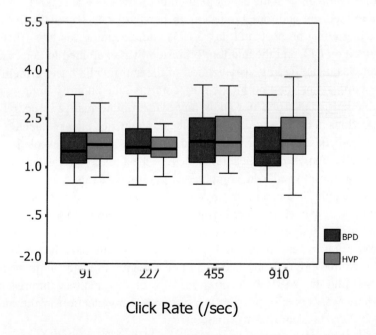

Figure 8. Means and standard errors of V/I amplitude ratio recorded at term age with 91-910/sec clicks. The amplitude ratio does not show any systematic change with varying click rate, and does not have any significant correlation with click rate in both HVP and BPD infants. The amplitude ratio in BPD infants is similar to those in HVP infants at all click rates, without any significant difference.

Neural conduction in the developing auditory brainstem is closely related to myelination in the auditory pathway. Myelination is one of the prominent morphological parameters to determine functional development in the central nervous system, including the auditory system. The brainstem auditory pathway, including rely nuclei and fibers, develops myelination in the fetal and early postnatal periods. The significant increase in the I-V and, in particular, III-V intervals in infants with BPD indicates impaired neural conduction and so impaired myelination in the more central regions of the auditory brainstem. The impairment is mainly related to or due to the chronic sublethal hypoxia associated with BPD. To test the hypothesis that chronic sublethal hypoxia affects myelination of the immature auditory brainstem, suggested by our electrophysiological study in infants with BPD, we carried out preliminary experiments in animal model of chronic sublethal hypoxia.

During the third trimester of gestation in human fetus or the first several weeks of postnatal life in very preterm infants, developmental events occurring in the immature brain is particularly susceptible to hypoxic episodes (Huttenlocher et al., 1982; Kostovic and Rakic, 1990). These events include the elaboration of axonal and dendritic arbors, the production and maintenance of synaptic contacts and the peak period of naturally occurring cell death (Dobbing 1971; Rothblat and Hayes, 1982; Olavarria and Van Sluyters, 1985; Ferrer et al, 1992; Malinak and Silverstein, 1996). Such events occurring during the period in the human brain are equivalent to those events occurring during the first 20 days of postnatal life in the developing rat brain. Therefore, the newborn rat provides a good model for studying the immature brain in very preterm infants who are at high risk of BPD. To mimic the chronic sublethal hypoxia that accompanies preterm birth, typically in BPD, newborn rats were reared in chronic sublethal hypoxia ($FiO_2$ 9.5%). Such newborn rat model of chronic sublethal hypoxia faithfully mimics the effect of preterm birth on the developing brain (Schwartz et al., 2004).

We examined the auditory brainstem in newborn rats reared in the environment with FiO2 9.5% beginning on postnatal day 3 (P3) and extending for day 10 (P13). The animals were sacrificed on P13, and the auditory brainstem was examined to detect any abnormalities. Myelination was quantified by visualization of the anti-myelin basic protein (MBP) antibody. Compared with age-matched normoxic rats (controls), the auditory brainstem in rats reared in chronic sublethal hypoxia did not show any evident abnormality in crysyl violet staining of brainstem sections at the levels of cochlear nucleus, superior olivary nucleus, lateral lemniscus, and inferior colliculus. However, electron microscopes analysis revealed striking changes in brainstem myelination. Axonal sheath thickness in the auditory brainstem of hypoxically reared animals was significantly reduced, compared with normoxic rats.

In the developing brainstem the myelination process is carried out by oligodendrocytes. Quantification of axonal number around oligodendrocytes showed less axonal sheath distribution in the auditory brainstem of animals reared in chronic sublethal hypoxia. The oligodendrocytes were less mature in hypoxically reared animals than in normoxically reared controls. There was a significant decrease in myelination in major white tracts of the auditory pathway. Staining for MBP in central regions of the auditory brainstem was markedly reduced. There was a patchy distribution of residual myelination in the auditory brainstem, with isolated discrete islands of myelination.

If myelination is affected by chronic sublethal hypoxia, there should be altered maturation in one or more oligodendrocyte linage stages in rats reared in chronic sublethal hypoxia. Thus, further work was carried out to address whether the poor or impaired myelination found in the auditory brainstem in rats reared in chronic sublethal hypoxia is related to abnormal oligodendrocyte lineage maturation. Staining with the O1 and O4 monoclonal antibodies demonstrated a significant reduction in the markers of premyelinating and early myelinating oligodendrocytes in the auditory brainstem. These findings suggest that hypoxia-induced poor myelination is due to abnormal oligodendrocyte lineage progression at the early oligodendrocyte progenitor stage.

Western analyses of MBP demonstrated that MBP expression was reduced in the auditory brainstem in hypoxically reared animals. It seems that chronic sublethal hypoxia inhibits the expression of MBP in the immature auditory brainstem. The reduced MBP expression verifies that chronic sublethal hypoxia damages myelination in the immature auditory brainstem and that chronic sublethal hypoxia damages the white matter. We further noticed that MBP expression was highest in the medulla, second in the pons, and lowest in the midbrain, which was basically similar in hypoxically and normoxically animals. This demonstrates that myelination in the auditory brainstem processes sequentially from caudal to rostral regions in developing animals, i.e. in a caudal-to-rostral fashion, but chronic sublethal hypoxia does not appear to affect the caudal-to-rostral fashion of myelination in the auditory brainstem.

Earlier reports regarding brain myelination in infants with BPD are somewhat controversial. Myelination was accelerated in some infants with BPD but delayed in the others (Takashima and Becker, 1984). Our results of animal experiments show clear evidence that neonatal chronic sublethal hypoxia reduces the extent of myelination in the auditory brainstem, and that the impaired myelination after chronic sublethal hypoxia is related to delayed pre-oligodendrocyte maturation.

## CONCLUSIONS

To date, our understanding of the influence of chronic sublethal hypoxia on the immature auditory system remains limited. In very preterm infants with BPD the significant abnormalities in the MLS BAER variables that mainly reflect central auditory function suggest a significant delay in neural conduction, mainly reflecting impaired myelination, in the more central regions of the auditory brainstem. These infants also had some abnormalities in click rate-dependent changes in MLS BAER central components, mainly reflecting a certain degree of decreased efficacy of synaptic transmission. In contrast, there is no major abnormality in peripheral neural function of the auditory pathway. Apparently, chronic sublethal hypoxia damages myelination and synaptic dysfunction in the immature central auditory system, with no major effect on neural function of the peripheral auditory system. In newborn rats reared in chronic sublethal hypoxia there is a significant reduction in myelination in major white tracts and staining of myelin basic protein in the auditory brainstem. Myelin basic protein expression was also reduced in the auditory brainstem. It appears that chronic sublethal hypoxia causes poor myelination and white matter injury and inhibits the expression of MBP in the auditory brainstem. These recent findings provide new insights into our understanding of the influence of chronic sublethal hypoxia on functional integrity of the very immature auditory system. These findings may have important clinical implications, particularly with regard to the study of therapeutic measures aimed at protecting the immature auditory system and improving auditory outcome in infants with chronic sublethal hypoxia resulting from various perinatal problems.

# REFERENCES

Bell, SL; Allen, R; Lutman, ME. The feasibility of maximum length sequences to reduce acquisition time of the middle latency response. *J Acoust Soc Am*, 2001, 109, 1073-1081.

Bell, SL; Allen, R; Lutman, ME. Optimizing the acquisition time of the middle latency response using maximum length sequences and chirps. *J Acoust Soc Am*, 2002, 112, 2065-2073.

Böhm, B; Katz-Salamon, M. Cognitive development at 5.5 years of children with chronic lung disease of prematurity. *Arch Dis Child Fetal Neonatal Ed*, 2003, 88, 101-105.

Brody, BA; Kinney, HC; Kloman, AS; Gilles, FH. Sequence of central nervous system myelination in human infancy. I. An autopsy study of myelinaion. *J Neuropathol Exp Neurol*, 1987, 46, 283-301.

Chiappa, KH. Brainstem auditory evoked potentials: Methodology. In: Chiappa KH, editor. Evoked Potentials in Clinical Medicine. New York: *Raven Press*, 1990. 173-221.

Curristin, SM; Cao, A; Stewart, WB; Zhang, H; Madri, JA; Morrow, JS; Ment, LR. Disrupted synaptic development in the hypoxic newborn brain. *Proc Natl Acad Sci USA*, 2002, 99, 15729-15734.

Dambska, M; Laure Kamionowska, M; Liebhart, M. Brainstem lesions in the course of chronic fetal asphyxia. *Clin Neuropathol*, 1987, 6, 110-115.

Dixon, G; Badawi, N; Kurinczuk, JJ; Keogh, JM; Silburn, SR; Zubrick, SR; Stanley, FJ. Early developmental outcomes after newborn encephalopathy. *Pediatrics* 2002, 109, 26–33.

Dobbing, J. The later growth of the brain and its vulnerability. *Pediatrics*, 1974, 53, 2-6.

Eysholdt, U; Schreiner, C. Maximum length sequences - a fast method for measuring brainstem evoked responses. *Audiology*, 1982, 21, 242-250.

Ferrer, I; Soriano, E; del Rio, JA; Alcántara, S; Auladell, C. Cell death and removal in the cerebral cortex during development. *Prog Neurobiol*, 1992, 39, 1-43.

Gonzalez, FF; Miller, SP. Does perinatal asphyxia impair cognitive function without cerebral palsy? *Arch Dis Child Fetal Neonatal Ed*, 2006, 91, F454–459.

GrandPré, T; Li, S; trittmatter, SM. Nogo-66 receptor antagonist peptide promotes axonal regeneration. *Nature*, 2002, 417, 547-551.

Greenough, A; Milner, AD. Pulmonary disease of the newborn: Chronic lung disease. In: Rennie JM; editor. Roberton's Textbook of Neonatology, 4th ed. Edinburgh, Schotland: *Elsevier Churchill Livingstone*, 2005. p. 554-572.

Gregoire, MC; Lefebvre, F; Glorieux, J. Health and developmental outcomes at 18 months in very preterm infants with bronchopulmonary dysplasia. *Pediatrics*, 1998, 101, 856-860.

Hack, M; Wright, LL; Shankaran, S; Tyson, JE; Horbar, JD; Bauer, CR; Younes, N. Very-low-birth-weight outcomes of the National Institute of Child Health and Human Development Neonatal Network, November 1989 to October 1990. *Am J Obstet Gynecol*, 1995, 172, 457-464.

Henderson-Smart, DJ; Pettigrew, AG; Edwards, DA; Jiang, ZD. Brain stem auditory evoked responses: physiological and clinical issues. In: Hanson MA, editor. The Fetal and Neonatal Brain Stem: developmental and clinical issues. Cambridge: *Cambridge University Press*, 1991. p. 211-29.

Hecox, K; Cone, B; Blaw, M: Brainstem auditory evoked response in the diagnosis of pediatric neurologic diseases. *Neurology*, 1981, 31, 832-839.

Huttenlocher, PR; De Courten, C; Garey, LJ; van der Loos, H. Synaptic development in human cerebral cortex. *Int J Neurol*, 1982-1983, 16-17, 144-154.

Hüppi, PS; Schuknecht, B; Boesch, C; Bossi, E; Felblinger, J; Fusch, C; Herschkowitz, N. Structural and neurobehavioral delay in postnatal brain development of preterm infants, *Pediatr Res*, 1996, 39, 895-901.

Hüppi, PS; Murphy, B; Maier, SE; Zientara, GP; Inder, TE; Barnes, PD; Kikinis, R; Jolesz, FA; Volpe, JJ. Microstructural brain development after perinatal cerebral white matter injury assessed by diffusion tensor magnetic resonance imaging. *Pediatrics*, 2001, 107, 455–460.

Inagaki, M; Kaga, M; Isumi, H; Hirano, S; Takashima, S; Nanba, E. Hypoxia-induced ABR changes and heat shock protein expression in the pontine auditory pathway of young rabbits. *Brain Res*, 1997, 757, 111-118.

Jiang, ZD. Long-term effect of perinatal and postnatal asphyxia on developing human auditory brainstem responses: peripheral hearing loss. *Int J Pediatr Otorhinolaryngol*, 1995, 33, 225-238.

Jiang,, ZD. Maturation of peripheral and brainstem auditory function in the first year following perinatal asphyxia - a longitudinal study. *J Speech Lang Hear Res*, 1998, 41, 83-93.

Jiang, ZD. Outcome of brainstem auditory electrophysiology in children who survived purulent meningitis. *Ann Otol Rhinol Laryngol*, 1999, 108, 429-434.

Jiang, ZD. Brainstem electrophysiological changes after perinatal hypoxia ischemia. In: Hämäläinen E; editor. New Trends in Brain Hypoxia Ischemia Research. New York: *Nova Science Publishers*, 2008. p. 203-220.

Jiang, ZD; Tierney, TS. Long-term effect of perinatal and postnatal asphyxia on developing human auditory brainstem responses: brainstem impairment. *Int J Pediatr Otorhinolaryngol*, 1996, 34, 111-127.

Jiang, ZD; Brosi, DM; Wilkinson, AR. Brainstem auditory evoked response recorded using maximum length sequences in term neonates. *Biol Neonat*, 1999, 76, 193-199.

Jiang, ZD; Brosi, DM; Shao, XM; Wilkinson, AR. Maximum length sequence brainstem auditory evoked response in infants after perinatal hypoxia-ischaemia. *Pediatr Res*, 2000, 48, 639-645.

Jiang, ZD; Brosi, DM; Wilkinson, AR. Comparison of brainstem auditory evoked responses recorded at different presentation rates of clicks in neonates after asphyxia. *Acta Paediatr*, 2001, 90, 1416-1420.

Jiang, ZD; Brosi, DM; Wilkinson, AR. Auditory neural responses to click stimuli of different rates in the brainstem of very preterm infants at term. *Pediatr Res*, 2002, 51, 454-459

Jiang, ZD; Brosi, DM; Wang, J; Xu, X; Chen, GQ; Shao, XM; Wilkinson, AR: Time course of brainstem pathophysiology during first month in term infants after perinatal asphyxia, revealed by MLS BAER latencies and intervals *Pediatr Res*, 2003, 54, 680 687.

Jiang, ZD; Yin, R; Shao, XM; Wilkinson, AR. Brainstem auditory impairment during the neonatal period in infants after asphyxia: dynamic changes in brainstem auditory evoked responses to different rate clicks. *Clin Neurophysiol*, 2004, 115, 1605-1615.

Jiang, ZD; Brosi, DM; Li, ZH; Chen, C; Wilkinson, AR. Brainstem auditory function at term in preterm babies with and without perinatal complications. *Pediatr Res*, 2005a, 58, 1164-1169.

Jiang, ZD; Woung, GM; Shao, XM. Dynamic changes in brainstem auditory electrophysiology in newborn piglets after ischaemia. *Pediatr Res*, 2005b, 58, 426.

Jiang, ZD; Brosi, DM; Wilkinson, AR. Brainstem auditory function in very preterm infants with chronic lung disease: Delayed neural conduction. *Clin Neurophysiol*, 2006a, 117, 1551-1559.

Jiang, ZD; Brosi, DM; Wilkinson, AR. Maximum length sequence BAER at term in low-risk babies born at 30-32 week gestation. *Brain Dev*, 2006b, 28, 1-7.

Jiang, ZD; Woung, JM; Shao, XM. Brainstem auditory conduction in hypoxic-ischaemic piglets treated with selective head cooling. *E-PAS*, 2006c, 59, 441.

Jiang, ZD; Shao, XM; Wilkinson, AR. Changes in BAER amplitudes after perinatal asphyxia during the neonatal period in term infants. *Brain Dev*, 2006d, 28, 554-559.

Jiang, ZD; Yin, R; Wilkinson, AR. Brainstem auditory evoked responses in very low birthweight infants with chronic lung disease. *Eur J Pediatr Neurol*, 2007a, 11, 153-159.

Jiang, ZD; Xu, X; Brosi, DM; Shao, XM; Wilkinson, AR. Sub-optimal function of the auditory brainstem in term neonates with transient low Apgar scores. *Clin Neurophysiol*, 2007b, 118, 1088-1096.

Jiang, ZD; Brosi, DM; Shao, XM; Wilkinson, AR. Sustained depression of brainstem auditory electrophysiology during the first month in term infants after perinatal asphyxia. *Clin Neurophysiol*, 2008, 119, 1496-1505.

Jiang, ZD; Brosi, DM; Wilkinson, AR. Brainstem auditory response amplitudes in neonatal chronic lung disease and comparison with perinatal asphyxia. *Clin Neurophysiol*, 2009a, 120, 967-973.

Jiang, ZD, Brosi, DM; Wilkinson, AR. Depressed brainstem auditory electrophysiology in preterm infants after perinatal hypoxia-ischemia. *J Neurolog Sci*, 2009b, 281, 28-33.

Jiang ZD, Brosi DM, Wilkinson AR. Impairment of perinatal hypoxia-ischaemia to the preterm brainstem. *J Neurolog Sci* 2009c;15:287:172-7.

Jiang, ZD; Brosi, DM; Wilkinson, AR. Changes in BAER wave amplitudes in relation to total serum bilirubin level in term neonates. *Eur J Pediatr*, 2009d, 168, 1243-1250.

Jiang ZD, Brosi D, Wu YY, Wilkinson AR. Relative maturation of the peripheral and central regions of the auditory brainstem from preterm to term and the influence of preterm birth. *Pediatr Res* 2009e, 65, 657-662.

Jiang, ZD; Brosi, DM; Wilkinson, AR. Differences in impaired brainstem conduction between neonatal chronic lung disease and perinatal asphyxia. *Clin Neurophysiol*, 2010 (in press).

Jirsa, RE. Maximum length sequences-auditory brainstem responses from children with auditory processing disorders. *J Am Acad Audiol*, 2001, 12, 155-164.

Johnston, MV; Trescher, WH; Taylor, GA. Hypoxic and ischaemic central nervous system disorders in infants and children. *Adv Ped*, 1995, 42, 1-5.

Johnston, M; Trescher, WH; Ishida, A; Nakajima W: Neurobiology of hypoxic-ischemic injury in the developing brain. *Pediatr Res*, 2001, 49, 735-741.

Katz-Salamon M; Gerner EM; Jonsson B; Lagercrantz H. Early motor and mental development in very preterm infants with chronic lung disease. Arch Dis Child 2000, 83, F1-6.

Ken-Dror, A; Pratt, H; Zeltzer, M; Sujov, P; Katzir, J; Benderley, A. Auditory brainstem evoked potentials to clicks at different presentation rates: estimating maturation of pre-term and full-term neonates. *Electroencephalog Clin Neurophysiol*, 1987, 68, 209-218.

Kileny, P; Connelly, C; Robertson, C. Auditory brainstem responses in perinatal asphyxia. *Int J Pediatr Otorhinolaryngol*, 1980, 2, 147-159.

Kim, JE; Li, S; GrandPré, T; Qiu, D; Strittmatter, SM. Axon regeneration in young adult mice lacking Nogo-A/B. *Neuron*, 2003, 38, 187-199.

Kostovic, I; Rakic, P. Developmental history of the transient subplate zone in the visual and somatosensory cortex of the macaque monkey and human brain. *J Comp Neurol*, 1990, 297, 441-470.

Krumholz, A; Felix, JK; Goldstein, PJ; McKenzie, E. Maturation of the brain stem auditory evoked potential in premature infants. *Electroenceph Clin Neurophysiol*, 1985, 62, 124-134.

Kurzner, SI; Garg, M; Bautista, DB; Sargent, CW; Bowman, M; Keens, TG. Growth failure in bronchopulmonary dysplasia, elevated metabolic rates and pulmonary mechanics. *J Pediatr*, 1988, 112, 73-80.

Lagercrantz, H; Ringstedt, T. Epigenetic and functional organization of the neuronal circuts in the CNS during development. In: Levene MI; Chervenak FA; Whittle M; editors. Fetal and neonatal neurology and neurosurgery, 4th ed. Edinburgh: Churchill-Livingstone, 2001, 3-9.

Lasky, RE. Rate and adaptation effects on the auditory evoked brainstem response in human newborns and adults. *Hear Res*, 1997, 11, 165-176.

Lasky, RE; Perlman, J; Hecox, K. Maximum length sequence auditory evoked brainstem responses in human newborns and adults. J Am Acad Audiol 1992, 3, 383-389.

Lasky, RE; Maier, MM; Hecox, K. Auditory evoked brain stem responses to trains of stimuli in human adults. *Ear Hear*, 1996, 17, 544-551.

Lasky, RE; Barry, D; Veen, V; Maier, MM. Nonlinear functional modelling of scalp recorded auditory evoked responses to maximum length sequences. *Hear Res*, 1998, 120, 133-142.

Leech, RW; Alvord, EC; Jr. Anoxic-ischemic encephalopathy in the human neonatal period: the significance of brain stem involvement. *Arch Neurol*, 1977, 34, 109-113.

Levene, MI. The newborn infant. In: Levene MI; Chervenak FA, Whittle M, editors. Fetal and neonatal neurology and neurosurgery, 4th ed. Edinburgh: Churchill-Livingstone, 2001, 471-504.

Levene, MI; Evans, DJ. Neurological problems in the newborn: Hypoxic-ischaemic brain injury. In: Rennie JM; editor. Roberton's Textbook of Neonatology, 4th ed. Edinburgh: *Elsevier Churchill Livingstone*, 2005, 1128-1148.

Lina Granade, G; Collet, L; Morgon, A. Auditory-evoked brainstem responses elicited by maximum-length sequences in normal and sensorineural ears. *Audiology*, 1994, 33, 218-236.

Majnemer, A; Rosenblatt, B; Riley, P. Prognostic significance of the auditory brainstem evoked response in high-risk neonates. *Dev Med Child Neurol*, 1988, 30, 43-52.

Malinak, C; Silverstein, FS. Hypoxic-ischemic injury acutely disrupts microtubule-associated protein 2 immunostaining in neonatal rat brain. *Biol Neonate*, 1996, 69, 257-267.

Marlow, N; Rose, AS; Rands, CE; Draper, ES. Neuropsychological and educational problems at school age associated with neonatal encephalopathy. *Arch Dis Child*, 2005, 90, 380-387.

Meisels, SJ; Plunkett, JW; Roloff, DW; Pasick, PL; Steifel, GS. Growth and development of preterm infants with respiratory distress syndrome and bronchopulmonary dysplasia. *Pediatrics*, 1987, 77, 345-352.

Ment, LR; Schwartz, M; Makuch, RW; Stewart, WB. Association of chronic sublethal hypoxia with ventriculomegaly in the developing rat brain. *Dev Brain Res*, 1998, 111, 197-203.

Moore, JK; Perazzo, LM; Braun, A. Time course of axonal myelination in the human brainstem auditory pathway. *Hear Res*, 1995, 87, 21-31.

Moore, JK; Guan, YL; Shi, SR. Axogenesis in the human fetal auditory system, demonstrated by neurofilament immunohistochemistry. *Anat Embryol Berl*, 1997, 195, 15-30.

Murphy, BP; Inder, TE; Huppi, PS; Warfield, S; Zientara, GP; Kikinis, R; Jolesz, FA; Volpe, JJ. Impaired cerebral cortical gray matter growth after treatment with dexamethasone for neonatal chronic lung disease. *Pediatrics*, 2001, 107, 217-221.

Myers, RE. Experimental models of perinatal brain damage: relevance to human pathology in intrauterine asphyxia and the developing fetal brain. In: Gluck L, editor. Asphyxia in the developing fetal brain. Chicago: *Year Book Publishers*, 1977. p. 39-97.

Natsume, J; Watanabe, K; Kuno, K; Hayakawa, F; Hashizume, Y. Clinical, neurophysiologic, and neuropathological features of an infant with brain damage of total asphyxia type (Myers). *Pediatr Neurol*, 1995, 13, 61-64.

Norman MG. Perinatal brain damage. Perspect Pediatric Pathol 1975, 4, 41-92.

Northway WH, Jr; Moss, RB; Carlisle, KB; Parker, BR; Popp, RL; Pitlick, PT; Eichler, I; Lamm, RL; Brown, BW; Jr. Late pulmonary sequelae of bronchopulmonary dysplasia. *N Engl J Med*, 1990, 323, 1793-1799.

Olavarria, J; Van Sluyters, RC. Organization and postnatal development of callosal connections in the visual cortex of the rat. *J Comp Neurol*, 1985, 239, 1-26.

Pasternak, JF. Hypoxic-ischemic brain damage in the term infants: lessons from the laboratory. *Pediatr Clin North Am*, 1993, 40, 1061-1072.

Paneth N. Classifying brain damage in preterm infants, J Pediatr 1999, 134, 527–529.

Perlman, JM. Neurobehavioral deficits in premature graduates of intensive care - potential medical and neonatal environmental risk factors. *Pediatrics.*, 2001, 108, 1339-1348.

Peterson, BS; Vohr, B; Staib, LH; Cannistraci, CJ; Dolberg, A; Schneider, KC; Katz, KH; Westerveld, M; Sparrow, S; Anderson, AW; Duncan, CC; Makuch, RW; Gore, JC; Ment, LR. Regional brain volume abnormalities and long-term cognitive outcome in preterm infants, *J Am Med Assoc*, 2000, 284, 1939-1947.

Pinto-Martin, JA; Whitaker, AH; Feldman, JF; Van Rossem, R; Paneth, N. Relation of cranial ultrasound abnormalities in low-birthweight infants to motor or cognitive performance at ages 2, 6 and 9 years. *Dev Med Child Neurol*, 1999 Dec, 41, 826-833.

Picton, TW; Champagne, SC; Kekkett, AJ. Human auditory evoked potentials recorded using maximum length sequences. *Electroencephalog Clin Neurophysiol*, 1992, 84, 90-100.

Poets, CF; Stebbens, VA; Richard, D; Southall, DP. Prolonged episodes of hypoxia in preterm infants indetectable by cardiorespiratory monitors. *Pediatrics*, 1995, 95, 860-863.

Ponton, CW; Moore, JK; Eggermont, JJ. Auditory brain stem response generation by parallel pathways: differential maturation of axonal conduction time and synaptic transmission. *Ear Hear*, 1997, 17, 402-410.

Psatta, DM; Matei, M. Age-dependent amplitude variation of brain-stem auditory evoked potentials. *Electroencephalogr Clin Neurophysiol*, 1988, 71, 27-32.

Rennie, JM; Hagmann, CF; Robertson, NJ. Outcome after intrapartum hypoxic ischaemia at term. *Semin Fetal Neonatal Med*, 2007, 12, 398-407.

Rothblat, LA; Hayes, LL. Age-related changes in the distribution of visual callosal neurons following monocular enucleation in the rat. *Brain Res*, 1982, 246, 146-149.

Scher, MS; Richardson, GA; Salerno, DG; Day, NL; Guthrie, RD. Sleep architecture and continuity measures of neonates with chronic lung disease. *Sleep.*, 1992, 15, 195-201.

Short, EJ; Klein, NK; Lewis, BA; Fulton, S; Eisengart, S; Kercsmar, C; Baley, J; Singer, LT; Cognitive and academic consequences of bronchopulmonary dysplasia and very low birth weight: 8-year-old outcomes. *Pediatrics*, 2003, 112, 359-9.

Singer, L; Yamashita, T; Linlien, L; Collin, M; Baley, J. A longitudinal study of developmental outcome of infants with bronchopulmonary dysplasia and very low birth weight. *Pediatrics*, 1997, 100, 987-993.

Skidmore, MD; Rivers, A; Hack, M. Increased risk of cerebral palsy among very low-birthweight infants with chronic lung disease. *Dev Med Child Neurol*, 1990, 32, 325-332.

Sohmer, H; Freeman, S; Gafni, M; Goitein, K. The depression of the auditory nerve-brainstem evoked response in hypoxemia - mechanism and site of effect. *Electroencephalog Clin Neurophysiol*, 1986a, 64, 334-338.

Sohmer, H; Freeman, S; Malachi, S. Multi-modal evoked potentials in hypoxemia. *Electroenceph Clin Neurophysiol*, 1986b, 64, 328-333.

Schwartz, MLS; Vaccarino, F; Chacon, M; Yan, WL; Ment, LR; Stewart, WB. Chronic neonatal hypoxia leads to long term decreases in the volume and cell number of the rat cerebral cortex. *Semin Perinatol*, 2004, 28, 379-388.

Stewart, WB; Ment, LR; Schwartz, M. Chronic postnatal hypoxia increases the numbers of cortical neurons. *Brain Res*, 1997, 760, 17-21.

Takashima, S; Becker, LE. Developmental neuropathology in bronchopulmonary dysplasia: alteration of glial fibrillary acidic protein and myelination. Brain Dev 1984, 6, 451-457.

Thompson, DK; Warfield, SK; Carlin, JB; Pavlovic, M; Wang, HX; Bcar, M; Kean, MJ; Doyle, LW; Egan, GF; Inder, TE. Perinatal risk factors altering regional brain structure in the preterm infant. *Brain*, 2007, 130, 667-677.

Urbani, L; Lucertini, M. Effects of hypobaric hypoxia on the human auditory brainstem responses. *Hear Res*, 1994, 76, 73-77.

Vannucci, RC. Experimental biology of cerebral hypoxia-ischemia: relation to perinatal brain damage. *Pediatr Res*, 1990, 27, 317-326.

Vohr, BR; Msall, ME. Neuropsychological and functional outcomes of very low birth weight infants, *Semin Perinatol*, 1997, 21, 202–220.

Vohr, BR; Wright, LL; Dusick, AM; Mele, L; Verter, J; Steichen, JJ; Simon, NP; Wilson, DC; Broyles, S; Bauer, CR; Delaney-Black, V; Yolton, KA; Fleisher, BF; Papile, LA; Kaplan, MD. Neurodevelopmental and functional outcomes of extremely low birth weight infants in the National Institute of Child Health and Human Development Neonatal Research Network, 1993-1994. *Pediatrics*, 2000, 105, 1216-1226.

Volpe, JJ. Neurologic outcome of prematurity, *Arch Neurol*, 1998, 55, 297-300.

Volpe, JJ. Perinatal brain injury. From pathogenesis to neuroprotection. *Ment Retard Dev Disabil Res Rev*, 2001, 7, 56–64.

Volpe, JJ: Hypoxic-ischemic encephalopathy: Clinical aspects. In: Volpe JJ, editor. Neurology of the Newborn. 4th ed, Philadelphia (PA): *WB Saunders*, 2001, 331-94.

Weber, BA; Roush, PA. Application of maximum length sequence analysis to auditory brainstem response testing of premature newborns. *J Am Acad Audiol*, 1993, 4, 157-162.

Weiss, J; Takizawa, B; McGee, A; Stewart, WB; Zhang, H; Ment, L; Schwartz, M; Strittmatter, S. Neonatal hypoxia suppresses oligodendrocyte Nogo-A and increases axonal sprouting in a rodent model for human prematurity. *Exp Neurol*, 2004, 189, 141-149.

Wilkinson, AR; Jiang, ZD. Brainstem auditory evoked response in neonatal neurology. *Semin Fet Neonatol Med*, 2006, 11, 444-451.

Wilkinson, AR; Brosi, DM; Jiang, ZD. Functional impairment of the brainstem in infants with bronchopulmonary dysplasia. *Pediatrics*, 2007, 120, 362-371.

Yakovlev, PI; Lecour, A. The myelogenetic cycles of regional maturation of the brain. In: Minkowski AFA, editor. Regional Development of the Brain in Early Life. Philadelphia: *Davis*, 1967, 3-69.

Yin, R; Wilkinson, AR; Chen, C; Brosi, DM; Jiang, ZD. No close correlation between brainstem auditory function and peripheral auditory threshold in preterm infants. *Clin Neurophysiol*, 2008, 119, 791-795.

In: Deafness, Hearing Loss and the Auditory System
Editors: D. Fiedler and R. Krause, pp.181-195

ISBN: 978-1-60741-259-5
©2010 Nova Science Publishers, Inc.

*Chapter 6*

# TREATMENT OF TINNITUS WITH TRANSCRANIAL MAGNETIC STIMULATION

## *Tobias Kleinjung[1,3]\* and Berthold Langguth[2,3]*

[1]Department of Otorhinolaryngology, University of Regensburg, Germany
[2]Department of Psychiatry and Psychotherapy, University of Regensburg, Germany
[3]Interdisciplinary Tinnitus Center, University of Regensburg, Germany

## ABSTRACT

The pathophysiology of tinnitus remains incompletely understood and treatment is elusive. Recent neurophysiological and neuroimaging data suggest that some forms of tinnitus are associated with synchronized hyperactivity in the auditory cortex. Therefore targeted modulation of tinnitus-related cortical hyperactivity has been considered as a new promising treatment strategy. Repetitive transcranial magnetic stimulation (rTMS) is a non-invasive method for modifying neural activity in the stimulated area and at a distance along functional anatomical connections. This chapter will summarize the effects of clinical studies using rTMS in tinnitus patients.

This technique can be applied in two different ways in diagnosing and treating tinnitus patients. One approach uses single sessions of high-frequency rTMS applied to the temporal cortex. This method has shown success in suppressing tinnitus transiently during the time of stimulation and has been suggested as a predictor for treatment outcome of direct electrical epidural stimulation with implanted electrodes. Low-frequency rTMS is an efficient method to selectively reduce the abnormally increased activity in cortical areas. Several small controlled studies demonstrated beneficial effects in tinnitus patients after repeated sessions of low-frequency rTMS. In some patients, treatment effects outlasted the stimulation period by twelve months and more. However, available studies are characterized by the high inter-individual variability of treatment effects and only moderate effect sizes. Basic research should focus on a better understanding of the neurobiological effects of this technique. Clinical studies with larger sample sizes can provide more information on the impact of patient-related (e.g. hearing

---

\* Corresponding author: Department of Otorhinolaryngology, University of Regensburg, Franz-Josef-Strauss-Allee 11, D-93053 Regensburg, Germany, E-mail: tobias.kleinjung@klinik.uni-regensburg.de, Phone: +49 941 944 9505, Fax: +49 941 944 9512.

loss, age, tinnitus-duration) and stimulation-related (e.g. frequency, target control) factors on treatment outcome.

## 1. TINNITUS: INTRODUCTION, EPIDEMIOLOGY AND CLASSIFICATION

Tinnitus is the perception of sound in the head or the ears in the absence of an external sound source. The word "tinnitus" derives from the Latin verb "tinnire", meaning to ring. With a prevalence of 10-15% in the adult population, tinnitus is a frequent condition [1,2]. In about 5% tinnitus is perceived as moderately or severely annoying and in 0.5% tinnitus severely affects the ability to lead a normal life [3].

Tinnitus can be divided into two categories, objective and subjective tinnitus. Objective tinnitus is relatively rare and is caused by sound generated in the body, usually in the ear, head or neck, reaching the cochlea through conduction in body tissues [4]. The sound source can either be turbulences in blood vessels or muscle contractions. In some cases these conditions can be heard by an observer using a stethoscope. Subjective tinnitus reflects meaningless sounds which are not associated with a physical sound and only the person who has the tinnitus can hear it. Auditory hallucinations are meaningful sounds like music or voices. These hallucinations occur not exclusively but most frequently in psychiatric disorders such as schizophrenia. In the following, this chapter will only be concerned with subjective tinnitus and will not discuss objective tinnitus or auditory hallucinations.

As a purely subjective phenomenon, tinnitus is difficult to measure and has many different clinical forms [5]. It can be localized to one ear or both ears and it can be heard in the center of the head. Subjective tinnitus often occurs in combination with hearing loss. The hearing loss can have different reasons such as noise trauma, presbyacusis, Meniere´s disease, acoustic neuroma or middle-ear disease. In fact any lesion along the auditory tract may cause tinnitus, but it may also occur in subjects with normal hearing. The different forms of tinnitus may vary in their pathophysiology and in the exact anatomical location of the physiological abnormalities, but central parts of the auditory nervous system seem to be involved in all cases [6]. A frequent comorbidity of tinnitus is hyperacusis, which is defined as an abnormal, lowered tolerance to (any) sound [7].

Even if tinnitus is a purely subjective phenomenon, there are several techniques available for the clinical assessment of tinnitus: psychoacoustical measurement of tinnitus loudness, pitch and maskability allow a quantitative evaluation [8]. In detail different tones and sounds are presented to the patient, who is asked to indicate what frequency and loudness best fits or masks his tinnitus. The subjective tinnitus intensity and loudness can be quantified by visual analogue scales or numeric rating scales [5]. Interestingly, even sounds that are rated as highly intensive or very loud are usually matched between 5 and 10 dB above hearing threshold, which complies with the intensity of a whisper [9]. There is only a poor correlation between the results obtained by psychoacoustical measurement procedures and the degree of annoyance the tinnitus creates [10]. Therefore the degree of tinnitus severity and distress is best evaluated by validated self-report tinnitus questionnaires [11]. This technique plays an important role in the evaluation of effects before, during and after tinnitus therapy.

Many patients learn to ignore the sounds and experience no major effects; others experience the tinnitus as very troublesome. In those patients tinnitus is frequently associated with anxiety, depression and insomnia [12, 13] and is very difficult to treat. Successful therapeutic strategies are obviously hampered by the heterogeneity of underlying mechanisms that can cause tinnitus. Therefore the most frequently used standard therapies like auditory stimulation and cognitive behavioural therapy attempt to manage the situation rather than cure the underlying symptom [14]. More causally oriented therapeutic strategies are lacking and need to be developed to relieve tinnitus and tinnitus-related distress.

## 2. TINNITUS PATHOPHYSIOLOGY

Subjective tinnitus is the perception of sound in the absence of an external stimulus. Even if it is natural to expect this symptom to originate in the ear, there is increasing evidence that many forms of auditory phantom perceptions are mainly due to alterations in the central auditory system. The fact that tinnitus can develop after transection of the auditory nerve was a first indicator for a possible central origin of the symptom [15]. Neural plasticity appears to play a central role in the development of the central abnormalities that can cause tinnitus [16]. Deprivation of input is a strong promoter of an expression of neural plasticity, which explains why tinnitus often appears together with hearing loss related to different otological pathologies [17]. Expression of neural plasticity can change the balance between excitation and inhibition in the nervous system, promote hyperactivity and cause reorganization [16]. Similar to phantom limb pain, it is suggested that most forms of tinnitus may be a maladaptive manifestation of cortical reorganisation after damage to peripheral auditory structures [18].

The auditory system consists of two main parallel pathways providing auditory information to the cerebral cortex: the tonotopically organized classical (lemniscal) system, and the non-tonotopic non-classical (extralemniscal) system. Whereas the classical pathways project directly to the primary auditory cortex, the non-classical pathways project to the secondary auditory cortex and association cortices, thus bypassing the primary cortex and representing a direct connection between the auditory tract and non-auditory brain areas. Presumably it is this non-classical pathway which mediates the influence of emotional state on neural activity in auditory pathways [19]. Studies have found signs that these pathways are active in subjects with severe tinnitus, indicating that these structures might be responsible for the degree of tinnitus-related distress [20].

Animal studies demonstrate that tinnitus is related to an increase of firing rate and neuronal synchrony in both classical and non-classical pathways [21-23], resulting in alterations of the tonotopic maps [24]. These changes occur as a consequence of neuroplastic reorganization due to an acute or chronic lack of auditory input [25]. Accordingly, studies of tinnitus patients with magnetoencephalography (MEG) have shown reorganisation of the auditory cortex with a shift in the tonotopic map of the auditory cortex at the tinnitus frequency [26]. The model of thalamocortical dysrhythmia, which has been elaborated by Llinas and co-workers [27], could provide an explanation for the changes of neural activity observed in tinnitus patients. According to this model, thalamic deafferentiation from auditory input, which is associated with hearing loss, may produce slow theta-frequency oscillations in thalamocortical ensembles due to changes in the firing pattern of thalamic relay cells. As an "edge effect", a reduced lateral inhibition at the cortical level was thought to generate high-frequency activity in the gamma band (30-50 Hz) that could be the neuronal correlate of the positive symptoms of tinnitus percept [28]. This in turn may participate in cortical reorganization via simple Hebbian mechanisms and neural plasticity phenomena that occur after sensorial deafferentation and finally result in alterations of the tonotopic maps [25]. However, even if this model of thalamocortical dysrhythmia can provide an explanation for some aspects of tinnitus generation, experimental data for its support are still very limited.

Recent advantages in functional imaging have offered new possibilities in visualizing cerebral areas of altered neuronal activity. Data coming from $[^{15}O]H_2O$ positron emission tomography (PET) in patients who could alter their tinnitus by movements of mouth, face or eyes demonstrated an association of tinnitus loudness with increased regional cerebral blood flow (rCBF) predominantly in temporoparietal areas of the cerebral cortex [29-31]. Accordingly, the transient reduction of tinnitus by intravenous lidocaine infusion showed increased rCBF in temporoparietal regions during the phase of loud tinnitus perception [32, 33]. In patients with unilateral tinnitus, functional resonance imaging (fMRI) revealed reduced blood oxygen level-dependent (BOLD) contrast in the contralateral auditory system after auditory stimulation [34, 35]. In patients with bilateral tinnitus, fMRI activation induced by auditory stimulation was symmetrical in the investigated areas of the auditory pathway (auditory cortex, thalamus, inferior colliculus) [34]. In contrast to fMRI, which only can visualize brain activity changes in response to a stimulus, Fluordeoxyglucose (FDG) PET allows experts to analyze the level of steady-state activity in the brain of tinnitus patients (see Figure 1). Several investigations using this technique have demonstrated asymmetrical FDG uptake with higher levels of spontaneous activity within the left auditory cortex, irrespective of tinnitus laterality [36-39]. In addition to alterations in the auditory system, imaging studies confirmed involvement of limbic and frontal areas (amygdala, hippocampus, anterior cingulate, orbitofrontal cortex). It is assumed that altered activity in these regions reflects tinnitus-related emotional distress [30, 40, 41].

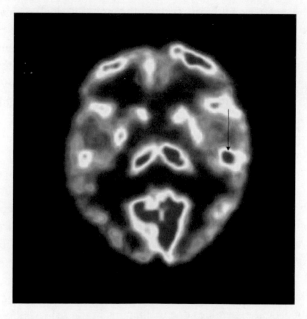

Figure 1. This axial slice from a FDG PET scan illustrates unilaterally increased metabolic activity in the left temporal cortex of a tinnitus patient.

## 3. THE RATIONALE FOR THE APPLICATION OF TRANSCRANIAL MAGNETIC STIMULATION (TMS) IN TINNITUS PATIENTS

Neuroimaging and electrophysiological studies clearly indicate that tinnitus is related to alterations of neuronal function on the cortical and subcortical levels. Consequently a technique which allows an interference of the neural activity in these regions should be able to influence tinnitus perception. Transcranial magnetic stimulation (TMS) is a non-invasive electromagnetic method for brain stimulation [42, 43]. The magnetic field passes almost without attenuation through the skull and induces neuronal depolarisation in superficial brain areas without causing pain. Magnetic coils can have different shapes. Round coils are relatively powerful. Figure-eight-shaped coils are more focal with a maximal current at the intersection of the two round components. The insulated coil is held over the region of particular interest by a mechanical arm. A brief, high electrical current in the coil produces a strong magnetic field (1.5-2 Tesla). An electrical field is induced perpendicular to the magnetic field and causes a flow of current in the superficial cortex and electric charges accumulate on neuronal membranes, resulting in neuronal depolarisation (see Figure 2). Whereas single magnetic pulses do not seem to have longer lasting effects, the application of multiple pulses in rhythmic session, called repetitive TMS (rTMS), can block or inhibit focal brain function and create a transient functional lesion in the immediate poststimulation period [44]. This can be used as a non-invasive approach to test whether tinnitus can be transiently interrupted by interfering with neural activity in specific superficial brain areas.

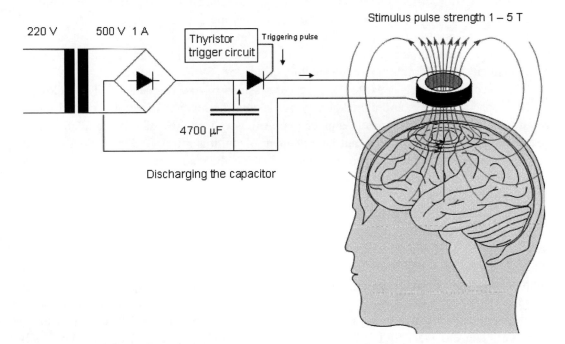

Figure 2. The basic principle of transcranial magnetic stimulation: short pulses of high amplitude current which are generated in a stimulator produce a magnetic field in the coil which passes largely undistorted through the skull and induces electric currents in superficial neurons of the brain (adapted with permission from: Jaako Malmivuo & Robert Plonsey: Bioelectromagnetism - Principles and Applications of Bioelectric and Biomagnetic Fileds, Oxford University Press, New York, 1995).

Furthermore rTMS can induce specific after-effects that outlast the stimulation period. In general, cortical excitability is decreased by low-frequency ($\leq 1$ Hz) rTMS [45, 46] and increased by high-frequency (5-20 Hz) rTMS [47, 48]. Moreover, the repetition of multiple pulses of rTMS on subsequent days can reinforce and prolong rTMS effects, which might represent a potential treatment method. Additional support for this rationale comes from the promising results of rTMS treatment of other pathological conditions with increased cortical activity such as auditory hallucinations, writer's cramp or obsessive compulsive disorders [49-51].

## 4. CRITICAL DISCUSSION OF CLINICAL EFFECTS OF rTMS IN TINNITUS

During the last decade the effect of r TMS in tinnitus patients has been investigated in several studies in different countries (for review see also [52, 53]). Single sessions of rTMS have been performed in order to transiently interrupt tinnitus perception [54-57]. In these types of studies, mainly trains of high-frequency rTMS (10-20 Hz) were administered. The largest study investigated the effect of single sessions of rTMS in 114 patients with unilateral tinnitus at frequencies between 1 and 20 Hz over the auditory cortex contralateral to the tinnitus [55]. In this study the amount of tinnitus suppression correlated with higher stimulation frequency and with shorter tinnitus duration, indicating the potential of TMS as a diagnostic tool for differentiating pathophysiologically distinct forms of chronic tinnitus. Furthermore, this approach has been used as a screening method to select patients for surgical implantation of cortical electrodes. Patients responding to this type of rTMS with a short-lasting suppression of tinnitus perception were considered good surgical candidates for a permanent electrical stimulation of the auditory cortex [58, 59].

The second approach consisted of repeated sessions of low-frequency (1 Hz) rTMS on several consecutive days and aimed at a longer lasting modulation of tinnitus related neural activity as a potential therapeutic application. Almost all studies of this stimulation type demonstrated statistically significant improvement of tinnitus after rTMS treatment [37, 60-66]. However, the amount of improvement varied across the studies and the average treatment effect was only moderate. This was reflected by a reduction of tinnitus perception, but not a complete suppression in most cases. Such positive treatment effects occurred on an average of about 50% of the subjects treated. Most rTMS treatment studies applied low-frequency rTMS in long trains of 1200-2000 pulses repeatedly over 5-10 days. Practically all studies addressed temporal or temporoparietal cortical areas. The methods for coil localisation varied across the studies, ranging from highly sophisticated neuronavigation based techniques to easily applied methods. The use of neuronavigational systems allows experts to localize the coil exactly over the area of increased activity based on individual imaging data. The target region for the camera system of the neuronavigation machine was defined by different functional imaging techniques such as FDG PET [37, 65], [$^{15}$O]H$_2$O PET [32, 60] or fMRI [66]. More easily applied techniques include coil localisation according to the 10-20 EEG coordinate system [62] or to anatomical landmarks as provided by structural MRI scans [61]. Even if comparison across the studies is difficult due to differences in the study design, there is no indication that any one of these techniques is superior to the others.

Tinnitus is a subjective condition, which might be susceptible to placebo effects. Therefore evaluation of treatment efficacy requires adequate methodology to check for unspecific treatment effects. The majority of controlled studies published so far has used placebo treatment either by coil angulations 45° or 90° away from the skull [65] or by the use of a so-called sham-coil system [37], which mimics the sound of the active coil without producing a magnetic field. Other techniques for the placebo condition consist of the stimulation of non-auditory brain areas [60, 64] or the stimulation of head or neck muscles without reaching brain areas. Due to limitations in the blinding of patient and operator to different stimulus conditions and the fact that TMS itself results in a multimodal sensory stimulation in addition to the actual brain site specific effect, the optimum placebo condition has not yet been determined precisely.

Whereas some studies demonstrated effects that outlasted the stimulation period by 3,4, 6 or 12 months [37, 64, 67], others were not able to observe lasting effects [32, 60, 63] at all. The number of daily sessions may be an important issue to achieve sustained results in tinnitus patients, as already seen in other TMS applications, like depression and auditory hallucinations [68, 69].

The high variability of treatment results, which is encountered in all studies, supports the notion of the neurobiological heterogeneity of distinct subtypes of tinnitus. This in turn implies that no single approach will be successful in every patient. In this context the identification of treatment predictors is of importance. Several rTMS studies indicate tinnitus duration as a robust predictor for treatment response. Tinnitus with shorter duration (less than 3-4 years) is related to better treatment outcome [55, 60, 61, 64]. Hearing impairment has been identified as a negative predictor in one study [61]. Deprivation from auditory input is assumed to induce disinhibition in the central auditory system, which in turn is believed to be critically involved in the generation of tinnitus. Thus a high degree of hearing impairment might attenuate rTMS effects by perpetually triggering neuroplastic changes in central auditory structures.

Another important issue is the choice of outcome measurements in rTMS studies. As there is still a lack of objective methods for the assessment of treatment-induced changes, validated tinnitus questionnaires and visual analogue scales (VAS) serve as a primary outcome measurement in the majority of studies [70, 71]. By quantifying treatment results, these methods allow experts to determine whether rTMS induced changes reach statistical significance, but it remains to be demonstrated which amount of change is of clinical relevance. The additional use of a clinical global impression scale (CGI) can be of further value in this context [60, 72]. Functional imaging techniques before and after treatment may contribute to a better understanding of rTMS effects in tinnitus treatment studies [65].

Recent research was seeking the optimization of treatment effects in different ways. First, stimulation parameters were modified. Based on preclinical findings that showed that the effects of 1 Hz might be enhanced by priming stimulation with 6 Hz [73], a standard protocol of 1 Hz has been compared with a priming stimulation protocol where 1Hz rTMS was administered after 6Hz rTMS. Both treatment protocols reduced tinnitus severity; however, there was no difference between the standard and the priming protocol [74]. Second, the coil position was subject to change. New insights into neurobiology of chronic tinnitus suggested that functional abnormalities are not limited to temporal and temporoparietal cortical areas, but can also occur in brain areas used for attentional and emotional processing, such as the dorsolateral prefrontal cortex [40]. A recently published study demonstrated a more pronounced long-term effect of a combined treatment protocol of rTMS applied to the temporal and dorsolateral prefrontral cortex as compared to an exclusive stimulation of the temporal cortex [75]. Third, recently it was suggested that the suppressing effect of low-frequency rTMS can be enhanced by pharmacologic activation of dopamine receptors [76]. However, in tinnitus patients the application of L-Dopa prior to each rTMS session did not enhance TMS effects [77]. Just recently a case report demonstrated the feasibility of maintenance rTMS for the management of chronic tinnitus [78]. In this patient, tinnitus was reduced repeatedly by one to three maintenance sessions and finally remained stable on a low level after the third stimulation round. The positive clinical effect of this maintenance stimulation was reflected by reduced cerebral metabolism in PET imaging after treatment.

## 5. NEUROBIOLOGICAL RFFECTS OF rTMS IN TINNITUS PATIENTS

In section 3 of this chapter we speculated about the rationale for rTMS as a causally oriented tinnitus therapy. This section will summarize the available knowledge about the mechanisms that underlie the clinical effects.

Even if there is increasing evidence that rTMS interferes with neuronal mechanisms involved in the pathophysiology of tinnitus, the exact mechanisms of action of the different applications are not clear. Animal data [47], and longitudinal imaging or electrophysiological data before and after temporal rTMS in control and tinnitus subjects are still very limited [65, 79, 80]. Therefore our knowledge of the underlying neurobiological effects remains speculative, since it is mainly based on analogies with direct electrical stimulation in animals or on data about rTMS effects on motor cortex excitability.

One possible mechanism is that low frequency rTMS evokes long-term-depression (LTD) like effects [45]. The prolongation of the cortical silent period after temporal rTMS may reflect LTD mediated enhancement of subcortical inhibition [79]. However, whereas LTD-like effects should be more pronounced when areas of increased excitability are stimulated [45, 81], in tinnitus patients enhanced activity of the stimulated area seems not to increase TMS effects [32, 38, 74]. Also the application of dopaminergic drugs known to facilitate LTD effects [76] did not enhance rTMS treatment effects [77].

An alternative explanation could be that rTMS disrupts the malfunctioning network involved in tinnitus generation and thereby facilitates the plastic reversal of maladaptive changes that led to tinnitus. This hypothesis is supported by the recent studies of Khedr et al., which indicates that rTMS effects in tinnitus treatment do not critically depend on stimulation frequency and show long-term effects up to one year [64, 67].

It also remains to be elucidated whether TMS exerts its effects primarily in the directly stimulated area or whether the clinical effects are mediated by changes in more remote areas. There is some electrophysiologic and imaging data which suggests that TMS over the temporal cortex interferes with tinnitus by modulating thalamocortical processing [79, 82].

Another possibility is that TMS over auditory areas modifies the connectivity between the auditory system and non-auditory areas. A recent magnetoencephalographic study suggests that tinnitus distress correlates with the degree of neuronal synchrony between temporal and frontal areas [83]. So it is conceivable that rTMS may exert its effects on tinnitus by interfering with this long range connectivity between thalamocortical auditory activity and neuronal activity related to emotional distress. Further support for this theory comes from the finding that combined frontal and temporal TMS revealed superior effects compared to temporal stimulation alone [75].

## 6. SAFETY AND SIDE EFFECTS OF TMS

The safety of rTMS is proven by an extensive body of data, especially if it is performed according to published safety guidelines [84]. It is essential that contraindications such as electronic implants (e.g. cardiac pace makers, cochlea implants), intracranial pieces of metal or previous epileptic seizures are considered. Most data is available from rTMS studies in depressed subjects. After 2- 4 weeks of daily prefrontal rTMS there was no sign of structural MRI changes [85], no significant changes in auditory thresholds and no significant electroencephalogram abnormalities [86]. Adverse auditory effects such as hearing loss or auditory hallucinations have not been reported after temporal rTMS so far. The risk of high-intensity and high-frequency rTMS induced epileptic seizures, which had been reported in individual cases, has been largely reduced since the introduction of safety guidelines [84]. Mild adverse effects such as light local sensation of pain on the skull beneath the coil during stimulation or transient headache after stimulation are reported by about 10-20% of the patients stimulated.

## 7. CONCLUSION

Almost all available studies have shown that TMS reduces tinnitus in a subgroup of patients, and that the effect reaches statistical significance for the whole group. This clearly demonstrates that TMS is a very promising new approach for the treatment of tinnitus. Even more important, TMS seems to represent a causally oriented treatment. In other words, whereas most other currently available treatments for tinnitus aim to "*learn to live with tinnitus*", the goal of TMS is to "*overlearn*" the neuronal changes which cause the perception of tinnitus.

However it has to be considered that at the moment TMS is still at an early stage of development. Applied for the first time in 2002, clinical and scientific experience is still relatively limited. Other important limitations are that the currently used stimulation procedures do not completely suppress tinnitus but only reduce it. The average treatment effect is only moderate. This is due to the fact that not every patient benefits from TMS. This in turn can be explained by the fact that there are different forms of tinnitus which probably differ in their underlying neuronal mechanisms. Most studies have shown that positive effects occur in about half of the patients stimulated. Here it seems that patients with a shorter duration of tinnitus have a higher chance for improvement. Further research is needed for identifying additional clinical and neurobiological predictors for treatment outcome. This might even result in more individualized treatment protocols. The monitoring of rTMS effects with electrophysiological and neuroimaging methods might contribute to a better understanding of neurobiological mechanisms that underlie the clinical effects.

In summary, the available clinical data has shown promise that rTMS has the potential to manage distinct forms of tinnitus. Replication of data in multicenter trials with long-term follow-up and more detailed knowledge of neurobiological mechanisms are essential before this technique can be considered the standard treatment in clinical routine.

## 8. ABBREVIATONS

| | |
|---|---|
| BOLD | Blood oxygen level dependent |
| EEG | Electroencephalography |
| FDG PET | Fluordeoxyglucose positron emission tomography |
| fMR | Functional magnetic resonance imaging |
| LTD | Long-term depression |
| MEG | Magnetoencephalography |
| MRI | Magnetic resonance imaging |
| PET | Positron emission tomography |
| rCBF | Regional cerebral blood flow |
| rTMS | Repetitive transcranial magnetic stimulation |
| TMS | Transcranial magnetic stimulation |

## REFERENCES

[1]     Axelsson, A. & Ringdahl, A. (1989). Tinnitus - a study of its prevalence and characteristics. *Br J Audiol.*, *23*, 53-62.

[2]     Davis, A. C. (1989). The prevalence of hearing impairment and reported hearing disability among adults in Great Britain. *Int J Epidemiol.*, *18*, 911-917.

[3]     Davis, A. C. & El Rafaie A. (2000). Epidemiology of tinnitus. In: R. S. Tyler, (Ed.), *Tinnitus Handbook* (1st edition, 1-23). Clifton Park, NY: Thomson Learning.

[4]     Møller, A. R. (2003). Pathophysiology of tinnitus. *Otolaryngol Clin North Am.*, *36*, 249-66.

[5]     Langguth, B., Goodey, R., Azevedo, A., Bjorne, A., Cacace, A., Crocetti, A., et al. (2007). Consensus for tinnitus patient assessment and treatment outcome measurement: Tinnitus Research Initiative meeting, Regensburg, July 2006. *Prog Brain Res.*, *166*, 525-536.

[6]     Møller, A. R. (2007). Tinnitus: presence and future. *Prog Brain Res.*, *166*, 3-16.

[7]     Baguley, D. M. (2003). Hyperacusis. *J R Soc Med.*, *96*, 582-585.

[8]     Henry, J. A. & Meikle, M. B. (2000). Psychoacoustic measures of tinnitus. *J Am Acad Audiol*, *11*, 138-155.

[9]     Andersson, G., Baguley, D. M., McKenna, L. & McFerran, D. (2005). *Tinnitus – a multidisciplinary approach* (1st edition). London, Great Britain: Whurr Publishers.

[10]   Hiller, W. & Goebel, G. (2006). Factors influencing tinnitus loudness and annoyance. *Arch Otolaryngol Head Neck Surg.*, *132*, 1323-1330

[11] Wilson, P. H. & Henry, J. A. (2000). Psychological Management of tinnitus. In: R. S. Tyler (Ed.), *Tinnitus Handbook* (1st edition, 263-279). Clifton Park, NY: Thomson Learning.

[12] Langguth, B., Kleinjung, T., Fischer, B., Hajak, G., Eichhammer, P. & Sand, P. G. (2007). Tinnitus severity, depression, and the five big personality traits. *Prog Brain Res., 166*, 221-225.

[13] Crönlein, T., Langguth, B., Geisler, P. & Hajak, G. (2007). Tinnitus and insomnia. *Prog Brain Res., 166*, 227-233.

[14] Jastreboff, P. & Hazell, J. W. P. (1993). A neurophysiological approach to tinnitus: clinical implications. *Br J. Audiol., 27*, 1-11.

[15] House, J. W. & Brackmann, D. E. (1981). Surgical treatment of tinnitus. *Ciba Found Symp., 85*, 204-216.

[16] Møller, A. R. (2007). The role of neural plasticity in tinnitus. *Prog Brain Res., 166*, 37-45.

[17] Henry, J. A., Dennis, K. C. & Schechter, M. A. (2005). General review of tinnitus: prevalence, mechanisms, effects, and management. *J Speech Lang Hear Res., 48*, 1204-1235.

[18] Møller, A. R. (2000). Similarities between severe tinnitus and chronic pain. *J Am Acad Audiol., 11*, 115-124.

[19] Møller, A. R. (2003). *Sensory Systems: Anatomy and Physiology* (1st edition). Amsterdam, The Netherlands: Academic Press.

[20] Møller, A. R., Møller, M. B. & Yokota, M. (1992). Some forms of tinnitus may involve the extralemniscal auditory pathway. *Laryngoscope, 102*, 1165-1172.

[21] Chen, M. J. & Jastreboff, P. (1995). Salicylate-induced abnormal activity in the inferior colliculus of rats. *Hear Res., 82*, 158-178.

[22] Eggermont, J. J. (2003). Central tinnitus. *Auris Nasus Larynx, 30 Suppl*, 7-12.

[23] Eggermont, J. J. & Kenmochi, M. (1998). Salicylate and quinine selectively increase spontaneous firing rates in secondary auditory cortex. *Hear Res., 117*, 149-160.

[24] Eggermont, J. J. (2007). Pathophysiology of tinnitus. *Prog Brain Res., 166*, 19-35.

[25] Eggermont, J. J. & Roberts, L. E. (2004). The neuroscience of tinnitus. *Trends Neurosci., 27*, 676-682.

[26] Muhlnickel, W. Elbert, T., Taub, E. & Flor, H. (1998). Reorganization of auditory cortex in tinnitus. *Proc Natl Acad Sci*, U S A., *95*, 10340-10343.

[27] Llinas, R. R., Ribary, U., Jeanmonod, D., Kronberg, E. & Mitra, P. P. (1999). Thalamocortical dysrhythmia: A neurological and neuropsychiatric syndrome characterized by magnetoencephalography. *Proc Natl Acad Sci*, U S A., *96*, 15222-15227.

[28] Weisz, N., Muller, S., Schlee, W., Dohrmann, K., Hartmann, T. & Elbert, T. (2007). The neural code of auditory phantom perception. *J Neurosci., 27*, 1479-1484.

[29] Lockwood, A. H., Wacks, D. S., Burkard, R. F., Coad, M. L., Reyes, S. A., Arnold S. A. & Salvi, R. J. (2001). The functional anatomy of gaze-evoked tinnitus and sustained lateral gaze. *Neurology, 56*, 472-480.

[30] Lockwood, A. H., Salvi, R. J., Coad, M. L., Towsley, M. L., Wack, D. S. & Murphy, B. W. (1998). The functional neuroanatomy of tinnitus: evidence for limbic system links and neural plasticity. *Neurology, 50*, 114-120.

[31]  Giraud, A. L., Chery-Coze, S., Fischer, F., Fischer, C:, Vighetto, A. Gregoire, M. C., Lavenne, F. & Collet, L. (1999). A selective imaging of tinnitus. *Neuroreport*, *10*, 1-5.

[32]  Plewnia, C., Reimold, M., Najib, A., Brehm, B., Reischl, G., Plontke, S. K. & Gerloff, C. (2007). Dose-dependent attenuation of auditory phantom perception (tinnitus) by PET-guided repetitive transcranial magnetic stimulation. *Hum Brain Mapp*, *28*, 238-246.

[33]  Mirz, F., Pedersen, B., Ishizu, K., Johannsen, P., Ovesen, T., Stodkilde-Jorgensen, H. & Gjedde, A. (1999). Positron emission tomography of cortical centers of tinnitus. *Hear Res.*, *134*, 133-144

[34]  Melcher, J. R., Sigalowsky, I. S., Guinan, J. J. & Levine, A. R. (2000). Lateralized tinnitus studied with functional magnetic resonance imaging: abnormal inferior colliculus activation. *J. Neurophysiol.*, *83*, 1058-1072.

[35]  Smits, M., Kovacs, S., De Ridder, D., Peeters, R. R., Van de Heyning, P. & Sunaert, S. (2007). Lateralization of functional magnetic resonance imaging (fMRI) activation in the auditory pathway of patients with lateralized tinnitus. *Neuroradiology*, *49*, 669-679

[36]  Arnold, W., Bartenstein, P., Oestreicher, E., Romer, W. & Schwaiger, M. (1996). Focal metabolic activation in the predominant left auditory cortex in patients suffering from tinnitus: a PET study with [18F]deoxyglucose. *ORL J Otorhinolaryngol Relat Spec*, *58*, 195-199.

[37]  Kleinjung, T., Eichhammer, P., Langguth, B., Jacob, P., Marienhagen, J., Hajak, G. Wolf, S. R. & Strutz, J. (2005). Long-term effects of repetitive transcranial magnetic stimulation (rTMS) in patients with chronic tinnitus. *Otolaryngol Head Neck Surg*, *132*, 566-569.

[38]  Langguth, B., Eichhammer, P., Kreutzer, A., Maenner, P., Marienhagen, J., Kleinjung, T., Sand, P. & Hajak, G. (2006). The impact of auditory cortex activity on characterizing and treating patients with chronic tinnitus - first results from a PET study. *Acta Otolaryngol Suppl*, *556*, 84-88.

[39]  Wang, H., Tian, J., Yin, D., Jiang, S., Yang, W., Han, D., Yao, S. & Shao, M. (2000). Regional glucose metabolic increases in left auditory cortex in tinnitus patients; a preliminary study with positron emission tomography. *Chin Med J.*, *114*, 848-851.

[40]  Muhlau, M., Rauschecker, J. P., Oestreicher, E., Gaser, C., Rottinger, M., Wohlschlager, A. M., Simon, F., Etgen, T., Conrad, B. & Sander, B. (2006). Structural brain changes in tinnitus. *Cereb Cortex.*, *16*, 1283-1288.

[41]  Schlee, W., Dohrmann, K., Hartmann, T. Lorenz, N., Mueller, N., Elbert, T. & Weisz, N. (2008). Assessment and modification of the tinnitus-related cortical networks. *Sem Hearing.*, *29*, 270-287.

[42]  Barker, A. T., Jalinous, R. & Freeston, I. L. (1985). Non-invasive stimulation of the human motor cortex. *Lancet*, *1(8437)*, 1106-1107.

[43]  George, M. S. & Belmaker, R. H. (2000). *Transcranial magnetic stimulation in neuropsychiatry* (1st edition). Washington DC, American Psychiatric Press.

[44]  Walsh, V. & Rushworth, M. (1999). A primer of magnetic stimulation as a tool for neuropsychology. *Neuropsychologia*, *37*, 125-35.

[45]  Chen, R., Classen, J., Gerloff, C., Celnik, P., Wassermann, E. M., Hallett, M. & Cohen, L. G. (1997). Depression of motorcortex excitability by low-frequency transcranial magnetic stimulation. *Neurology*, *48*, 1398-03,

[46] Hoffman, R. E. & Cavus, I. (2002). Slow transcranial magnetic stimulation, long-term depotentiation, and brain hyperexcitability disorders. *Am J Psychiatry.*, *159*, 1093-1102.

[47] Pascual-Leone, A., Valls-Solle, J., Wassermann, E. M. & Hallett, M. (1994). Responses to rapid-rate transcranial magnetic stimulation of the human motor cortex. *Brain*, *117*, 847-58.

[48] Wang, H., Wang, X. & Scheich, H. (1996). LTD and LTP induced by transcranial magnetic stimulation in auditory cortex. *Neuroreport, 7*, 521-525.

[49] Hoffman, R. E., Hawkins, K. A., Gueorguieva, R., Boutros, N. N., Rachid, F., Carroll, K. & Krystal, J. H. (2003). Transcranial magnetic stimulation of left temporoparietal cortex and medication-resistant auditory hallucinations. *Arch Gen Psychiatry*, *60*, 49-56.

[50] Mantovani, A., Lisanby, S. H., Pieraccini, F., Ulivelli, M., Castrogiovanni, P. & Rossi, S. (2006). Repetitive transcranial magnetic stimulation (rTMS) in the treatment of obsessive-compulsive disorder (OCD) and Tourette's syndrome (TS). *Int J Neuropsychopharmacol.*, *9*, 95-100.

[51] Siebner, H. R., Tormos, J. M., Ceballos-Baumann, A. O., Auer, C., Catala, M. D., Conrad, B. & Pascual-Leone, A. (1999). Low-frequency repetitive transcranial magnetic stimulation of the motor cortex in writer's cramp. *Neurology*, *52*, 529-537.

[52] Kleinjung, T., Vielsmeier, V., Landgrebe, M., Hajak, G. & Langguth, B. (2008). Transcranial magnetic stimulation: a new diagnostic and therapeutic tool for tinnitus patients. *Int Tinnitus J.*, *14*, 112-118.

[53] Langguth, B., De Ridder, D., Dornhoffer, J., Eichhammer, P., Folmer, R. L., Frank, E., et al. (2008). Controversy: Does repetitive transcranial magnetic stimulation/ transcranial direct current stimulation show efficacy in treating tinnitus patients? *Brain Stimulation*, *1*, 192-205.

[54] Plewnia, C. Bartels, M. & Gerloff, C. (2003). Transient suppression of tinnitus by transcranial magnetic stimulation. *Ann Neurol.*, *53*, 263-266.

[55] De Ridder, D., Verstraeten, E., Van der Kelen, K., De Mulder, G., Sunaert, S., Verlooy, J., Van de Heyning, P. & Møller, A. R. (2005). Transcranial magnetic stimulation for tinnitus: influence of tinnitus duration on stimulation parameter choice and maximal tinnitus suppression. *Otol Neurotol.*, *26*, 616-619.

[56] Folmer, R. L., Carroll, J. R., Rahim, A., Shi, Y. & Martin, W. H. (2006). Effects of repetitive transcranial magnetic stimulation (rTMS) on chronic tinnitus. *Acta Otolaryngol Suppl.*, *556*, 96-101.

[57] Fregni, F., Marcondes, R., Boggio, P. S., Marcolin, M. A., Rigonatti, S. P., Sanchez, T. G., Nitsche, A. & Pascual-Leone, A. (2006). Transient tinnitus suppression induced by repetitive transcranial magnetic stimulation and transcranial direct current stimulation. *Eur J Neurol.*, *13*, 996-1002.

[58] De Ridder, D., De Mulder, G., Verstraeten, E., Van der Kelen, K., Sunaert, S, Smits, M., Kovacs, S., Verlooy, J., Van de Heyning, P. & Møller, A. (2006). Primary and secondary auditory cortex stimulation for intractable tinnitus. *ORL J Otorhinolaryngol Relat Spec.*, *68*, 48-54.

[59] De Ridder, D., De Mulder, G., Verstraeten, E., Seidman, M., Elisevich, K., Sunaert, S., Kovacs, S., Van der Kelen, K., Van der Heyning, P. & Møller A. (2007). Auditory cortex stimulation for tinnitus. *Acta Neurochir Suppl.*, *97*, 451-462.

[60] Plewnia, C., Reimold, M., Najib, A., Reischl, G., Plontke, S. K. & Gerloff, C. (2007). Moderate therapeutic efficacy of positron emission tomography-navigated repetitive transcranial magnetic stimulation for chronic tinnitus: a randomised, controlled pilot study. *J Neurol Neurosurg Psychiatry*, *78*, 152-156.

[61] Kleinjung, T., Steffens, T., Sand, P., Murthum, T., Hajak, G., Strutz, J., Langguth, B. & Eichhammer, P. (2007). Which tinnitus patients benefit from transcranial magnetic stimulation? *Otolaryngol Head Neck Surg.*, *137*, 589-95.

[62] Langguth, B., Zowe, M., Landgrebe, M., Sand, P., Kleinjung, T., Binder, H., Hajak, G. & Eichhammer, P. (2006). Transcranial Magnetic Stimulation for the treatment of tinnitus: A new coil positioning method and first results. *Brain Topogr.*, *18*, 241-247.

[63] Rossi, S., De Capua, A., Ulivelli, M., Bartalini, S., Falzarano, V., Filippone, G. & Passero, S. (2007). Effects of repetitive transcranial magnetic stimulation on chronic tinnitus. A randomised, cross over, double blind, placebo-controlled study. *J Neurol Neurosurg Psychiatry.*, *78*, 857-863.

[64] Khedr, E., Rothwell, J. C., Ahmed, M. A. & El-Atar, A. (2008). Effect of daily repetitive transcranial magnetic stimulation for treatment of tinnitus: comparison of different stimulus frequencies. *J Neurol Neurosurg Psychiatry.*, *79*, 212-5

[65] Smith, J. A., Mennemeier, M., Bartel, T., Chelette, K. C., Kimbrell, T., Triggs, W. & Dornhoffer, J. (2007). Repetitive transcranial magnetic stimulation for tinnitus: a pilot study. *Laryngoscope 117*, 529-534.

[66] Londero, A., Lefaucheur, J. P., Malinvaud, D., Brugieres, P., Peignard, P., Nguyen, J. P., Avan, P. & Bonfils, P. (2006). Magnetic stimulation of the auditory cortex for disabling tinnitus: preliminary results. *Presse Med.*, *35*, 200-206.

[67] Khedr, E. M., Rothwell, J. C. & El-Atar, A. (2009). One-year follow-up of patients with chronic tinnitus treated with temporoparietal rTMS. *Eur J Neurol.*, *16*, 404-408.

[68] Gershon, A. A., Dannon, P. N. & Grunhaus, L. (2003). Transcranial magnetic stimulation in the treatment of depression. *Am J Psychiatry.*, *160*, 835-45.

[69] Hoffman, R. E., Gueorguieva, R., Hawkins, K.A., Varanko, M., Boutros, N. N., Wu, Y. T., Carroll, K. & Krystal, J. H. (2005). Temporoparietal transcranial magnetic stimulation for auditory hallucinations: safety, efficacy and moderators in a fifty patient sample. *Biol Psychiatry*, *58*, 97-104.

[70] Newman, C. W., Jacobson, G. P. & Spitzer, J. B. (1996). Development of the Tinnitus Handicap Inventory. *Arch Otolaryngol Head Neck Surg.*, *122*, 143-148.

[71] Hallam, R. S. (1996). *Manual of the Tinnitus Questionnaire*. London, Great Britain: The Psychological Corporation.

[72] Zaider, T. I., Heimberg, R. G., Fresco, D. M., Schneier, F. R. & Liebowitz, M. R. (2003). Evaluation of the clinical global impression scale among individuals with social anxiety disorders. *Psychol Med.*, *33*, 611-622.

[73] Iyer, M. B., Schleper, N. & Wassermann, E. M. (2003). Priming stimulation enhances the depressant effect of low-frequency repetitive transcranial magnetic stimulation. *J Neurosci.*, *23*, 10867-10872.

[74] Langguth, B., Kleinjung, T., Frank, E., Landgrebe, M., Sand, P., Dvorakova, J. Frick, U., Eichhammer, P. & Hajak, G. (2008). High-frequency priming stimulation does not enhance the effect of low-frequency rTMS in the treatment of tinnitus. *Exp Brain Res.*, *184*, 587-591.

[75] Kleinjung, T., Eichhammer, P., Landgrebe, M., Sand, P., Hajak, G., Steffens, T., Strutz, J. & Langguth B. (2008). Combined temporal and prefrontal transcranial magnetic stimulation for tinnitus treatment: A pilot study. *Otolaryngol Head Neck Surg.*, *138*, 497-501.

[76] Lang, N., Speck, S., Harms, J., Rothkegel, H., Paulus, W. & Sommer, M. (2008). Dopaminergic potentiation of rTMS-induced motor cortex inhibition. *Biol Psychiatry.*, *63*, 231-233.

[77] Kleinjung, T., Steffens, T., Landgrebe, M., Vielsmeier, V., Frank, E., Hajak, G., Strutz, J. & Langguth, B. (2009). Levodopa does not enhance the effect of low-frequency transcranial magnetic stimulation in tinnitus treatment. *Otol Head Neck Surg.*, *140*, 92-95.

[78] Mennemeier, M., Chelette, K. C., Myhill, J., Taylor-Cooke, P., Bartel, T., Triggs, W., Kimbrell, T. & Dornhoffer, J. (2008). Maintenance repetitive transcranial magnetic stimulation can inhibit the return of tinnitus. *Laryngoscope*, *118*, 1228-1232.

[79] Eichhammer, P., Kleinjung, T., Landgrebe, M., Hajak, G. & Langguth, B. (2007). TMS for treatment of chronic tinnitus: neurobiological effects. *Prog Brain Res.*, *166*, 369-375.

[80] Langguth, B., Kleinjung, T., Marienhagen, J., Binder, Hajak, G. & Eichhammer, P. (2007). Transcranial magnetic stimulation for the treatment of chronic tinnitus: Effects on cortical excitability. *BMC Neurosci.*, *8*, 45.

[81] Siebner H. R., Lang, N., Rizzo, V., Nitsche, M. A., Paulus, W., Lemon, R. N. & Rothwell, J. C. (2004). Preconditioning of low-frequency repetitive transcranial magnetic stimulation with transcranial direct current stimulation: evidence for homeostatic plasticity in the human motor cortex. *J Neurosci.*, *24*, 3379-3385.

[82] May, A., Hajak, G., Ganssbauer, S., Steffens, T., Langguth, B., Kleinjung, T. & Eichhammer, P. (2007). Structural brain alterations following 5 days of intervention: dynamic aspects of neuroplasticity. *Cereb Cortex.*, *17*, 205-210.

[83] Weisz, N., Dohrmann, K. & Elbert, T. (2007). The relevance of spontaneous activity for the coding of the tinnitus sensation. *Prog Brain Res.*, *166*, 61-70.

[84] Wassermann, E. M. (1998). Risk and safety of repetitive transcranial magnetic stimulation: report and suggested guidelines from the International Workshop on the Safety of Repetitive Transcranial Magnetic Stimulation, June 5-7, 1996. *Electroencephalogr Clin Neurophysiol.*, *108*, 1-16.

[85] Nahas, Z., DeBrux, C., Chandler, V., Lorberbaum, J. P,, Speer, A. M., Molloy, M. A., Liberatos, C., Risch, S. C. & George, M. S. (2000). Lack of significant changes on magnetic resonance scans before and after 2 weeks of daily prefrontal transcranial magnetic stimulation for depression. *J ECT.*, *16*, 380-390.

[86] Loo, C. K., Sachdev, P. S., Elsayed, H., McDarmont, B. N., Mitchell, P. B., Wilkinson, M , Parker, G. & Gandevia, S. C. (2000). Effects of a 2- to 4-week course of repetitive transcranial magnetic stimulation (rTMS) on neuropsychological functioning, electroencephalogram and auditory threshold in depressed patients. *Biol Psychiatry.*, *49*, 615-623.

In: Deafness, Hearing Loss and the Auditory System    ISBN: 978-1-60741-259-5
Editors: D. Fiedler and R. Krause, pp.197-210    ©2010 Nova Science Publishers, Inc.

*Chapter 7*

# AN INFORMATICS APPROACH TO STUDYING THE ROLE OF MYOSINS IN THE INNER EAR

## *Christopher M. Frenz*[*]

Department of Computer Engineering Technology,
New York City College of Technology (CUNY), Brooklyn, NY, USA

## ABSTRACT

The ear is a complex organ system that contains a diversity of cell and tissue types and as such the elucidation of the various biological factors that can contribute to deafness can be quite challenging. The starting point for any such investigation is generally a comprehensive search of the biomedical literature to see what factors have already been determined to play a role and in what ways. The overwhelming volume of biomedical literature available, however, can often make uncovering such information difficult as standard keyword based search techniques often fail to narrow down search results into readily manageable quantities. This study will demonstrate the use of the informatics technique of text mining via regular expression based pattern matching as a means of uncovering the various genetic causes of deafness described in the biomedical literature. Several genetic causes of deafness can be linked to genes encoding proteins of the myosin family. As such, a text mining technique is illustrated that will match the expression of myosin variants to various parts of the ear in an effort to better elucidate the roles of myosins in the normal and aberrant function of the ear.

## INTRODUCTION

The present era is often referred to as an information age in that much of today's economy is shifting its focus from the production of physical goods and services and is instead focused on the manipulation and utilization of vast amounts of information. These radical economic shifts have largely been made possible by the rapid development and adoption of computer systems and networks that make the storage, retrieval, and processing

---

[*] Corresponding author: E-mail: cfrenz@citytech.cuny.edu.

of large amounts of information a now feasible task. To witness this phenomenon one need only type a query into a search engine like Google and take note of how even the most mundane terms return thousands of hits. In fact, information sources have often times become so abundant that the challenge lies not in finding relevant information, but in trying to isolate the information that is of quality from the information that is not. For example, in a typical Google search are all of those thousands of hits really pertinent to your needs or are a few useful while most are not? It is these new challenges in information processing that has given birth to the fields of informatics which try to process these vast arrays of information and extract useful patterns or other data.

The field of biology has been no exception to the rule and parallels have been drawn between current approaches to the biological sciences and the information sciences. For the typical biological researcher one of the most frequently used informatics tools is that of Pubmed since this service provides access to an index of over 17 million biomedical articles (Wheeler et al., 2008). It is this vast number of indexed articles that makes the resource so valuable, because the initial stages of any research project generally entails taking an in depth look at what related work has already been done, as means of refining your own hypothesis in the context of others results as well determining the novelty of the research contribution you intend to make. Even at the later stages of a project such a resource is of great value as the findings of other researchers often provide a great tool for aiding in the interpretation of your own results. Yet as with the Google example above, the vastness of the information repository can often make finding pertinent information challenging. This is especially true when one is involved in researching medical conditions such as deafness that can not only have a diversity of causes but also occurs in a complex organ system comprised of numerous cell and tissue types. Using Pubmed alone, there is no way to readily determine what factors contribute to deafness in what cell and tissue types short of manually processing returned search results by reading through the set of returned abstracts. Yet, without some insight into a given research area, narrowing down a search so that you need to read through only abstracts that are likely relevant can be difficult. For example, a Pubmed search for deafness, as of the time of August 2008, returns in excess of 27,400 indexed articles.

Difficulties in researching biomedical information can be further compounded by the fact that Pubmed uses a keyword based approach to searching in which returned search results are index entries that contain the keyword(s) entered as the search query. Many types of biological data/terms can be difficult to express in the form of a keyword. For example, suppose a researcher was interested in mutations in a protein such as connexin 26, which plays a role in the development of the inner ear and whose mutation has been demonstrated to result in deafness (Frenz & Van de Water, 2000; Evirgen et al., 2008). As individuals performing such a search we might skim through abstracts containing the keywords "connexin 26" and "deafness" looking for mutations by scanning for a recognizable mutation nomenclature, such as the one that provides the amino acid typically found at a given position, the position in the protein, and the amino acid that is substituted in the mutant form of the protein, but there is no natively supported way to perform such a search directly using keywords. One approach to dealing with this issue is to use regular expressions, a syntax for defining a textual pattern, as a part of a search query in order to better match biological nomenclatures that follow a predetermined pattern but are hard to quantify using keywords (Frenz, 2005). In a study conducted by Horn et al. (2004) the regular expression

[ARNDCEQGHILKMFPSTWYV]\d+[ ARNDCEQGHILKMFPSTWYV]|
[A-Z][a-z][a-z]\d+[A-Z][a-z][a-z]

was used to match mutations written in either the single letter amino acid notation or the three letter amino acid notation. This expression was able to lead to the extraction of 2736 true point mutations from a body of 914 articles on G protein-coupled receptors. This chapter will discuss how similar text mining techniques have been applied to the study of deafness and will expand upon this existing body of work by demonstrating how such informatics techniques can be used to assign the expression of biological factors that play a role in deafness to the parts of the inner ear they affect, via the application of text mining to studying the role of myosins in the inner ear.

## CURRENT APPLICATIONS OF REGULAR EXPRESSIONS TO THE STUDY OF DEAFNESS

To date, regular expression based pattern matching has been used to generate a comprehensive listing of the DFN classes of deafness mutations contained in Pubmed abstracts. Pattern matching lends itself well to uncovering such data because deafness mutations are typically named according to a nomenclature that begins with the letters DFN, followed by another letter, followed by a number, such as the DFNA15 mutation which affects the POU4F3 transcription factor and results in non-syndromic hearing loss (Hertzano et al., 2004). As with the biochemical mutation notation example provided above, this nomenclature lends itself well to description in the form of a regular expression, but is difficult to quantify in terms of keywords. The regular expression DFN[A-Z]\d+ was utilized in conjunction with the PREP.pl Perl program to search for the DFN mutation pattern in all Pubmed abstracts that contain the keywords "human ear". The PREP.pl program is available from http://bioinformatics.org/project/?group_id=494 (Frenz, 2007).

This program processed 61,371 Pubmed records and matched the DFN mutation pattern in 117 of those records. This type of refinement is indicative that regular expression based pattern matching can be a useful tool for biomedical researchers, since the Perl script was able to reduce the list of relevant Pubmed records to slightly less 0.2% of the "human ear" records contained in Pubmed. This approach was highly successful at generating a comprehensive listing of the varying types of deafness mutations and the mutations uncovered by this approach are listed in Table 1 (Frenz, 2007).

This approach was able to uncover 45 different types of deafness mutations illustrating the utility of such search techniques (Frenz, 2007). There are some caveats that users of such techniques do need to take into consideration, however, when using such text mining techniques. One is that the choice of keywords used to acquire data for processing by the PREP program is highly important. For example, the DFNB35 mutation was not picked up by the PREP program, because the Pubmed record in which the mutation is discussed did not appear in a search for the keywords "human ear" (Ansar et al., 2003). Another caveat is in the construction of the regular expressions used to perform pattern matching on the data. The regular expression needs to be general enough to match all of the pattern variants, but specific enough to limit the number of false positives (Frenz, 2005). In a study conducted by Horn et al (2004) in which they searched for point mutations in proteins, they encountered certain false positives such as the abbreviation for the cell line T47D, which is patterned in a manner similar to the biochemical notation for mutations. In order to combat this, filters were used to reduce the number of common false positives. Despite these caveats, for data that can be expressed in the form of a textual pattern, regular expression based pattern matching can greatly enhance the speed at which biomedical literature can be effectively processed.

**Table 1. Deafness mutations uncovered by the PREP program.**

| Mutation Name | Mutation Effect | Representative Source |
|---|---|---|
| DFNA1 | Diaphonous gene mutation associated with autosomal dominant non-syndromic hearing loss | Lalwani et al., 1998 |
| DFNA10 | Mutation in EYA4 causes late onset deafness | Zou et al., 2006 |
| DFNA11 | MYO7A mutation that results in progressive loss of mechanotransduction | Bolz et al., 2004 |
| DFNA12 | TECTA mutation resulting in hearing impairment | Veerhoeven et al., 1998 |
| DFNA13 | Mutation leading to cochlear conductive loss | De Leenheer et al, 2004 |
| DFNA14 | wolframin mutation cauisng non-syndromic dominant low frequency hearing loss | McHugh & Friedman, 2006 |
| DFNA15 | Mutation in POU4F3 that leads to autosomal dominant non-syndromic hearing loss | Hertzano et al., 2004 |
| DFNA17 | Mutation in myosin heavy chain IX linked to hearing impairment | Parker et al., 2006 |
| DFNA2 | KCNQ4 potassium channel mutation leading to progressive hearing loss | Kharkovets et al., 2006 |
| DFNA20 | ACTG1 mutation causing autosomal dominant heairng loss | van Wijk et al., 2003 |
| DFNA24 | Caspase 3 mutation associated with autosomal dominant non-syndromic hearing loss | Morishita et al., 2001 |
| DFNA26 | ACTG1 mutation causing autosomal dominant heairng loss | van Wijk et al., 2003 |
| DFNA36 | Mutation in transmembrane cochlear expressed gene 1 causing progressive deafness | Marcotti et al., 2006 |
| DFNA38 | wolframin mutation cauisng non-syndromic dominant low frequency hearing loss | McHugh & Friedman, 2006 |
| DFNA39 | Hearing loss associated with Dentinogenesis imperfecta | Xiao et al., 2001 |
| DFNA4 | MYH14 mutation leading to autosomal dominant hearing loss | Donaudy et al., 2004 |
| DFNA48 | MYO1A mutation resulting in autosomal dominant hearing loss | Donaudy et al., 2003 |
| DFNA5 | Mutation causing autosomal dominant hearing impairment | Van Laer et al., 2005 |
| DFNA6 | wolframin mutation cauisng non-syndromic dominant low frequency hearing loss | McHugh & Friedman, 2006 |

**Table 1. (Continued)**

| Mutation Name | Mutation Effect | Representative Source |
|---|---|---|
| DFNA8 | TECTA mutation resulting in hearing impairment | Veerhoeven et al., 1998 |
| DFNA9 | Coagulation factor C homology gene mutations causing sensioneural hearing loss | Robertson et al., 2006 |
| DFNB1 | Connexin 26 mutation leading to non-syndromic hearing loss | Palmada et al., 2006 |
| DFNB11 | Mutation in transmembrane cochlear expressed gene 1 causing congenital deafness | Marcotti et al., 2006 |
| DFNB12 | Cadherin 23 mutation causing prelingual hearing loss | McHugh & Friedman, 2006 |
| DFNB13 | Mutations causing autosomal recessive non-syndromic deafness | Masmoudi et al., 2004 |
| DFNB14 | Hearing loss associated with split hand/split foot malformation | Fukushima et al., 2003 |
| DFNB16 | Stereocilan mutation leading to autsomal recessive non-syndromic deafness | Verpy et al., 2001 |
| DFNB17 | FAM3C mutation causing autosomal recessive non-syndromic hearing loss | Pilipenko et al., 2004 |
| DFNB18 | Deafness associated with Usher syndrome 1C | Johnson et al., 2003 |
| DFNB2 | Deafness associated with mutations in myosin VIIA gene | Ernest et al., 2000 |
| DFNB22 | Otoancorin mutation resulting in autosmal recessive deafness | Zwaenepoel et al., 2003 |
| DFNB23 | Usher Syndrome 1F related deafness | Ahmed et al., 2006 |
| DFNB25 | Chromosome 5 mutation that effects sensory mechanotransduction | Odeh et al., 2004 |
| DFNB28 | TRIOBP mutation resulting in recessive prelingual sensioneural hearing loss | Shahin et al., 2006 |
| DFNB29 | CLDN14 mutations resulting in autosomal recessive non-syndromic deafness | Wilcox et al., 2001 |
| DFNB3 | Myo15a related non-syndromic deafness | Kanzaki et al., 2006 |
| DFNB30 | Mutation in myosin IIIA resulting in progressive hearing loss | Walsh et al., 2002 |
| DFNB31 | Whirlin mutation resulting in hearing loss | van Wijk et al., 2006 |
| DFNB4 | Mutation in PDS gene causing congenital deafness | Albert et al., 2006 |
| DFNB59 | Autosomal recessive auditory neuropathy | Delmaghani et al., 2006 |
| DFNB6 | Mutation causing autosomal recessive deafness | Cho et al., 2003 |
| DFNB67 | Mutation in THMS causing recessive non-syndromic hearing loss | Shabbir et al., 2006 |
| DFNB7 | Mutation in transmembrane cochlear expressed gene 1 causing congenital deafness | Marcotti et al., 2006 |
| DFNB8 | TMPRSS3 mutation associated with non-syndromic autosommal recessive hearing loss | Guiponni et al., 2002 |
| DFNB9 | Mutation in otoferlin causing prelingual hearing loss | Rodriguez-Bellesteros et al., 2003 |

This approach was able to uncover 45 different types of deafness mutations illustrating the utility of such search techniques (Frenz, 2007). There are some caveats that users of such techniques do need to take into consideration, however, when using such text mining techniques. One is that the choice of keywords used to acquire data for processing by the PREP program is highly important. For example, the DFNB35 mutation was not picked up by the PREP program, because the Pubmed record in which the mutation is discussed did not appear in a search for the keywords "human ear" (Ansar et al., 2003). Another caveat is in the construction of the regular expressions used to perform pattern matching on the data. The regular expression needs to be general enough to match all of the pattern variants, but specific enough to limit the number of false positives (Frenz, 2005). In a study conducted by Horn et al (2004) in which they searched for point mutations in proteins, they encountered certain false positives such as the abbreviation for the cell line T47D, which is patterned in a manner similar to the biochemical notation for mutations. In order to combat this, filters were used to reduce the number of common false positives. Despite these caveats, for data that can be expressed in the form of a textual pattern, regular expression based pattern matching can greatly enhance the speed at which biomedical literature can be effectively processed.

## FURTHERING THE APPLICATION OF SUCH TECHNIQUES TO THE STUDY OF DEAFNESS

Given the utility shown by text mining techniques in enhancing the searching of biomedical literature, the question that arises is how these techniques can be further expanded upon to enhance the efficacy of deafness related research. An examination of the various mutations that can cause deafness provided in Table 1 demonstrates that multiple variants of the protein myosin are linked with differing deafness variants. Myosin proteins are a diverse class of motor proteins found within the cells of eukaryotes, and over 40 myosin expressing genes are believed to exist within the human genome (Berg et al., 2001). The various known types of myosin are listed in Table 2.

**Table 2. A listing of myosin variants by class.**

| Class | Variants | | | | | | | |
|---|---|---|---|---|---|---|---|---|
| I | MYO1A | MYO1B | MYO1C | MYO1D | MYO1E | MYO1F | MYO1G | MYO1H |
| II | MYH1 | MYH2 | MYH3 | MYH4 | MYH6 | MYH7 | MYH7B | MYH9 |
| | MYH10 | MYH11 | MYH13 | MYH14 | MYH15 | MYH16 | | |
| III | MYO3A | MYO3B | | | | | | |
| V | MYO5A | MYO5B | MYO5C | | | | | |
| VI | MYO6 | | | | | | | |
| VII | MYO7A | MYO7B | | | | | | |
| IX | MYO9A | MYO9B | | | | | | |
| X | MYO10 | | | | | | | |
| XV | MYO15A | | | | | | | |
| XVIII | MYO18A | MYO18B | | | | | | |
| Light Chain | MYL1 | MYL2 | MYL3 | MYL4 | MYL5 | MYL6 | MYL6B | MYL7 |
| | MYL9 | MYLIP | MYLK | MYLK2 | | | | |

Using an informatics based approach, this study will outline a method that seeks to address the questions of 1) what myosins are expressed within the inner ear and 2) where in the inner are these mysoins expressed, as means of better elucidating the role of myosins in both hearing and deafness. The first step in this process is to develop a regular expression capable of matching all of the various types of myosins described in Table 2, and as such the following regular expression was derived:

$$MY[OHL]\backslash d+[A-H]?|MYLIP|MYLK2?|[Mm]yosin$$

This expression allows for all of the above myosin variants to be matched as well as the word myosin itself, in case any abstracts discuss myosin in the context of the inner ear but fail to mention a specific variant.

Now that the ability to match all myosin variants has been established, the next step was to develop a listing of all of the parts of the inner ear to also try to match against an article abstract. For purposes of this study a regular expression containing such a list was developed and is described below:

Cochlea|Organ of Corti|inner hair cell|outer hair cell|hair cell|Hensen\'s cell|Dieter\'s cell|Cells of Claudius|Cells of Boettcher|Pillar cell|Tectorial membrane| Endolymphatic duct| Endolymphatic sac|Semicircular ducts|cristae ampullaris|Vestibule|Utricle|Saccule| Macula|Spiral limbus|Stria Vascularis|Reissner\'s membrane|Basilar membrane|Spiral ganglion|Vestibular ganglion

Now that the required regular expressions for pattern matching have been derived, the next step was to modify the PREP.pl script (Frenz, 2007) to first enable matches to the myosin regular expression to be made. If a Pubmed record successfully matches the myosin pattern the record is then matched against the parts of the inner ear regular expression in an attempt to classify where that particular type of myosin is expressed within the inner ear. This modified script was then utilized to perform the described pattern matching against the results returned by a Pubmed keyword search for the words "inner ear".

## RESULTS

The Pubmed search for the keywords "inner ear" returned 40,961 at the time of execution from which the modified PREP script was able to find myosin pattern matches in 258 records. Of these matches, the majority consisted of matches of the word myosin to the inner ear parts of cochlea, Organ of Corti, or hair cell (Figure 1).

Yet, in addition to these generic myosin matches the modified PREP script was also able to match 9 myosin variants and assign 7 of them to parts of the inner ear. For the MYO7A, MYO6, MYO15A, MYO1C, and MYH9 variants, numerous pattern matches occurred and only a representative result is listed in Table 3. Moreover the ear part that is most specific is listed for each variant in the interest of limiting the table length. Thus, for example, even though MYO7A was found in both conjunction with studies in the cochlea and in the hair cells, it is listed as matching to the hair cells, since this provides the most specificity in terms of the location of expression.

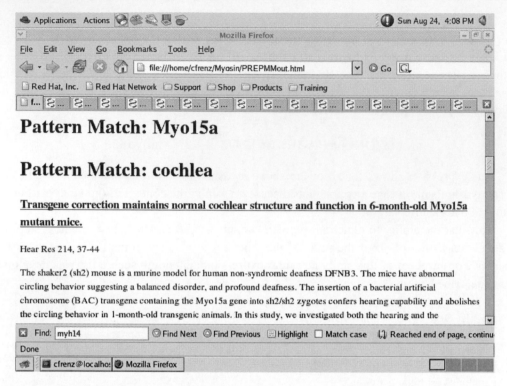

Figure 1. A sampling of the modified PREP script output.

**Table 3. Myosin patterns matched with their corresponding inner ear parts.**

| Patterned Matched | Inner Ear Part | Representative Source |
|---|---|---|
| Myosin | Cochlea | Furness et al, 2008 |
| Myosin | Organ of Corti | Pagedar et al, 2006 |
| Myosin | hair cells | Dose et al, 2008 |
| Myosin | Outer hair cell | Waguespacket al, 2007 |
| MYO1A | Cochlea | Donaudy et al, 2003 |
| MYO1B |  | Mencarelli et al, 2007 |
| MYO1C | hair cells | Adamek et al, 2008 |
| MYH9 | Cochlea | Lalwani et al, 2008 |
| MYO3A |  | Dose et al, 2003 |
| MYO6 | hair cells | Hilgert et al, 2008 |
| MYO7A | hair cells | Riazuddin et al, 2008 |
| MYH14 | Cochlea | Donaudy et al, 2004 |
| MYO15A | hair cells | Nal et al, 2007 |

## DISCUSSION

Overall the text mining approach was able to successfully pick out a diversity of Myosin types that are expressed in the inner ear and was successfully able to assign the expression of these myosin variants to the cochlear region of the inner ear and in particular the hair cells where myosins form components of the stereocilia and are involved in the mechanotransduction of sound. For MYO1B the script was unable to assign a part of the inner ear where the myosin plays a role, because the abstract texts only references the myosin in the context of the inner ear but does not go on to specify the specific locale in any greater depth (Mencarelli et al., 2007). MYO3A was also not assigned to a specific location within the inner ear and that is because the article that contains the pattern match mentions MYO3A in the context of the sacculus which was not a term that was listed in the inner ear parts regular expression making matching to it impossible. The regular expression used contained the word saccule and did not account for this spelling variant. MYO3A also demonstrates the potential utility of the myosin regular expression being adapted to also match the older format Myosin nomenclature of Myosin IIIA and the like, since a number of articles still made use of this nomenclature. It is noteworthy, however, that such an adaptation would not have increased the number of myosin variants found to play a role in the inner ear, but it would have allowed for a definitive assignment of MYO3A to the hair cells and reduced the number of matches to "Myosin" by allowing many of these matches to match to more specific variants.

It is also noteworthy that two false positives were discovered among the results which linked Myosin to the tectorial membrane (Friedman et al., 2007) and the basilar membrane (Harvey et al. 2001). Upon reading the abstracts of these articles, however, it would be clear that these results were false positives and that mention of myosin was not in relation to the inner ear part mentioned. The incidence of false positives, however, was low and thus does not diminish the utility of such an approach.

## CONCLUSION

The number and differing types of myosin variants able to be successfully associated with their corresponding part of the inner ear illustrates the utility of such text mining approaches to studying complex organ and disease systems such as the inner ear and deafness. The script was able to rapidly process over 40,000 abstracts in a period of only a few hours and thus was able to determine such associations and provide Pubmed records backing up such associations in far less time than would be possible using standard Pubmed searches with a human having to read through all such records. Given the crucial role knowledge discovery plays in any biomedical research project the ability to rapidly and reliably process such information would be of great benefit to biomedical researchers in all fields, and one mechanism of doing so is via regular expression based pattern matching. The true potential for such techniques, however, lies not is better ascertaining the role of a single family of protein within a given organ system, but in generating a regular expression capable of matching a vast array of proteins, growth factors, transcription factors, and genes of interest and using these pattern matching techniques to create expression profiles of the types of biological factors expressed within each type of cell/tissue that comprises an organ system of interest and thereby enhance the understanding of the entire organ system and its underlying functionality.

# REFERENCES

Adamek, N., Coluccio, L. M. & Geeves, M. A. (2008). Calcium sensitivity of the cross-bridge cycle of Myo1c, the adaptation motor in the inner ear. *Proc. Natl. Acad. Sci.*, USA, *105*, 5710-5715.

Ahmed, Z. M., Goodyear, R., Riazuddin, S., Lagziel, A., Legan, P. K., Behra, M., Burgess, S. M., Lilley, K. S., Wilcox, E. R., Riazuddin, S., Griffith, A. J., Frolenkov, G. I., Belyantseva, I. A., Richardson, G. P. & Friedman, T. B. (2006). The tip-link antigen, a protein associated with the transduction complex of sensory hair cells, is protocadherin-15. *J.Neurosci.*, *26*, 7022-7034.

Albert, S., Blons, H., Jonard, L., Feldmann, D., Chauvin, P., Loundon, N., Sergent-Allaoui, A., Houang, M., Joannard, A., Schmerber, S., Delobel, B., Leman, J., Journel, H., Catros, H., Dollfus, H., Eliot, M.M., David, A., Calais, C., Drouin-Garraud, V., Obstoy, M. F., Tran Ba Huy P., Lacombe, D., Duriez, F., Francannet, C., Bitoun, P., Petit, C., Garabédian, E. N., Couderc, R., Marlin, S. & Denoyelle, F. (2006). SLC26A4 gene is frequently involved in nonsyndromic hearing impairment with enlarged vestibular aqueduct in Caucasian populations. *Eur. J. Hum. Genet.*, *14*, 773-779.

Ansar, M., Din, M. A., Arshad, M., Sohail, M., Faiyaz-Ul-Haque, M., Haque, S., Ahmad, W. & Leal, S. M. (2003). A novel autosomal recessive non-syndromic deafness locus (DFNB35) maps to 14q24.1-14q24.3 in large consanguineous kindred from Pakistan. *Eur.J.Hum.Genet.*, *11*, 77-80.

Berg, J. S., Powell, B. C. & Cheney, R. E. (2001). A millennial myosin census. *Mol. Biol. Cell*, *12*, 780-794.

Bolz, H., Bolz, S. S., Schade, G., Kothe, C., Mohrmann, G., Hess, M. & Gal, A. (2004). Impaired calmodulin binding of myosin-7A causes autosomal dominant hearing loss (DFNA11). *Hum.Mutat.*, *24*, 274-275.

Cho, K. I., Lee, J. W., Kim, K. S., Lee, E. J., Suh, J. G., Lee, H. J., Kim, H. T., Hong, S. H., Chung, W. H., Chang, K. T., Hyun, B. H., Oh, Y. S. & Ryoo, Z. Y. (2003). Fine mapping of the circling (cir) gene on the distal portion of mouse chromosome 9. *Comp Med.*, *53*, 642-648.

De Leenheer, E. M., Bosman, A. J., Kunst, H. P., Huygen, P. L. & Cremers, C. W. (2004). Audiological characteristics of some affected members of a Dutch DFNA13/COL11A2 family. *Ann.Otol.Rhinol.Laryngol.*, *113*, 922-929.

Delmaghani, S., del Castillo, F. J., Michel, V., Leibovici, M., Aghaie, A., Ron, U., Van, Laer L., Ben-Tal, N., Van, Camp G., Weil, D., Langa, F., Lathrop, M., Avan, P. & Petit, C. (2006). Mutations in the gene encoding pejvakin, a newly identified protein of the afferent auditory pathway, cause DFNB59 auditory neuropathy. *Nat.Genet.*, *38*, 770-778.

Donaudy, F., Ferrara, A., Esposito, L., Hertzano, R., Ben-David, O., Bell, R. E., Melchionda, S., Zelante, L., Avraham, K. B. & Gasparini, P. (2003). Multiple mutations of MYO1A, a cochlear-expressed gene, in sensorineural hearing loss. *Am.J.Hum.Genet.*, *72*, 1571-1577.

Donaudy, F., Snoeckx, R., Pfister, M., Zenner, H. P., Blin, N., Di, Stazio M., Ferrara, A., Lanzara, C., Ficarella, R., Declau, F., Pusch, C. M., Nurnberg, P., Melchionda, S., Zelante, L., Ballana, E., Estivill, X., Van, Camp G., Gasparini, P. & Savoia, A. (2004). Nonmuscle myosin heavy-chain gene MYH14 is expressed in cochlea and mutated in patients affected by autosomal dominant hearing impairment (DFNA4). *Am.J.Hum.Genet.*, *74*, 770-776.

Dosé, A. C., Ananthanarayanan, S., Moore, J. E., Corsa, A.C., Burnside, B. & Yengo, C. M. (2008). The kinase domain alters the kinetic properties of the myosin IIIA motor. *Biochemistry*, *47*, 2485-2496.

Dosé, A. C., Hillman, D. W., Wong, C., Sohlberg, L., Lin-Jones, J. & Burnside, B. (2003). Myo3A, one of two class III myosin genes expressed in vertebrate retina, is localized to the calycal processes of rod and cone photoreceptors and is expressed in the sacculus. *Mol. Biol. Cell*, *14*, 1058-1073.

Ernest, S., Rauch, G. J., Haffter, P., Geisler, R., Petit, C. & Nicolson, T. (2000). Mariner is defective in myosin VIIA: a zebrafish model for human hereditary deafness. *Hum.Mol.Genet.*, *9*, 2189-2196.

Evirgen, N., Solak, M., Dereköy, S., Erdoğan, M., Yildiz, H., Eser, B., Arikan, S. & Erkoc, A. (2008). Genotyping for Cx26 and Cx30 mutations in cases with congenital hearing loss. *Genet. Test.*, *12*, 253-256.

Frenz, C. M. & Van De Water, T. R. (2000). Immunolocalization of connexin 26 in the developing mouse cochlea. *Brain Res. Brain Res. Rev.*, *32*, 172-180.

Frenz, C. M. (2005). *Pro Perl Parsing*, Berkeley, CA; Apress.

Frenz, C. M. (2007). Deafness mutation mining using regular expression based pattern matching. *BMC Medical Informatics and Decision Making*, *7*, 3.

Friedman, L. M., Dror, A. A. & Avraham, K. B. (2007). Mouse models to study inner ear development and hereditary hearing loss. *Int. J. Dev. Biol.*, *51*, 609-631.

Fukushima, K., Nagai, K., Tsukada, H., Sugata, A., Sugata, K., Kasai, N., Kibayashi, N., Maeda, Y., Gunduz, M. & Nishizaki, K. (2003). Deletion mapping of split hand/split foot malformation with hearing impairment: a case report. *Int.J.Pediatr.Otorhinolaryngol.*, *67*, 1127-1132.

Furness, D. N., Mahendrasingam, S., Ohashi, M., Fettiplace, R. & Hackney, C. M. (2008). The dimensions and composition of stereociliary rootlets in mammalian cochlear hair cells: comparison between high- and low-frequency cells and evidence for a connection to the lateral membrane. *J. Neurosci.*, *28*, 6342-6353.

Guipponi, M., Vuagniaux, G., Wattenhofer, M., Shibuya, K., Vazquez, M., Dougherty, L., Scamuffa, N., Guida, E., Okui, M., Rossier, C., Hancock, M., Buchet, K., Reymond, A., Hummler, E., Marzella, P. L., Kudoh, J., Shimizu, N., Scott, H. S., Antonarakis, S. E. & Rossier, B. C. (2002). The transmembrane serine protease (TMPRSS3) mutated in deafness DFNB8/10 activates the epithelial sodium channel (ENaC) in vitro. *Hum.Mol.Genet.*, *11*, 2829-2836.

Harvey, S. J., Mount, R., Sado, Y., Naito, I., Ninomiya, Y., Harrison, R., Jefferson, B., Jacobs, R. & Thorner, P. S. (2001). The inner ear of dogs with X-linked nephritis provides clues to the pathogenesis of hearing loss in X-linked Alport syndrome. *Am. J. Pathol.*, *159*, 1097-1104.

Hertzano, R., Montcouquiol, M., Rashi-Elkeles, S., Elkon, R., Yucel, R., Frankel, W. N., Rechavi, G., Moroy, T., Friedman, T. B., Kelley, M. W. & Avraham, K. B. (2004). Transcription profiling of inner ears from Pou4f3 (ddl/ddl) identifies Gfi1 as a target of the Pou4f3 deafness gene. *Hum. Mol. Genet.*, *13*, 9-15.

Hilgert, N., Topsakal, V., van Dinther, J., Offeciers, E., Van de Heyning, P. & Van Camp, G. (2008). A splice-site mutation and overexpression of MYO6 cause a similar phenotype in two families with autosomal dominant hearing loss. *Eur. J. Hum. Genet.*, *16*, 593-602.

Horn, F., Lau, A. L. & Cohen, F. E. (2004). Automated extraction of mutation data from the literature application of MuteXt to G protein-coupled receptors and nuclear hormone receptors. *Bioinformatics*, *20*, 557-568.

Johnson, K. R., Gagnon, L. H., Webb, L. S., Peters, L. L., Hawes, N. L., Chang, B. & Zheng, Q. Y. (2003). Mouse models of USH1C and DFNB18: phenotypic and molecular analyses of two new spontaneous mutations of the Ush1c gene. *Hum.Mol.Genet.*, *12*, 3075-3086.

Kanzaki, S., Beyer, L., Karolyi, I. J., Dolan, D. F., Fang, Q., Probst, F. J., Camper, S. A. & Raphael, Y. (2006). Transgene correction maintains normal cochlear structure and function in 6-month-old Myo15a mutant mice. *Hear.Res.*, *214*, 37-44.

Kharkovets, T., Dedek, K., Maier, H., Schweizer, M., Khimich, D., Nouvian, R., Vardanyan, V., Leuwer, R., Moser, T. & Jentsch, T. J. (2006). Mice with altered KCNQ4 K+ channels implicate sensory outer hair cells in human progressive deafness. *EMBO J.*, *25*, 642-652.

Lalwani, A. K., Atkin, G., Li, Y., Lee, J. Y., Hillman, D. E. & Mhatre, A. N. (2008). Localization in stereocilia, plasma membrane, and mitochondria suggests diverse roles for NMHCC-IIa within cochlear hair cells. *Brain Res.*, *1197*, 13-22.

Lalwani, A. K., Jackler, R. K., Sweetow, R. W., Lynch, E. D., Raventos, H., Morrow, J., King, M. C. & Leon, P. E. (1998). Further characterization of the DFNA1 audiovestibular phenotype. *Arch. Otolaryngol. Head Neck Surg.*, *124*, 699-702.

Marcotti, W., Erven, A., Johnson, S. L., Steel, K. P. & Kros, C. J. (2006). Tmc1 is necessary for normal functional maturation and survival of inner and outer hair cells in the mouse cochlea. *J.Physiol.*, *574*, 677-698.

Masmoudi, S., Charfedine, I., Rebeh, I. B., Rebai, A., Tlili, A., Ghorbel, A. M., Belguith, H., Petit, C., Drira, M. & Ayadi, H. (2004). Refined mapping of the autosomal recessive non-syndromic deafness locus DFNB13 using eight novel microsatellite markers. *Clin.Genet.*, *66*, 358-364.

McHugh, R. K. & Friedman, R. A. (2006). Genetics of hearing loss: Allelism and modifier genes produce a phenotypic continuum. *Anat.Rec.A Discov.Mol.Cell Evol.Biol.*, *288*, 370-381.

Mencarelli, M. A., Caselli, R., Pescucci, C., Hayek, G., Zappella, M., Renieri, A. & Mari, F. (2007). Clinical and molecular characterization of a patient with a 2q31.2-32.3 deletion identified by array-CGH. *Am. J. Med. Genet. A.*, *143A*, 858-865.

Morishita, H., Makishima, T., Kaneko, C., Lee, Y. S., Segil, N., Takahashi, K., Kuraoka, A., Nakagawa, T., Nabekura, J., Nakayama, K. & Nakayama, K. I. (2001). Deafness due to degeneration of cochlear neurons in caspase-3-deficient mice. *Biochem. Biophys. Res. Commun.*, *284*, 142-149.

Nal, N., Ahmed, Z. M., Erkal, E., Alper, O. M., Lüleci, G., Dinc, O., Waryah, A. M., Ain, Q., Tasneem, S., Husnain, T., Chattaraj, P., Riazuddin, S., Boger, E., Ghosh, M., Kabra, M., Riazuddin, S., Morell, R. J. & Friedman, T. B. (2007). Mutational spectrum of MYO15A: the large N-terminal extension of myosin XVA is required for hearing. *Hum. Mutat.*, *28*, 1014-1019.

Odeh, H., Hagiwara, N., Skynner, M., Mitchem, K. L., Beyer, L. A., Allen, N. D., Brilliant, M. H., Lebart, M. C., Dolan, D. F., Raphael, Y. & Kohrman, D. C. (2004). Characterization of two transgene insertional mutations at pirouette, a mouse deafness locus. *Audiol.Neurootol.*, *9*, 303-314.

Pagedar, N.A., Wang, W., Chen, D. H., Davis, R. R., Lopez, I., Wright, C. G. & Alagramam, K. N. (2006). Gene expression analysis of distinct populations of cells isolated from mouse and human inner ear FFPE tissue using laser capture microdissection – a technical report based on preliminary findings. *Brain Res.*, *1091*, 289-299.

Palmada, M., Schmalisch, K., Bohmer, C., Schug, N., Pfister, M., Lang, F. & Blin, N. (2006). Loss of function mutations of the GJB2 gene detected in patients with DFNB1-associated hearing impairment. *Neurobiol.Dis.*, *22*, 112-118.

Parker, L. L., Gao, J. & Zuo, J. (2006). Absence of hearing loss in a mouse model for DFNA17 and MYH9-related disease: the use of public gene-targeted ES cell resources. *Brain Res.*, *1091*, 235-242.

Pilipenko, V. V., Reece, A., Choo, D. I. & Greinwald, J. H. Jr. (2004). Genomic organization and expression analysis of the murine Fam3c gene. *Gene*, *335*, 159-168.

Riazuddin, S., Nazli, S., Ahmed, Z. M., Yang, Y., Zulfigar, F., Shaikh, R. S., Zafar, A. U., Khan, S. N., Sabar, F., Javid, F. T., Wilcox, E. R., Tsilou, E., Boger, E. T., Sellers, J. R., Belyantseva, I. A., Riazuddin, S. & Friedman, T. B. (2008). Mutation spectrum of MYO7A and evaluation of a novel nonsyndromic deafness DFNB2 allele with residual function. *Hum. Mutat.*, *29*, 502-511.

Robertson, N. G., Cremers, C. W., Huygen, P. L., Ikezono, T., Krastins, B., Kremer, H., Kuo, S. F., Liberman, M. C., Merchant, S. N., Miller, C. E., Nadol, J. B. Jr., Sarracino, D. A., Verhagen, W. I. & Morton, C. C. (2006). Cochlin immunostaining of inner ear pathologic deposits and proteomic analysis in DFNA9 deafness and vestibular dysfunction. *Hum.Mol.Genet.*, *15*, 1071-1085.

Rodriguez-Ballesteros, M., del Castillo, F. J., Martin, Y., Moreno-Pelayo, M. A., Morera, C., Prieto, F., Marco, J., Morant, A., Gallo-Teran, J., Morales-Angulo, C., Navas, C., Trinidad, G., Tapia, M. C., Moreno, F. & Del, Castillo, I. (2003). Auditory neuropathy in patients carrying mutations in the otoferlin gene (OTOF). *Hum.Mutat.*, *22*, 451-456.

Shabbir, M. I., Ahmed, Z. M., Khan, S. Y., Riazuddin, S., Waryah, A. M., Khan, S. N., Camps, R. D., Ghosh, M., Kabra, M., Belyantseva, I. A., Friedman, T. B. & Riazuddin, S. (2006). Mutations of human TMHS cause recessively inherited non-syndromic hearing loss. *J.Med.Genet.*, *43*, 634-640.

Shahin, H., Walsh, T., Sobe, T., Abu, Sa'ed J., Abu, Rayan A., Lynch, E. D., Lee, M. K., Avraham, K. B., King, M. C. & Kanaan, M. (2006). Mutations in a novel isoform of TRIOBP that encodes a filamentous-actin binding protein are responsible for DFNB28 recessive nonsyndromic hearing loss. *Am.J.Hum.Genet.*, *78*, 144-152.

Van Wijk, E., van der Zwaag, B., Peters, T, Zimmermann, U., Te Brinke, H., Kersten, F. F., Märker, T., Aller, E., Hoefsloot, L. H., Cremers, C. W., Cremers, F. P., Wolfrum, U., Knipper, M., Roepman, R. & Kremer, H. (2006). The DFNB31 gene product whirlin connects to the Usher protein network in the cochle and retina by direct association with USH2A and VLGR1. *Hum. Mol. Genet.*, *15*, 751-765.

Van, Laer L., Pfister, M., Thys, S., Vrijens, K., Mueller, M., Umans, L., Serneels, L., Van, Nassauw L., Kooy, F., Smith, R. J., Timmermans, J. P., Van Leuven, F. & Van Camp, G.

(2005). Mice lacking Dfna5 show a diverging number of cochlear fourth row outer hair cells. *Neurobiol.Dis.*, *19*, 386-399.

van, Wijk E., Krieger, E., Kemperman, M. H., De Leenheer, E. M., Huygen, P. L., Cremers, C. W., Cremers, F. P. & Kremer, H. (2003). A mutation in the gamma actin 1 (ACTG1) gene causes autosomal dominant hearing loss (DFNA20/26). *J.Med.Genet.*, *40*, 879-884.

Verhoeven, K., Van Laer, L., Kirschhofer, K., Legan, P. K., Hughes, D. C., Schatteman, I., Verstreken, M., Van Hauwe, P., Coucke, P., Chen, A., Smith, R. J., Somers, T., Offeciers, F. E., Van de Heyning, P., Richardson, G. P., Wachtler, F., Kimberling, W. J., Willems, P. J., Govaerts, P. J. & Van Camp, G. (1998). Mutations in the human alpha-tectorin gene cause autosomal dominant non-syndromic hearing impairment. *Nat.Genet.*, *19*, 60-62.

Verpy, E., Masmoudi, S., Zwaenepoel, I., Leibovici, M., Hutchin, T. P., Del Castillo, I, Nouaille, S., Blanchard, S., Laine, S., Popot, J. L., Moreno, F., Mueller, R. F. & Petit, C. (2001). Mutations in a new gene encoding a protein of the hair bundle cause non-syndromic deafness at the DFNB16 locus. *Nat.Genet.*, *29*, 345-349.

Waguespack, J., Salles, F.T., Kachar, B. & Ricci, A. J. (2007). Stepwise morphological and functional maturation of mechanotransduction in rat outer hair cells. *J. Neurosci.*, *27*, 13890-13902.

Walsh, T., Walsh, V., Vreugde, S., Hertzano, R., Shahin, H., Haika, S., Lee, M. K., Kanaan, M., King, M. C. & Avraham, K. B. (2002). From flies' eyes to our ears: mutations in a human class III myosin cause progressive nonsyndromic hearing loss DFNB30. *Proc.Natl.Acad.Sci.*, U.S.A., *99*, 7518-7523.

Wheeler, D. L., Barrett, T., Benson, D. A., Bryant, S. H., Canese, K., Chetvernin, V., Church, D. M., Dicuccio, M., Edgar, R., Federhen, S., Feolo, M., Geer, L. Y., Helmberg, W., Kapustin, Y., Khovayko, O., Landsman, D., Lipman, D. J., Madden, T. L., Maglott, D. R., Miller, V., Ostell, J., Pruitt, K. D., Schuler, G. D., Shumway, M., Sequeira, E., Sherry, S. T., Sirotkin, K., Souvorov, A., Starchenko, G., Tatusov, R. L., Tatusova, T. A., Wagner, L. & Yaschenko, E. (2008). Database resources of the National Center for Biotechnology Information. *Nucleic Acids Res.*, *36*, D13-21.

Wilcox, E. R., Burton, Q. L., Naz, S., Riazuddin, S., Smith, T. N., Ploplis, B., Belyantseva, I., Ben-Yosef, T., Liburd, N. A., Morell, R. J., Kachar, B., Wu, D. K., Griffith, A. J., Riazuddin, S. & Friedman, T. B. (2001). Mutations in the gene encoding tight junction claudin-14 cause autosomal recessive deafness DFNB29. *Cell*, *104*, 165-172.

Xiao, S., Yu, C., Chou, X., Yuan, W., Wang, Y., Bu, L., Fu, G., Qian, M., Yang, J., Shi, Y., Hu, L., Han, B., Wang, Z., Huang, W., Liu, J., Chen, Z., Zhao, G. & Kong, X. (2001). Dentinogenesis imperfecta 1 with or without progressive hearing loss is associated with distinct mutations in DSPP. *Nat.Genet.*, *27*, 201-204.

Zou, D., Silvius, D., Rodrigo-Blomqvist, S., Enerback, S. & Xu, P. X. (2006). Eya1 regulates the growth of otic epithelium and interacts with Pax2 during the development of all sensory areas in the inner ear. *Dev.Biol.*, *298*, 430-441.

Zwaenepoel, I., Mustapha, M., Leibovici, M., Verpy, E., Goodyear, R., Liu, X. Z., Nouaille, S., Nance, W. E., Kanaan, M., Avraham, K. B., Tekaia, F., Loiselet, J., Lathrop, M., Richardson, G. & Petit, C. (2002). Otoancorin, an inner ear protein restricted to the interface between the apical surface of sensory epithelia and their overlying acellular gels, is defective in autosomal recessive deafness DFNB22. *Proc.Natl.Acad.Sci.*, U.S.A., *99*, 6240-6245.

In: Deafness, Hearing Loss and the Auditory System
Editors: D. Fiedler and R. Krause, pp.211-225
ISBN: 978-1-60741-259-5
©2010 Nova Science Publishers, Inc.

*Chapter 8*

# TIGHT JUNCTION PROTEINS AND THE ETIOLOGY OF HEREDITARY HEARING LOSS IN HUMANS AND ANIMAL MODELS

## *Tamar Ben-Yosef*\*

Department of Genetics, The Rappaport Family Institute for Research in the Medical Sciences, Faculty of Medicine, Technion-Israel Institute of Technology, Haifa, Israel

## ABSTRACT

Multicellular organisms have separate compartments of different compositions. In the cochlea of the inner ear separation between endolymph and perilymph, two compartments with very different sodium and potassium ion concentrations, is necessary for normal hearing. This compartmentalization is achieved by tight junctions (TJs), which form the major selective barrier of the paracellular pathway between epithelial cells. TJ strands contain at least five types of membrane-spanning proteins. To date, mutations in five different TJ membrane integral proteins have been associated with hearing loss. Mutations in claudin 14 and in tricellulin are associated with hereditary hearing loss in humans. Claudin 9-, claudin 11- and claudin 14-mutant mice are deaf. In zebrafish, a mutation of the *cldnj* gene leads to abnormal auditory and vestibular functions. There are different etiologies for hearing loss associated with each of these proteins, including hair cell loss, reduced endocochlear potentials, and abnormal embryonic development of the inner ear. Nevertheless, in all cases the underlying cause is dysfunction of the paracellular barrier. These findings elucidate the crucial role played by TJs in the auditory apparatus, and enhance our understanding of the hearing process. This knowledge will be further enhanced by identification of hearing-related phenotypes associated with additional TJ proteins and generation of additional animal models in years to come.

\* Corresponding author: Phone: 972-4-829-5228. Fax: 972-4-829-5225. E-mail: benyosef@tx.technion.ac.il.

## INTRODUCTION

A basic physiological requirement in multicellular organisms is the existence of separate compartments of different compositions. For example, in the cochlea of the inner ear the perilymph of the scala vestibuli and scala tympani has very different ionic composition as compared to the endolymph of the scala media (Figure 1) [1, 2]. Maintenance of different compartments is performed by epithelial or endothelial cells, which adhere to each other by forming different types of intercellular junctions [3], including desmosomes [4], adherens junctions [5], gap junctions [6] and tight junctions (TJs) [7, 8]. The movement of solutes, ions and water through epithelia occurs both across and between individual cells, and is referred to as the transcellular and the paracellular routes, respectively. Both routes display cell-specific and tissue-specific variations in permeability, and together account for the distinct transport properties of each tissue.

The major barrier in the paracellular pathway is created by TJs. TJs can be found in various epithelial tissues, in which they form regions of intimate contact between the plasma membranes of adjacent cells [3]. In freeze-fracture replicas of epithelial cells TJs appear as a band-like network of branching and interconnecting thin ridges or complementary grooves, known as TJ strands [3]. TJs between two adjacent cells are called bicellular TJs, while at tricellular contacts, where there are three epithelial cells, structurally specialized TJs, referred to as tricellular TJs, are formed [9-11].

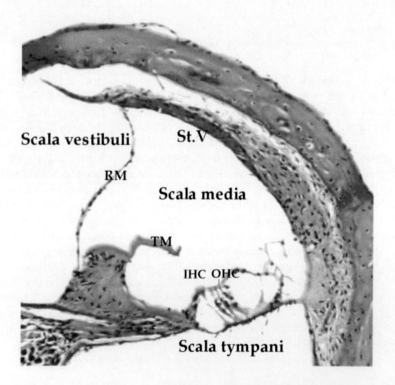

Figure 1. Hematoxylin and eosin staining of paraffin embedded sections (8 μm thick) of the organ of Corti of a two months old wt mouse (10X magnification). OHC, outer hair cells; IHC, inner hair cells; TM, tectorial membrane; RM, Reissner's membrane; St.V, stria vascularis.

**Table 1. Auditory phenotypes associated with mutations in TJ membrane integral proteins**

| Protein | Auditory Phenotype in Humans | Auditory Phenotype in Animal Models | References |
|---|---|---|---|
| Claudin 9 | | Severe hearing loss (mutant mice) | [56] |
| Claudin 11 | | Severe hearing loss (knockout mice) | [61, 62] |
| Claudin 14 | Autosomal recessive, congenital, bilateral, severe to profound sensorineural hearing loss DFNB29 | Severe hearing loss (knockout mice) | [46, 47] |
| Claudin j | | Hearing loss, vestibular dysfunction (zebrafish) | [66] |
| Tricellulin | Autosomal recessive, congenital, bilateral, moderate to profound sensorineural hearing loss DFNB49 | | [23] |

TJs close or seal the space between cells and thus set up a semi-permeable barrier which prevents or reduces paracellular diffusion ('barrier function') [12]. Depending on the functional requirements of an epithelium, there may be small or large amounts of water and small solutes flowing passively through the TJ [13]. The paracellular permeability of different epithelia was found to correlate with the number of TJ strands along the apical-basal axis [14]. The morphological pattern of the strands also varies among tissues, however the physiological correlate of these ultra structural differences is yet unknown. There is also some evidence that TJs form an intramembrane diffusion barrier that restricts the lateral diffusion of apical and basolateral membrane components, thus maintaining cellular polarity ('fence function') [15-18].

TJ strands are composed of several types of membrane-spanning proteins: occludin [19], members of the junction adhesion molecule (JAM) family [20], the coxsackievirus and adenovirus receptor (CAR) [21], tricellulin [22, 23], and more than 20 members of the claudin family [24, 25]. Here I review the contribution of TJ proteins to hereditary hearing loss in human beings and in animal models.

## TIGHT JUNCTION MEMBRANE INTEGRAL PROTEINS

Occludin was the first identified TJ protein. It is exclusively localized to TJs of both epithelial and endothelial cells. It spans the membrane four times with cytoplasmic amino and carboxy termini and forms two extracellular loops that are composed mostly of glycine and tyrosine [19]. Initially occludin was thought to be the main TJ sealing protein. However, several studies, including analyses of an occludin knockout mouse, revealed that TJ strands can be formed and function normally in the absence of occludin [26-29].

JAMs are immunoglobulin superfamily proteins expressed at cell junctions in epithelial and endothelial cells, particularly at the apical-most part of the lateral membrane near the TJ. JAM proteins have been shown to bind to various TJ-associated cytoplasmic proteins. Despite compelling data implicating JAM proteins in formation of intercellular junctions, their direct role in the TJ has not been identified yet [20].

CAR is a 46-kDa integral membrane protein with atypical transmembrane region, a long cytoplasmic domain, and an extracellular region composed of two Ig-like domains. In polarized epithelial cells CAR is expressed at the TJ, where it contributes to the barrier function [21].

The claudins are a family of more than 20 TJ proteins, which are the primary components responsible for the physiological and structural paracellular barrier function of TJs [30]. All members of the claudin family share the same membrane topology: they span the membrane four times with cytoplasmic amino and carboxy termini, and form two extracellular loops [31]. Claudins have various tissue distribution patterns, and many tissues express several different claudins which can interact with each other in both homotypic and heterotypic manners [32, 33]. Particular combinations and quantities of claudins modulate the charge selective permeability of the paracellular pathway and, hence, take part in the regulation of the ionic makeup of extracellular fluids [25].

Tricellulin is the most recently identified TJ integral membrane protein. Like claudins and occludin, it spans the membrane four times with cytoplasmic amino and carboxy termini and forms two extracellular loops. Interestingly, the carboxy terminus of tricellulin (approximately 130 amino acids) is 32% identical to the carboxy terminus of occludin. Tricellulin is concentrated at the vertically oriented TJ strands of tricellular contacts. Down-regulation of tricellulin expression lead to compromised epithelial barrier function, and both bicellular and tricellular contacts were disorganized [22, 23].


## TJs in the Inner Ear

The cochlea of the inner ear has two compartments with different ionic compositions. The perilymph of the scala vestibuli and scala tympani has low $K^+$ and high $Na^+$ concentrations (4 mM and 140 mM, respectively), similar to cerebrospinal fluid [2]. The ionic composition of the endolymph of the scala media is similar to that of an intracellular microenvironment, which has high $K^+$ (150-180 mM) and low $Na^+$ (1 mM) concentrations (reviewed in [1]). This large $K^+$ gradient contributes to an 80-100 mV endocochlear potential (EP), attributed in part to $Na^+$- $K^+$ ATPase activity in the stria vascularis (SV) [34-37]. This electrochemical gradient is critical for the depolarization of sensory hair cells, increasing the sensitivity of the mechanically activated transduction channels located at the top of stereocilia [38, 39].

Well-developed TJs have been observed in ultrastructural analyses of the cochlea and are necessary for compartmentalization within the inner ear. To maintain the high resting potential in the endolymph, epithelial tissues bordering the scala media, including the organ of Corti, Reissner's membrane, the spiral limbus, and the SV (Figure 1), are sealed with various types of TJs. For example, TJs between non-sensory cells that line the scala media, such as the epithelial cells in Reissner's membrane, are "intermediate to tight", while TJs between hair cells and in certain parts of the SV are "very tight" [14, 40-42].

In accordance with the wide spread existence of TJs in the inner ear, multiple TJ proteins are found in this organ, including JAM [43], CAR [44], occludin [45], tricellulin [23], and at least ten members of the claudin family [45]. In recent years mutations in some of these proteins were found to be associated with hereditary hearing loss in human beings and in animal models (Table 1).

# CLAUDIN 14

## Claudin 14 Expression in the Inner Ear

The developmental profile and cell-specific expression pattern of claudin 14 in the mouse inner ear were initially investigated using *in situ* hybridization and immunocytochemistry to detect claudin 14 mRNA and protein, respectively. No expression was detected by *in situ* hybridization at embryonic days 15 (E15) or 17 (E17), but it was detected at postnatal days 4 (P4) and 8 (P8). At P4, claudin 14 expression was apically located in the inner and outer hair cell region of the entire organ of Corti. At P8, the highest claudin 14 expression was detected in the supporting cells of the organ of Corti, including the pillar, Deiters' and inner sulcus cells [46].

In *Cldn14* knockout mice a *lacZ* reporter gene was placed under control of the endogenous *Cldn14* promoter. This feature was used to study *Cldn14* expression pattern in *Cldn14*$^{+/-}$ mice. At P0, ß-galactosidase activity was detected by X-gal staining in outer hair cells (OHCs) at the basal turn of the cochlea. At P4 ß -galactosidase activity was also found in inner hair cells (IHCs) and, to a lesser extent, in supporting cells, of the middle and apical turns. By P7 ß -galactosidase activity was observed in IHCs, OHCs and supporting cells throughout the cochlea, from base to apex. Low ß -galactosidase activity was observed in some spiral prominence cells adjacent to the SV and in the sensory epithelium of the vestibular system [47]. These data are in agreement with previous findings, which were based on *in situ* hybridization and immunostaining [46].

## Mutations in the Human *CLDN14* Gene Cause Autosomal Recessive Deafness DFNB29

The *DFNB29* locus on chromosome 21q22.1 was defined by two large consanguineous Pakistani families segregating prelingual, bilateral, severe to profound sensorineural hearing loss, in an autosomal recessive mode. DFNB29 affected individuals in these families showed no signs of vestibular dysfunction or any other symptoms beside deafness. The *DFNB29* 2.3 Mb interval included three genes, one of which was *CLDN14* [46]. Mutations of gap junction proteins encoded by *GJB2* (*Cx26*) and *GJB3* (*Cx31*) are significant causes of deafness [48]. It was therefore hypothesized that other proteins with functions important for inner ear intercellular junctions might be essential for hearing. This hypothesis made *CLDN14*, encoding for the TJ protein claudin 14, an excellent candidate gene for DFNB29. Sequencing of *CLDN14* single coding exon (exon 3) lead to the identification of two distinct mutations which co-segregated with deafness in both *DFNB29*-linked families. One of the families co-segregated c.398delT, a single nucleotide deletion within codon Met133, located in the third transmembrane domain. This frameshift mutation is predicted to cause premature translation termination 69 nucleotides later, after the incorporation of 23 incorrect amino acids and the loss of almost half of the predicted claudin 14 protein. The second *DFNB29*-linked family co-segregated a missense mutation, p.V85D (aspartic acid substituted for valine), due to a transversion of T to A at position 254 of *CLDN14* cDNA [46]. p.V85D was later identified in an additional consanguineous Pakistani family with similar characteristics [49]. Valine 85 is conserved among 12 of 20 claudins. Aspartic acid at position 85 is predicted to affect hydrophobicity and disrupt the predicted secondary structure in the second transmembrane domain. Neither of the two *CLDN14* mutations was detected in 300 normal control chromosomes from Pakistani individuals, indicating that these two variants are not common polymorphisms in the Pakistani population [46].

In 2005 Wattenhofer *et al.* reported the identification of a third putative pathogenic mutation of *CLDN14*, through a screen of 183 Greek and Spanish patients affected with nonsyndromic severe to profound congenital deafness. A heterozygous G to A transition at position 301 of *CLDN14* cDNA was identified in a Greek patient. This transition leads to the substitution of arginine for glycine at position 101 of claudin 14 (p.G101R). Glycine at position 101 is located in the second transmembrane domain and is conserved in 19 of 21 human claudin proteins. The affected child inherited this putative pathogenic missense mutation from his father. A maternal mutation was not found [50].

To investigate the effect of claudin 14 mutations on protein localization and function, a myc-GFP tagged claudin 14 was expressed in cultured cells. Staining of the wild type (wt) protein was observed both at the plasma membrane and in cytoplasmic compartments of MDCK cells. In LM cells, which do not endogenously express TJ components, expression of wt claudin 14 lead to formation of TJ strands. In the same experimental system, a claudin 14 expressed protein harboring the p.V85D mutation showed a difuzed cytoplasmic localization and did not localize at the plasma membrane of transfected cells. In contrast, the p.G101R mutant localized to both the plasma membrane and to cytopasmic compartments, like the wt protein. Nevertheless, it failed to form TJs in LM cells [50].

The finding of two mutant alleles of *CLDN14* (c.398delT and p.V85D) co-segregating with recessive deafness in three consanguineous families demonstrated the significant role of claudin 14 in the cochlea and its importance in the hearing process. However, the very small number of *CLDN14* mutant alleles and affected families identified to date indicate that mutations of *CLDN14* probably account for only a small portion of recessive nonsyndromic deafness worldwide.

### *Cldn14 knockout mice are deaf: a mouse model for autosomal recessive deafness DFNB29*

To explore the role of claudin 14 in the inner ear and in other organs and tissues a targeted deletion of *Cldn14* was used to create *Cldn14*-null mice [47]. *Cldn14*-null homozygous mice are viable, healthy and fertile, with normal vestibular function. However, these mice were found to be deaf, with auditory brainstem response (ABR) thresholds elevated by 50 dB-SPL or more over all frequencies tested, while thresholds of heterozygous and wt mice were indistinguishable from each other. *Cldn14* knockout mice are therefore a valuable model for studying the pathophysiology of autosomal recessive deafness DFNB29.

Hearing loss in *Cldn14*-null mice was not caused by reduction or absence of EP, as indicated by normal EP values which were measured in *Cldn14*$^{-/-}$ mice at five and ten weeks of age. However, rapid degeneration of cochlear OHCs, followed by slower degeneration of the IHCs, was detected during the first three weeks of life [47]. The onset of OHC loss in

*Cldn14*-null mice, at 8-9 days after birth, coincides with several important developmental processes which occur in inner ears of normal mice, including increase in endolymph $K^+$ concentration, onset of the EP, and formation of a fluid-filled space between OHCs, referred to as the space of Nuel. We assumed that the process of OHC loss in *Cldn14*-null mice was due to an altered ionic composition within the space of Nuel, which surrounds the basolateral membranes of OHCs. Specifically, it was demonstrated that claudin 14 is highly selective against cations. These properties are precisely what would be required to maintain the high cation gradients between perilymph and endolymph. Presumably, in the absence of claudin 14 the ability to maintain the paracellular barrier against cations at the reticular lamina is lost, and perhaps results in elevated $K^+$ concentration in the space of Nuel. This environment is probably toxic to the basolateral membrane of OHCs [47].

In the organ of Corti the apical parts of hair cells and supporting cells form the reticular lamina, which maintains the ion barrier between endolymph and perilymph. This barrier is necessary for normal hearing [51]. Occasional loss of hair cells occurs under normal conditions, while more pronounced OHC loss is observed after aminoglycoside treatment or noise trauma. Under these conditions the integrity of the reticular lamina is preserved by supporting cells, which provide a mechanism for maintenance of inner ear permeability barriers during structural reorganization [52-54]. In *Cldn14*-null mice the absence of claudin 14 from TJs in the reticular lamina leads to rapid and massive death of OHCs, which provides insight into the pathogenesis of human deafness due to *CLDN14* mutations, and further demonstrates the important role of claudins in control of the paracellular barrier.

# CLAUDIN 9

## Claudin 9 Expression in the Inner Ear

Of all the claudin family members, claudin 9 is the most highly expressed in the inner ear [55], and it is present in all of the major epithelial cell types that line the endolymphatic space, including the organ of Corti, marginal cells of the SV, Reissner's membrane, and the spiral limbus [45]. In the intercellular junctions between hair cells and supporting cells in the organ of Corti, claudin 9 and claudin 6 are located together in subdomains that are distinguishable from claudin 14-containing subdomains by strand morphology. Surprisingly, canonical adherens junction proteins (p120ctn, α- and β-catenins) co-localize with the claudin 9/6 subdomain, and form a hybrid TJ with adherens junction organization [55].

### *Cldn9 mutant mice are deaf*

Ethylnitrosourea (ENU)–mutagenesis has been a valuable approach for generating new animal models of deafness and discovering previously unrecognized gene functions. The nmf329 ENU–induced mouse mutant exhibits recessively inherited deafness. At P28 ABR thresholds of *nmf329/nmf329* mice were elevated by ~60 dB-SPL compared to that of wt littermates, whereas the ABR thresholds of heterozygous and wt animals were indistinguishable from each other. The hearing loss of *nmf329/nmf329* mice was equally severe at high- and low-frequencies, as indicated by the uniformly high ABR thresholds at 8, 16, and 32 kHz. This hearing loss was already severe at P16. A widespread loss of sensory hair cells was found in the organ of Corti of nmf329 mice after the second week of life. Positional cloning revealed that the nmf329 strain carries a missense mutation (p.F35L) in the *Cldn9* gene, encoding claudin 9. The affected amino acid (F35) is conserved among all claudin 9 orthologs that have been identified thus far. Moreover, F35 is conserved amongst many members of the claudin protein family [56].

In an epithelial cell line, heterologous expression of wt claudin 9 reduced the paracellular permeability to $Na^+$ and $K^+$, and the *nmf329* mutation eliminated this ion barrier function without affecting the plasma membrane localization of claudin 9. In the nmf329 mouse line, the perilymphatic $K^+$ concentration was found to be elevated, suggesting that the cochlear TJs were dysfunctional. Furthermore, the hair cell loss in the claudin 9–defective cochlea was rescued *in vitro* when the explanted organs of Corti were cultured in a low-$K^+$ milieu and *in vivo* when the endocochlear $K^+$-driving force was diminished by deletion of the *pou3f4* gene. Overall, these findings indicate that claudin 9 is required for the preservation of sensory cells in the organ Corti because claudin 9–defective TJs fail to shield the basolateral side of hair cells from the $K^+$-rich endolymph [56].

In addition to claudin 9, several other claudins have been detected in the junctional complexes of the organ of Corti [45]. Most notably, claudin 14 has been localized to the junctional complexes of hair cells and supporting cells [47, 55]. As described previously, mutations in the murine *Cldn14* gene have been shown to cause extensive hair-cell loss and deafness [47]. Thus, the phenotypes of *Cldn9* mutant mice and *Cldn14* knockout animals are similar. In the junctional complexes of OHCs, claudin 14 and claudin 9 are sorted into two separate subdomains; claudin 14 is found only in the most apical TJ strands, whereas claudin 9 is detected solely in the deeper (subapical) strands [55]. In addition, both claudin 9 and claudin 14 form paracellular ion permeability barriers for $K^+$ [47, 56]. Analysis of the nmf329 mice suggests that not only the apical TJ strands, but also those that are subapical, contribute significantly to the ion barrier capacity of junctional complexes [56].

In addition to being expressed in the cochlea, *Cldn9* has been detected in the vestibular system, liver, and developing kidney, yet *Cldn9* mutant mice exhibited no signs of vestibular, hepatic, or renal defects. Thus, the ion barrier function of claudin 9 is essential in the cochlea, but appears to be dispensable in other organs [56].

# CLAUDIN 11

## Claudin 11 Expression in the Inner Ear

Claudin 11 was first identified as a transmembrane protein highly expressed in central nervous system (CNS) myelin and in testis [57-59]. In the mouse embryo (E14.5) *Cldn11* is expressed in several tissues, including the cochlea and surrounding mesoderm of the ear [60]. In the inner ear of the adult mouse *Cldn11* is expressed in epithelial cells lining the vestibulocochlear apparatus, including the semicircular canals, ampulas, utricle and saccule, suprastrial zone, lateral wall of the cochlear duct, and CNS myelin in the eight cranial nerve. Within the cochlear duct expression is localized primarily to the basal cell layer of the SV, where claudin 11 is incorporated into TJ strands. Notably, while marginal cells of the SV express several claudin species, only claudin 11 was detectable in basal cells [61, 62].

### Cldn11 knockout mice are deaf

*Cldn11* knockout mice exhibited male sterility and neurological abnormalities, including slowed CNS nerve conduction, fine body tremor and persistant hindlimb weakness. These findings were explained by the lack of TJs in the CNS myelin and between Sertoli cells in the testis [60]. In addition, these mice have severe hearing impairment, with ABR thresholds elevated by 40-60 dB-SPL at the age of two months. No gross morphological malformations were observed in inner ears of *Cldn11*-null mice, except for an edematous appearance of the SV, which may reflect changes in ion composition of the intrastrial space, caused by infusion of perilymph from surrounding regions. Hearing loss is the result of markedly reduced EP, due to the lack of TJs from the basal cells of the SV [61, 62]. The SV is where the electrogenic machinery that generates the EP is located [63]. In *Cldn11*-null mice the absence of a paracellular barrier between basal cells renders the intrastrial space open to perilymph, and abolishes its electrical isolation [61, 62].

# CLAUDIN J

## The Zebrafish *Cldnj* Gene is Essential for Normal Ear Function and Important for Formation of Otoliths

The fish ear begins to develop as a two-cell thick ectodermal structure lateral to the hindbrain, called the otic placode. The layers cavitate creating a hollow fluid-filled cavity called the otocyst. Shortly thereafter, the first two hair cells appear. The kinocilia from these hair cells serve as the seed point for the calcium carbonate and protein deposits called otoliths, which are necessary for sound amplification. Creation of the otoliths requires the establishment of a sealed compartment containing a unique protein and ion composition. The boundaries of this compartment are defined by the cells of the otic placode and the TJs between them [64].

In 1999 Amsterdam *et al.* performed a large scale insertional mutagenesis screen in zebrafish, using the F5 retrovirus [65]. A screen for embryonic defects lead to the identification of a mutant allele, initially named Hi340. Fish which were homozygotes for this mutation displayed reduced otoliths, and impaired hearing and balance, as indicated by the lack of response to tapping stimulus and by the inability to orient in space. The mutation was caused by an insertion in the zebrafish *cldnj* gene. Phylogenetic analysis revealed that *cldnj* falls into a cluster of six zebrafish claudin genes, which appear to be related to human claudins 3, 4, 5, 6, and 9. In the zebrafish embryo *cldnj* was expressed in the otic placode and then in the otic vesicle. In *cldnj* mutant embryos the epithelial structure of the otocyst did not seem to be disrupted, therefore implicating that the cause for inner ear dysfunction is not simply a profound loss of epithelial integrity, but rather a deficiency in some barrier function for specific ions [66].

# TRICELLULIN

## Tricellulin Expression in the Inner Ear

Tricellulin expression in the mouse inner ear was studied by immunostaining with an anti- tricellulin antibody. At P5, P10, P16 and P90 tricellulin was found to be concentrated at tricellular points of contact in the majority of epithelial cells of the cochlea and vestibule, with a weaker punctate signal along bicellular TJs. At the junctions of OHCs with two adjacent supporting cells tricellulin was located along the entire depth of tricellular TJs, extending in near-perpendicular orientation to the reticular lamina. Tricellulin also spans the entire depth of tricellular TJs of other epithelial cell types, although the tricellular TJs of the nonsensory epithelium do not appear as deep as the tricellular TJs of the sensory epithelium of the organ of Corti [23].

## Mutations in the Human *TRIC* Gene Cause Autosomal Recessive Deafness DFNB49

The *DFNB49* locus on chromosome 5q12.3-q14.1 was initially defined by genetic linkage analysis of two large consanguineous Pakistani families segregating congenital, bilateral, moderate to profound sensorineural hearing loss, in an autosomal recessive mode [67]. Later on, six additional *DFNB49*-linked families were identified [23]. Both inter- and intrafamilial variability in the severity of hearing loss were observed in these families, which may be caused by genetic modifiers and/or environmental factors. Based on meiotic information from all affected families, the *DFNB49*-linked interval was refined to 2.4 Mb. This interval contained 33 annotated genes. A total of four pathogenic mutations were eventually found in one of these genes, *TRIC*, encoding for tricellulin, a novel TJ protein [23]. These include three splice-site mutations (IVS3-1G>A, IVS4+2delTGAG, and IVS4+2T>C), and a nonsense mutation (c.1498C>T; p.R500X). None of these mutations were detected in a total of 443 normal hearing individuals from Pakistan, India, and the Human Variation Panel.

*TRIC* mRNA has at least four alternatively-spliced isoforms in humans (*TRIC-a, TRIC-a1, TRIC-b,* and *TRIC-c*). Most isoforms contain an occludin-ELL domain in their carboxy terminus, while the shortest isoform, *TRIC-b*, lacks this domain [22, 23]. The carboxy terminus of occludin is known to bind the scaffolding protein ZO-1, which controls its targeting to cell-cell junctions [68]. A GST-fusion protein encoding the cytosolic C-terminal domain of wt tricellulin, including the occludin ELL-domain, was able to bind directly to ZO-1 *in vitro*. In contrast, binding of the p.R500X mutant tricellulin to ZO-1 was significantly compromised [23].

A common feature of the four identified *TRIC* mutant alleles is that they encode predicted truncated proteins that lack the ability to bind ZO-1. It is therefore possible that at least one underlying cause of cellular dysfunction in the cochlea is the inability to incorporate these mutant proteins into the cytosolic scaffold formed by ZO proteins. Given the ubiquitous expression pattern of tricellulin in epithelial junctions of tissues throughout the body, the limited phenotype associated with *TRIC* mutations is surprising. It is possible that some other molecule compensates for the absence of wt tricellulin in other epithelial cell types but not in the inner ear. Alternatively, the wt short isoform of tricellulin (*TRIC-b*) may be present in these mutants and may be sufficiently functional for tricellular junctions in tissues other than the ear. Generation of a mouse model for DFNB49 will be of much importance for elucidating the exact function of tricellulin in the auditory apparatus and the etiology of DFNB49-related deafness.

# CONCLUSION

In the cochlea of the inner ear separation between endolymph and perilimph is necessary for normal hearing. This compartmentalization is achieved by TJs, which form the major selective barrier of the paracellular pathway between epithelial cells. TJ strands contain at least five types of membrane-spanning proteins (occluding, claudins, JAM, CAR, and tricellulin). To date, mutations in five different TJ membrane integral proteins (claudin 9, claudin 11, claudin 14, claudin j, and tricellulin) have been associated with hearing loss in humans and/or in animal models (Table 1). There are different etiologies for hearing loss associated with each of these proteins, including hair cell loss, reduced EP, and abnormal embryonic development of the inner ear. Nevertheless, in all cases the underlying cause is dysfunction of the paracellular barrier. These findings elucidate the crucial role played by TJs in the auditory apparatus, and enhance our understanding of the hearing process. This knowledge will be further enhanced by identification of hearing-related phenotypes associated with additional TJ proteins and generation of additional animal models in years to come.

# ACKNOWLEDGMENTS

I thank Thomas Friedman for critical reading of this manuscript. This work was supported by a research grant from the Israel Science Foundation (grant number 24/05).

# REFERENCES

[1] Ferrary, E. & Sterkers, O. (1998) Mechanisms of endolymph secretion. *Kidney Int Suppl*, *65*, S98-103.

[2] Ryan, A. F., Wickham, M. G. & Bone, R. C. (1979) Element content of intracochlear fluids, outer hair cells, and stria vascularis as determined by energy-dispersive roentgen ray analysis. *Otolaryngol Head Neck Surg*, *87*, 659-665.

[3] Farquhar, M. G. & Palade, G. E. (1963) Junctional complexes in various epithelia. J Cell Biol, *17*, 375-412.

[4] Kowalczyk, A. P., Bornslaeger, E. A., Norvell, S. M., Palka, H. L. & Green, K. J. (1999) Desmosomes: intercellular adhesive junctions specialized for attachment of intermediate filaments. *Int Rev Cytol*, *185*, 237-302.

[5] Nagafuchi, A. (2001) Molecular architecture of adherens junctions. *Curr Opin Cell Biol*, *13*, 600-603.

[6]  Goodenough, D. A., Goliger, J. A. & Paul, D. L. (1996) Connexins, connexons, and intercellular communication. *Annu Rev Biochem*, *65,* 475-502.

[7]  Anderson, J. M. (2001) Molecular structure of tight junctions and their role in epithelial transport. *News Physiol Sci*, *16,* 126-130.

[8]  Tsukita, S., Furuse, M. & Itoh, M. (2001) Multifunctional strands in tight junctions. *Nat Rev Mol Cell Biol*, *2,* 285-293.

[9]  Staehelin, L. A. (1974) Structure and function of intercellular junctions. *Int Rev Cytol*, *39,* 191-283.

[10] Walker, D. C., MacKenzie, A. & Hosford, S. (1994) The structure of the tricellular region of endothelial tight junctions of pulmonary capillaries analyzed by freeze-fracture. *Microvasc Res*, *48,* 259-281.

[11] Walker, D. C., MacKenzie, A., Hulbert, W. C. & Hogg, J. C. (1985) A re-assessment of the tricellular region of epithelial cell tight junctions in trachea of guinea pig. *Acta Anat (Basel)*, *122,* 35-38.

[12] Madara, J. L. (1998) Regulation of the movement of solutes across tight junctions. *Annu Rev Physiol*, *60,* 143-159.

[13] Fromter, E. & Diamond, J. (1972) Route of passive ion permeation in epithelia. *Nat New Biol*, *235,* 9-13.

[14] Claude, P. & Goodenough, D. A. (1973) Fracture faces of zonulae occludentes from "tight" and "leaky" epithelia. *J Cell Biol*, *58,* 390-400.

[15] Cereijido, M., Valdes, J., Shoshani, L. & Contreras, R. G. (1998) Role of tight junctions in establishing and maintaining cell polarity. *Annu Rev Physiol*, *60,* 161-177.

[16] Dragsten, P. R., Blumenthal, R. & Handler, J. S. (1981) Membrane asymmetry in epithelia: is the tight junction a barrier to diffusion in the plasma membrane? *Nature*, *294,* 718-722.

[17] van Meer, G., Gumbiner, B. & Simons, K. (1986) The tight junction does not allow lipid molecules to diffuse from one epithelial cell to the next. *Nature*, *322,* 639-641.

[18] van Meer, G. & Simons, K. (1986) The function of tight junctions in maintaining differences in lipid composition between the apical and the basolateral cell surface domains of MDCK cells. *Embo J*, *5,* 1455-1464.

[19] Furuse, M., Hirase, T., Itoh, M., Nagafuchi, A., Yonemura, S., Tsukita, S. & Tsukita, S. (1993) Occludin: a novel integral membrane protein localizing at tight junctions. *J Cell Biol*, *123,* 1777-1788.

[20] Mandell, K. J. & Parkos, C. A. (2005) The JAM family of proteins. *Adv Drug Deliv Rev*, *57,* 857-867.

[21] Cohen, C. J., Shieh, J. T., Pickles, R. J., Okegawa, T., Hsieh, J. T. & Bergelson, J. M. (2001) The coxsackievirus and adenovirus receptor is a transmembrane component of the tight junction. *Proc Natl Acad Sci U S A*, *98,* 15191-15196.

[22] Ikenouchi, J., Furuse, M., Furuse, K., Sasaki, H., Tsukita, S. & Tsukita, S. (2005) Tricellulin constitutes a novel barrier at tricellular contacts of epithelial cells. *J Cell Biol*, *171,* 939-945.

[23] Riazuddin, S., Ahmed, Z. M., Fanning, A. S., Lagziel, A., Kitajiri, S., Ramzan, K., Khan, S. N., Chattaraj, P., Friedman, P. L., Anderson, J. M., Belyantseva, I. A., Forge, A., Riazuddin, S. & Friedman, T. B. (2006) Tricellulin is a tight-junction protein necessary for hearing. *Am J Hum Genet*, *79,* 1040-1051.

[24] Tsukita, S. & Furuse, M. (2000) The structure and function of claudins, cell adhesion molecules at tight junctions. *Ann N Y Acad Sci, 915,* 129-135.

[25] Van Itallie, C. M. & Anderson, J. M. (2006) Claudins and epithelial paracellular transport. *Annu Rev Physiol, 68,* 403-429.

[26] Hirase, T., Staddon, J. M., Saitou, M., Ando-Akatsuka, Y., Itoh, M., Furuse, M., Fujimoto, K., Tsukita, S. & Rubin, L. L. (1997) Occludin as a possible determinant of tight junction permeability in endothelial cells. J Cell Sci, 110 ( Pt 14), 1603-1613.

[27] Moroi, S., Saitou, M., Fujimoto, K., Sakakibara, A., Furuse, M., Yoshida, O. & Tsukita, S. (1998) Occludin is concentrated at tight junctions of mouse/rat but not human/guinea pig Sertoli cells in testes. *Am J Physiol, 274,* C1708-1717.

[28] Saitou, M., Fujimoto, K., Doi, Y., Itoh, M., Fujimoto, T., Furuse, M., Takano, H., Noda, T. & Tsukita, S. (1998) Occludin-deficient embryonic stem cells can differentiate into polarized epithelial cells bearing tight junctions. *J Cell Biol, 141,* 397-408.

[29] Wong, V. & Gumbiner, B. M. (1997) A synthetic peptide corresponding to the extracellular domain of occludin perturbs the tight junction permeability barrier. *J Cell Biol, 136,* 399-409.

[30] Tsukita, S. & Furuse, M. (2000) Pores in the wall: claudins constitute tight junction strands containing aqueous pores. *J Cell Biol, 149,* 13-16.

[31] Furuse, M., Fujita, K., Hiiragi, T., Fujimoto, K. & Tsukita, S. (1998) Claudin-1 and -2: novel integral membrane proteins localizing at tight junctions with no sequence similarity to occludin. *J Cell Biol, 141,* 1539-1550.

[32] Furuse, M., Sasaki, H. & Tsukita, S. (1999) Manner of interaction of heterogeneous claudin species within and between tight junction strands. *J Cell Biol, 147,* 891-903.

[33] Morita, K., Furuse, M., Fujimoto, K. & Tsukita, S. (1999) Claudin multigene family encoding four-transmembrane domain protein components of tight junction strands. *Proc Natl Acad Sci U S A, 96,* 511-516.

[34] Gratton, M. A., Smyth, B. J., Lam, C. F., Boettcher, F. A. & Schmiedt, R. A. (1997) Decline in the endocochlear potential corresponds to decreased Na,K-ATPase activity in the lateral wall of quiet-aged gerbils. *Hear Res, 108,* 9-16.

[35] Marcus, D. C. & Chiba, T. (1999) K+ and Na+ absorption by outer sulcus epithelial cells. *Hear Res, 134,* 48-56.

[36] Souter, M. & Forge, A. (1998) Intercellular junctional maturation in the stria vascularis: possible association with onset and rise of endocochlear potential. *Hear Res, 119,* 81-95.

[37] Stankovic, K. M., Brown, D., Alper, S. L. & Adams, J. C. (1997) Localization of pH regulating proteins H+ATPase and Cl-/HCO3- exchanger in the guinea pig inner ear. *Hear Res, 114,* 21-34.

[38] Hudspeth, A. J. (1989) How the ear's works work. *Nature, 341,* 397-404.

[39] Milhaud, P. G., Nicolas, M. T., Bartolami, S., Cabanis, M. T. & Sans, A. (1999) Vestibular semicircular canal epithelium of the rat in culture on filter support: polarity and barrier properties. *Pflugers Arch, 437,* 823-830.

[40] Anniko, M. & Wroblewski, R. (1984) The freeze fracture technique in inner ear research. *Scan Electron Microsc,* 2067-2075.

[41] Gulley, R. L. & Reese, T. S. (1976) Intercellular junctions in the reticular lamina of the organ of Corti. *J Neurocytol, 5,* 479-507.

[42] Jahnke, K. (1975) The fine structure of freeze-fractured intercellular junctions in the guinea pig inner ear. *Acta Otolaryngol Suppl, 336,* 1-40.

[43]Parris, J. J., Cooke, V. G., Skarnes, W. C., Duncan, M. K. & Naik, U. P. (2005) JAM-A expression during embryonic development. *Dev Dyn*, *233*, 1517-1524.

[44]Venail, F., Wang, J., Ruel, J., Ballana, E., Rebillard, G., Eybalin, M., Arbones, M., Bosch, A. & Puel, J. L. (2007) Coxsackie adenovirus receptor and alpha nu beta3/alpha nu beta5 integrins in adenovirus gene transfer of rat cochlea. *Gene Ther*, *14*, 30-37.

[45]Kitajiri, S. I., Furuse, M., Morita, K., Saishin-Kiuchi, Y., Kido, H., Ito, J. & Tsukita, S. (2004) Expression patterns of claudins, tight junction adhesion molecules, in the inner ear. *Hear Res*, *187*, 25-34.

[46]Wilcox, E. R., Burton, Q. L., Naz, S., Riazuddin, S., Smith, T. N., Ploplis, B., Belyantseva, I., Ben-Yosef, T., Liburd, N. A., Morell, R. J., Kachar, B., Wu, D. K., Griffith, A. J., Riazuddin, S. & Friedman, T. B. (2001) Mutations in the gene encoding tight junction claudin-14 cause autosomal recessive deafness DFNB29. *Cell*, *104*, 165-172.

[47]Ben-Yosef, T., Belyantseva, I. A., Saunders, T. L., Hughes, E. D., Kawamoto, K., Van Itallie, C. M., Beyer, L. A., Halsey, K., Gardner, D. J., Wilcox, E. R., Rasmussen, J., Anderson, J. M., Dolan, D. F., Forge, A., Raphael, Y., Camper, S. A. & Friedman, T. B. (2003) Claudin 14 knockout mice, a model for autosomal recessive deafness DFNB*29*, are deaf due to cochlear hair cell degeneration. *Hum Mol Genet*, *12*, 2049-2061.

[48]Nickel, R. & Forge, A. (2008) Gap junctions and connexins in the inner ear: their roles in homeostasis and deafness. *Curr Opin Otolaryngol Head Neck Surg*, *16*, 452-457.

[49]Ahmed, Z. M., Riazuddin, S., Friedman, T. B., Riazuddin, S., Wilcox, E. R. & Griffith, A. J. (2002) Clinical manifestations of DFNB29 deafness. *Adv Otorhinolaryngol*, *61*, 156-160.

[50]Wattenhofer, M., Reymond, A., Falciola, V., Charollais, A., Caille, D., Borel, C., Lyle, R., Estivill, X., Petersen, M. B., Meda, P. & Antonarakis, S. E. (2005) Different mechanisms preclude mutant CLDN14 proteins from forming tight junctions in vitro. *Hum Mutat*, *25*, 543-549.

[51]Tasaki, I., Davis, H. & Eldredge, D. H. (1954) Exploration of cochlear potentials in guinea pig with a microelectrode. *J Acoust Soc Am*, *26*, 765-773.

[52]Forge, A. (1985) Outer hair cell loss and supporting cell expansion following chronic gentamicin treatment. *Hear Res*, *19*, 171-182.

[53]Leonova, E. V. & Raphael, Y. (1997) Organization of cell junctions and cytoskeleton in the reticular lamina in normal and ototoxically damaged organ of Corti. *Hear Res*, *113*, 14-28.

[54]Raphael, Y. & Altschuler, R. A. (1991) Reorganization of cytoskeletal and junctional proteins during cochlear hair cell degeneration. *Cell Motil Cytoskeleton*, *18*, 215-227.

[55]Nunes, F. D., Lopez, L. N., Lin, H. W., Davies, C., Azevedo, R. B., Gow, A. & Kachar, B. (2006) Distinct subdomain organization and molecular composition of a tight junction with adherens junction features. *J Cell Sci*, *119*, 4819-4827.

[56]Nakano, Y., Kim, S. H., Kim, H. M., Sanneman, J. D., Zhang, Y., Smith, R. J., Marcus, D. C., Wangemann, P., Nessler, R. A. & Banfi, B. (2009) A claudin-9-based ion permeability barrier is essential for hearing. *PLoS Genet*, *5*, e1000610.

[57]Bronstein, J. M., Chen, K., Tiwari-Woodruff, S. & Kornblum, H. I. (2000) Developmental expression of OSP/claudin-11. *J Neurosci Res*, *60*, 284-290.

[58]Bronstein, J. M., Micevych, P. E. & Chen, K. (1997) Oligodendrocyte-specific protein (OSP) is a major component of CNS myelin. *J Neurosci Res*, *50*, 713-720.

[59]Morita, K., Sasaki, H., Fujimoto, K., Furuse, M. & Tsukita, S. (1999) Claudin-11/OSP-based tight junctions of myelin sheaths in brain and Sertoli cells in testis. *J Cell Biol, 145,* 579-588.

[60]Gow, A., Southwood, C. M., Li, J. S., Pariali, M., Riordan, G. P., Brodie, S. E., Danias, J., Bronstein, J. M., Kachar, B. & Lazzarini, R. A. (1999) CNS myelin and sertoli cell tight junction strands are absent in Osp/claudin-11 null mice. *Cell, 99,* 649-659.

[61]Gow, A., Davies, C., Southwood, C. M., Frolenkov, G., Chrustowski, M., Ng, L., Yamauchi, D., Marcus, D. C. & Kachar, B. (2004) Deafness in Claudin 11-null mice reveals the critical contribution of basal cell tight junctions to stria vascularis function. *J Neurosci, 24,* 7051-7062.

[62]Kitajiri, S., Miyamoto, T., Mineharu, A., Sonoda, N., Furuse, K., Hata, M., Sasaki, H., Mori, Y., Kubota, T., Ito, J., Furuse, M. & Tsukita, S. (2004) Compartmentalization established by claudin-11-based tight junctions in stria vascularis is required for hearing through generation of endocochlear potential. *J Cell Sci, 117,* 5087-5096.

[63]Salt, A. N., Melichar, I. & Thalmann, R. (1987) Mechanisms of endocochlear potential generation by stria vascularis. *Laryngoscope, 97,* 984-991.

[64]Kimmel, C. B., Ballard, W. W., Kimmel, S. R., Ullmann, B. & Schilling, T. F. (1995) Stages of embryonic development of the zebrafish. *Dev Dyn, 203,* 253-310.

[65]Amsterdam, A., Burgess, S., Golling, G., Chen, W., Sun, Z., Townsend, K., Farrington, S., Haldi, M. & Hopkins, N. (1999) A large-scale insertional mutagenesis screen in zebrafish. *Genes Dev, 13,* 2713-2724.

[66]Hardison, A. L., Lichten, L., Banerjee-Basu, S., Becker, T. S. & Burgess, S. M. (2005) The zebrafish gene claudinj is essential for normal ear function and important for the formation of the otoliths. *Mech Dev, 122,* 949-958.

[67]Ramzan, K., Shaikh, R. S., Ahmad, J., Khan, S. N., Riazuddin, S., Ahmed, Z. M., Friedman, T. B., Wilcox, E. R. & Riazuddin, S. (2005) A new locus for nonsyndromic deafness DFNB49 maps to chromosome 5q12.3-q14.1. *Hum Genet, 116,* 17-22.

[68]Li, Y., Fanning, A. S., Anderson, J. M. & Lavie, A. (2005) Structure of the conserved cytoplasmic C-terminal domain of occludin: identification of the ZO-1 binding surface. J Mol Biol, *352,* 151-164.

In: Deafness, Hearing Loss and the Auditory System    ISBN: 978-1-60741-259-5
Editors: D. Fiedler and R. Krause, pp.227-248    ©2010 Nova Science Publishers, Inc.

*Chapter 9*

# A SYSTEMATIC REVIEW OF HEARING PROTECTIVE DEVISES: TYPES, USES AND SAFETY

## *Regina P. El Dib*[*]

McMaster University, St. Joseph's Healthcare Hamilton, Ontario, Canada

## ABSTRACT

*Introduction:* Noise-induced hearing loss is one of the most common occupational diseases. Approximately 30 million workers in the USA alone are exposed to hazardous noise at work (WHO 2002). There is no effective treatment for permanent hearing loss resulting from excessive noise exposure. The condition can be easily prevented using preventative measures such as personal hearing protection devices or hearing protector (i.e., earplugs, earmuffs).

*Objective:* To summarize the evidence for the effectiveness and safety of different types of hearing protective devices among workers exposed to noise in the workplace.

*Methods:* A systematic review of the literature was conducted. We searched the Cochrane Central Register of Controlled Trials (CENTRAL); Pubmed; EMBASE; LILACS and; Current Controlled Trials for ongoing trials. The date of the last search was 16th February 2009. Studies were included if they had a randomized or quasi-randomized design, if they were among noise exposed (> 80 dB($\Lambda$)) workers and, if there was at least two hearing protectors to be compared. The reviewer selected relevant trials, assessed methodological quality and extracted data.

*Results:* Two studies were included with a total of 46 participants. It was not possible to combine the included studies in a meta-analysis. Both included studies evaluated earplugs as hearing protectors. The representations of meta-analysis with only one study showed that participants that worn HL SmartFit had fewer number of difficulties per number of conversations compared to E-A-R Push-Ins earplugs. In addition, participants

---

[*] Corresponding author: Post-doctoral Fellow, McMaster University, St. Joseph's Healthcare Hamilton, 50 Charlton Ave East, Hamilton, ON, Canada L8N 4A. Emails: re.lucci@terra.com.br

reported higher rate of satisfaction wearing HL SmartFit when compared to E-A-R Push-Ins or Sonomax SonoCustoms.

*Conclusion:* The evidence found in this review showed that the HL SmartFit earplug is more effective compared to E-A-R Push-Ins foam earplug and Sonomax SonoCustoms regarding the number of difficulties per number of conversations and satisfaction. Future trials should have standardized outcomes measures such as attenuation, speech intelligibility and audibility (hear communication) in the noise environment, worker acceptance of HPDs and the likelihood that workers will wear them consistently, hearing loss thresholds by audiometric test, costs and others.

# 1. INTRODUCTION

Noise-induced hearing loss is one of the most common occupational diseases. Approximately 30 million workers in the USA alone are exposed to hazardous noise at work (WHO 2002) and an annual worldwide incidence of noise-induced hearing loss of 1,628,000 cases (Leigh 1999). With a worldwide population of 6.525 billion this is equal to 25 per 100,000 per year (El Dib 2009). The condition is permanent and irreversible. Early damage is typically sustained in the basal turn of the cochlea and affects hearing in the frequency range from 3000 to 6000 hertz (Hz) (the frequency of speech) (El Dib 2009). Long-term exposure to noise levels beyond 80 dB(A) carries an increased risk of hearing loss which increases exponentially with the noise level. The risk of hearing impairment (average hearing loss > 35 dB(A) at 1, 2 and 3 kHz) at age 60 due to 40 years of exposure to noise levels of 100 dB(A) has been estimated at 55% (Malchaire 1997).

There is no effective treatment for permanent hearing loss resulting from excessive noise exposure. The ideal situation for preventing hearing loss would be the reduction of noise level at the source and, in most cases this is hard to obtain. Therefore, the condition can be easily prevented using preventative measures such as personal hearing protection devices or hearing protector (i.e., earplugs, earmuffs) and hearing conservation programmes or hearing loss prevention programme. The effectiveness of personal protective measures at preventing hearing loss from accumulated noise exposure depends mainly on how regularly they are used by workers. Studies have shown that if workers do not wear hearing protection 100% of the time its effectiveness will quickly diminish. For example, wearing hearing protection for only 90% of the time will decrease effectiveness to less than one third (Arezes 2002). Educational or behavioural interventions to promote its use are therefore important preventative measures.

A systematic review of the literature evaluated the effectiveness of interventions to influence workers to wear hearing protection to decrease their exposure to noise. The evidence found in this review showed that tailored interventions (the use of communication or other types of treatments that are specific for an individual or a group to change behavior) improve the mean use of hearing protective device versus non-intervention. Tailored education was more effective in the use of HPDs compared with target education programmes. However, the authors concluded that future trials should be performed with standard outcomes and interventions to allow the combining of results in a meta-analysis (El Dib 2009).

Intention to use the devices, perceived benefits and barriers to the use of hearing protection, proper training, fit the hearing protection devices (HPDs) properly to achieve a optimum attenuation are important variables to help workers on the permanent use of personal protective measures in the noise working environment. The HPDs should be in the ear far enough to satisfy a cursory visual compliance check (Brad 2007). The difference between a good insertion and a poor insertion is enough to cause a 30-40 dB improvement in attenuation at various frequencies when the personal protective measures is deeply inserted and achieves a good seal in the ear (Brad 2007).

There are different fit test methods available to measure the attenuation of hearing protectors and, thereby the effectiveness of HPDs through audiograms with and without their HPDs both before and after HPD insertion, before and after HPD removal during the work shifts. How much attenuation a hearing protector provides depends on its characteristics and how the worker wears it. The noise attenuation of hearing protectors as they are worn in the occupational environment is usually different from that realized in the laboratory. Hearing protectors often make communication difficult by reducing and distorting sounds.

The main types of hearing protectors: (i) formable earplugs (such as silicon or spun mineral fiber) made of expandable foam; (ii) pre-molded and custom-molded earplugs made from flexible plastics; (iii) semi-aural devices, or canal caps (semi-inserts) , consisting of flexible tips on a lightweight headband; and (iv) earmuffs having rigid cups with soft plastic cushions that seal around the ears. Figures 1, 2, 3 and 4 show the different types of earmuffs and earplugs.

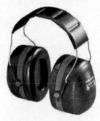

Figure 1. Over-the-Head earmuff.

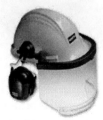

Figure 2. Earmuff helmet mounted.

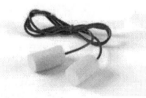

Figure 3. Foam earplugs.

Figure 4. Pre-formed earplugs.

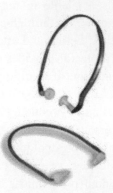

Figure 5. Semi-inserted (canal caps).

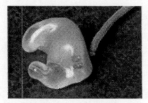

Figure 6. Earplug dB blocker vented.

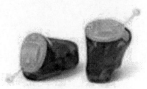

Figure 7. Custom-devices.

Usually the foam earplug is the most comfortable hearing protector, however requires more time to fit and requires good hygiene. The pre-former earplugs have an easier insertion, but can be uncomfortable to some for long wear. The semi-insert device is convenient and lightweight, but it is usually indicated for intermittent exposure. The earmuffs have different electronic models available for enhanced communication and special applications, but also are indicated for intermittent exposure; and the custom-devices are customized with easy insertion; however have a high initial cost (Alaska Occupational Audiology and Health Services).

Despite the fact that earplugs and earmuffs have been widely used, its effectiveness and safety with regards a higher attenuation; better communication between workers while on the use of HPDs, comfort, convenience and good seal was never determined, mainly, which hearing protector presents better performance for workers exposure to noise levels use it.

## 2. OBJECTIVES

To summarize the evidence for the effectiveness and safety of different types of hearing protective devices among workers exposed to noise in the workplace.

## 3. CRITERIA FOR CONSIDERING STUDIES FOR THIS REVIEW

### Types of Studies

All randomized and quasi-randomized controlled trials and cluster randomized controlled trials which fulfilled the criteria outlined below were included.

### Types of Participants

All workers exposed to noise levels above 80 dB(A) and who had the opportunity to wear ear protection because of occupational exposure to noise.

### Types of Interventions

This review considered all types of personal hearing protection devices or hearing protector (earmuffs, earplugs and canal caps).

We also considered different types of earmuffs such as helmet mounted and over the head as well as different types of earplugs (custom-molded silicone, expandable foam earplug, etc). We also considered the combination of different types of hearing protection devices (e.g. earmuffs in conjunction with earplugs).

Interventions were to be compared against each other.

The workers should be preliminary trained on how to correctly wear the hearing protective device and its adjustments, as would it be in a laboratory study, to allow a better definition of its attenuation and consequently, a better evaluation of the hearing protection performance.

### Types of Outcome Measures

*Primary outcome measure*
- Attenuation, using the real ear attenuation at threshold – REAT – test, which is based on the difference between the open and occluded hearing level of a subject;
- Speech intelligibility and audibility (hear communication) in the noise environment, analyzed by videotape during the worker's activities through various signs of speech communication difficulties such as removal of earplugs, distance between communicating people at less than one arm's length, cupping ear with the hand,

place ear next to the mouth of the speaker, increased use of hand gestures, writing, requests for clarification, repeated phrases in conversation, etc.

- Elimination of threshold shift (caused by continuous noise of high intensity).

## *Secondary outcome measures*

- Worker acceptance of HPDs and the likelihood that workers will wear them consistently (intention to use the devices): comfort and convenience, awareness of risk, ease of fit/good seal (self-reported use of hearing protection);
- Perceived benefits and barriers to use of hearing protection (self-reported use of hearing protection);
- Hearing loss thresholds by audiometric test;
- Costs (as a narrative analysis).

There were no specific exclusion criteria.

## Search Strategy for Identification of Studies

There was no language restriction. Trials were obtained from the following sources:

We searched the Cochrane Central Register of Controlled Trials (CENTRAL, The Cochrane Library, Issue 1 2009), PUBMED (1966 to February 2009), EMBASE (1980 to February 2009), LILACS (1982 to February 2009), and Current Controlled Trials to identify ongoing trials. The date of the last search was 16th February 2009.

The search strategy was composed only of terms for hearing protection in order to maximize sensitivity. As we searched with both subject headings and free text words, it was expected that all studies of hearing protection would be identified. The following exhaustive list of synonyms for hearing protective devices was identified:

((Ear Protective Device) OR (Ear Protective Devices) OR Earplugs OR Earplug OR (Hearing Protective Devices) OR (Hearing Protective Device) OR Earmuffs OR Earmuff OR (hearing protector) OR (hearing protection) OR (ear muff) OR (ear muffs) OR (ear plug) OR (ear plugs) OR (ear defender) OR (ear defenders)) **AND** ((Occupational Noise) OR (Occupational Noises))

We modeled subject strategies for databases on the search strategy designed for CENTRAL. Where appropriate, we combined subject strategies with adaptations of the highly sensitive search strategy for identifying randomized controlled trials and controlled clinical trials.

Search strategies for the type of study (randomized clinical trials) for each databases including PubMed are shown in Appendix 1.

Reference lists of the identified relevant studies were scrutinized for additional citations. Specialists in the field and authors of the included trials were contacted for unpublished data.

# 4. Methods of the Review

The author screened the trials identified by the literature search, extracted the data, assessed trial quality and analyzed the results.

## 4.1. Quality Assessment

The methodological quality of the included trials in this review was measured using the criteria described in the Cochrane Handbook (Higgins 2008), since scales and checklists are not a reliable method to assess the validity of a primary study (Jüni 1999):

Selection bias – Was allocation concealment adequate?
MET: adequate concealment of allocation;
UNCLEAR: not described, not reported;
NOT MET: inadequate;
Not used.

Selection bias - Was the generation of allocation sequence adequate?
MET: Adequate generation (random);
UNCLEAR: Unclear, not described in the paper or by contacting authors;
NOT MET: Inadequate generation of allocation;
Not used.

Detection bias – Was there a blinded assessment of outcomes?
MET: assessor unaware of the assigned treatment when collecting outcome measures;
UNCLEAR, not reported: blinding of assessor not reported and cannot be verified by contacting investigators;
NOT MET: assessor aware of the assigned treatment when collecting outcome measures.

Attrition bias – Were any withdrawals described?
MET: lesser than 20% and equally for both comparison groups;
UNCLEAR: not reported in paper or by authors;
NOT MET: greater than 20% or/and not equally for both comparison groups.

## 4.2. Data Extraction

A standard form was used to extract the following information: characteristics of the study (design, methods of randomisation); participants; interventions; outcomes (types of outcome measures, continuous or dichotomous) (Appendix 2).

## 4.3. Data Analysis

For dichotomous data, risk relative (RR) was used as the effect measure. For continuous data the weighted mean difference (WMD), in which the effect estimates of individual studies are weighted by dispersion measures, was used.

### 4.3.1. Heterogeneity
It was not necessary to measure heterogeneity in this version of the review. Inconsistency among the pooled estimates should be quantified using the i-squared statistic. This illustrates the percentage of the variability in effect estimates resulting from heterogeneity rather than sampling error (Higgins 2003; Higgins 2005). I2 = [(Q - df)/Q] x 100% test, where Q is the chi-squared statistic and df its degrees of freedom.

### 4.3.2. Sensitivity analysis
Sensitivity analysis to assess the effect of including or not including studies based on their methodological quality was not carried out in this review due to the low number of included studies.

### 4.3.3. Addressing publication bias
Again, due to the small number of studies included in this review we were not able to assess publication bias by preparing a funnel plot (trial effect versus trial size).

# 5. RESULTS

## 5.1. Description of Studies

### 5.1.1. Study selection
The search strategy identified approximately 585 titles (see Figure 8). Following assessment of 47 full text articles only 21 publications were considered for inclusion in this review. 19 studies were subsequently excluded (Nakao 2008; Abel 2006; Neitzel 2006; Lin 2005; Pääkkönen 2005; Ong 2004; Horie 2002; Wagstaff 2001; Pääkkönen 1998; Bhattacharya 1993; Dancer 1992; Sataloff 1986; Royster 1984; Chung 1983; Erlandsson 1980; Ivarsson 1980; Royster 1980; Smith 1980; Taniewski 1978). Two studies which met the minimal methodological requirements were included in the review (Wagoner 2007 and Lempert 1983).

### 5.1.2. Included studies
Two studies were included in this review (Wagoner 2007 and Lempert 1983) with a total of 46 participants.

### 5.1.3. Design of the studies
Wagoner 2007 study was a cross-over multicenter randomized controlled trial which subjects were recruited from the maintenance area of two airports (American Trans Air and Purdue University).

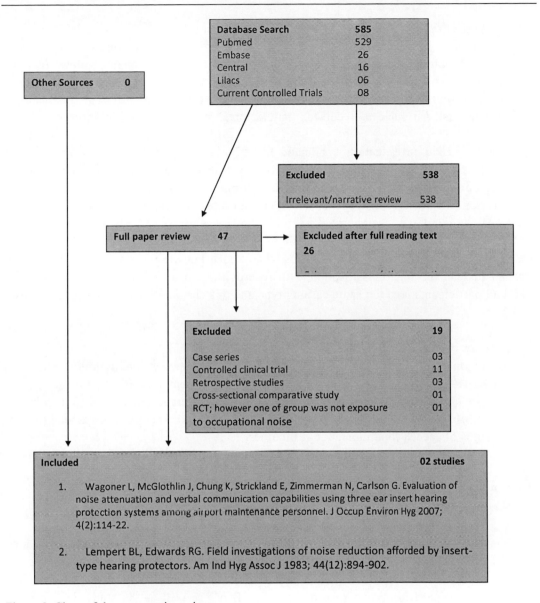

Figure 8. Chart of the systematic review.

Lempert 1983 study was a multicenter cluster randomized controlled trial at fifteen different industrial plants. There were two field investigations, one conducted in 1977 and the second in 1981.

### 5.1.4. Participants and duration of trials

In Wagoner 2007 study a total of 28 subjects participated in the study. All subjects were male and had an average of 41.3 years. The follow-up period was not described.

In Lempert 1983 study seven workers were selected randomly from each of four groups (high-active, high-passive, low-active and low-passive; please see description under types of intervention session), for a total of 28 workers at each plant. The authors did not report the follow-up period.

### 5.1.5. Types of intervention

In Wagoner 2007 each subject wore all three HPDs types: Sonomax SonoCustoms (Sonomax, Montreal, Canada) (custom-device), E-A-R Push-Ins foam earplugs (E-A-R, Indianapolis, Ind.) (user-molded), and Howard Leight SmartFits (HLS, Smithfield, R.I.) (adaptable shape). The subjects wore each of the three earplugs at different times and in different orders. All subjects received manufactures' directions for the insertion of the earplugs.

The first field investigation conducted in 1977 in Lempert 1983 study included an evaluation of three types of earplugs (one performed twin-flanged type, one performed single-flaged type known as V-51R, and one user-formed acoustic type. The second field investigation included also acoustic wool, custom-molded, and user-molded expandable foam. All workerd were categorized by the following variables: physical activity (either active e.g. production-line worker or passive e.g. supervisor) and by noise exposure (either high e.g. greater than 90dB or low e.g. less than 90dB. For the purpose of this review we focused just on the high classification with regards the noise exposure category. At each plant, all participants used the same earplug type and this characterized this study as a cluster design.

### 5.1.6. Types of outcome measures

In Wagoner 2007 study the outcomes of interest were: speech intelligibility (whether a difficulty was present during a conversation), and average attenuation results for each HPDs. The authors also analyzed the length of conversation and average noise level to help on the assessment of speech intelligibility. The videotape of the worker's activities was analyzed for various signs of speech communication difficulties.

The only outcome evaluated in Lempert 1983 study was the real-ear noise attenuation.

### 5.1.7. Notes

Wagoner 2007 study:

1. The study performed the trial as a laboratory and field studies and in both situation there was the randomization process;
2. As the subjects were recruited from the maintenance area of airports we hypothesized that all participants were exposed (> 80 dB(A)) as well as the study described the occurrence of communication abilities in noisy environments;
3. The authors did not report the study period or the justification of the sample size.

Lempert 1983 study:

1. One of the plants included in the first field investigation in 1977 was repeated in 1981, but the authors of the study just included the 1981 data from this plant in the paper to avoid repeat the same participants in their analysis;
2. The authors did not report the justification of the sample size, the setting of the study, neither the sex nor age of the participants.

### 5.1.8. Excluded studies

19 studies are described in the table 1 (Nakao 2008; Abel 2006; Neitzel 2006; Lin 2005; Pääkkönen 2005; Ong 2004; Horie 2002; Wagstaff 2001; Pääkkönen 1998; Bhattacharya 1993; Dancer 1992; Sataloff 1986; Royster 1984; Chung 1983; Erlandsson 1980; Ivarsson 1980; Royster 1980; Smith 1980; Taniewski 1978). The main reason for exclusion was that the studies were not randomized or quasi-randomized controlled trials.

### 5.1.9. Awaiting assessment

No study is awaiting assessment.

## 5.2. Methodological Quality of Included Studies

### 5.2.1. Allocation (sequence generation and allocation concealment)

Wagoner 2007 study described the method of allocation as 'table of random digits', therefore it was considered 'adequate'. However, allocation concealment was not reported ('unclear').

Lempert 1983 study did not report the generation of allocation neither the allocation concealment making this study classified as 'unclear'.

### Table 1. Characteristics of excluded studies.

| Study ID | Reason for exclusion |
|---|---|
| Nakao 2008 | Case series |
| Abel 2006 | Controlled clinical trial |
| Neitzel 2006 | Controlled clinical trial (the subjects were only randomized to four test groups of five workers to facilitate testing; they were not randomized to the interventions) |
| Lin 2005 | Case series |
| Pääkkönen 2005 | Controlled clinical trial |
| Ong 2004 | Cross-sectional comparative study |
| Horie 2002 | Case series |
| Wagstaff 2001 | Controlled clinical trial |
| Pääkkönen 1998 | Controlled clinical trial |
| Bhattacharya 1993 | Randomized controlled trial; however one of the group was not exposure to occupational noise |
| Dancer 1992 | Controlled clinical trial |
| Sataloff 1986 | Controlled clinical trial |
| Royster 1984 | Controlled clinical trial |
| Chung 1983 | Controlled clinical trial |
| Erlandsson 1980 | Retrospective study |
| Ivarsson 1980 | Retrospective study |
| Royster 1980 | Controlled clinical trial |
| Smith 1980 | Retrospective study |
| Taniewski 1978 | Controlled clinical trial |

### 5.2.2. Blinding

Both studies (Wagoner 2007 and Lempert 1983) did not report whether investigators and patients were blinded to the treatment allocation ('unclear').

### 5.2.3. Description of drop-outs/withdrawals

Wagoner 2007 study had withdrawals of less than 20% and therefore the assessment of attrition bias was recorded as 'met' (just two subjects dropped out). The intention-to-treat analysis was not used.

In Lempert 1983 study there was replacement of participants for those who chose not to participate after the randomization process, therefore, we considered it as withdrawal, however the authors did not described the number of participants who were replaced. This study was classified as 'unclear'.

## 5.3. Effect of Interventions

It was not possible to combine the included studies (Wagoner 2007 and Lempert 1983) in a meta-analysis. Furthermore, it was not possible to perform representation of meta-analysis from Lempert 1983 study due to the fact that the authors did not present the data from high versus low noise exposure separately.

### 5.3.1. Attenuations and speech intelligibility

The mean attenuations at each octave band were not statistically different among the HPDs testes in Wagoner 2007 laboratory study. In addition, the type of HPDs and the sequence in each the plug was testes were not significantly different from each other regarding the speech intelligibility (Wagoner 2007 laboratory study).

### 5.3.2. Elimination of threshold shift

The included studies did not report this outcome.

### 5.3.3. Hearing loss thresholds by audiometric test

The included studies did not report this outcome.

### 5.3.4. Costs (as a narrative analysis)

The included studies did not report this outcome.

## 6. DISCUSSION

The ideally way to prevent noise-induced hearing loss for workers is the removal of hazardous noise from the workplace. However, when engineering controls and work practices are not feasible for reducing noise exposures to safe levels, the best solution is the wearing of hearing protectors consistently.

(1) Sonomax SonoCustoms versus E-A-R Push-Ins foam earplugs (field study)

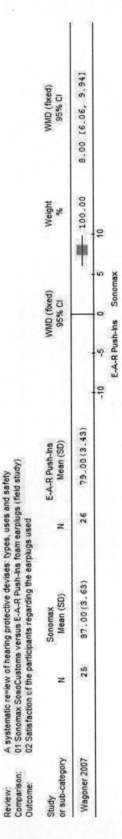

Review: A systematic review of hearing protective devises: types, uses and safety
Comparison: 01 Sonomax SonoCustoms versus E-A-R Push-Ins foam earplugs (field study)
Outcome: 01 Number of difficulties per number of conversations (type of Sonomax used in this outcome was full block)

| Study or sub-category | Sonomax n/N | E-A-R Push-Ins n/N | RR (fixed) 95% CI | Weight % | RR (fixed) 95% CI |
|---|---|---|---|---|---|
| Wagoner 2007 | 18/73 | 28/89 | | 100.00 | 0.78 [0.47, 1.30] |

Figure 9. Representation of meta-analysis from Wagoner 2007 field study that compared Sonomax SonoCustoms versus E-A-R Push-Ins foam earplugs. There was no statistically significant difference between the earplugs regarding the number of difficulties per number of conversations (RR 0.78 [95% Confidential Interval (CI) 0.47 to 1.30]). Note: the type of Sonomax used in this outcome was the full block.

Review: A systematic review of hearing protective devises: types, uses and safety
Comparison: 01 Sonomax SonoCustoms versus E-A-R Push-Ins foam earplugs (field study)
Outcome: 02 Satisfaction of the participants regarding the earplugs used

| Study or sub-category | N | Sonomax Mean (SD) | N | E-A-R Push-Ins Mean (SD) | WMD (fixed) 95% CI | Weight % | WMD (fixed) 95% CI |
|---|---|---|---|---|---|---|---|
| Wagoner 2007 | 25 | 87.00(3.63) | 26 | 79.00(3.43) | | 100.00 | 8.00 [6.06, 9.94] |

Figure 10. Representation of meta-analysis from Wagoner 2007 field study that compared Sonomax SonoCustoms versus E-A-R Push-Ins foam earplugs. There was a statistically significant difference favouring participants wearing the Sonomax regarding the satisfaction of earplugs (WMD 8.00 [95% CI 6.06 to 9.94]).

## (2) Sonomax SonoCustoms versus HL SmartFit (field study)

Review: A systematic review of hearing protective devises: types, uses and safety
Comparison: 02 Sonomax SonoCustoms versus HL SmartFit (field study)
Outcome: 01 Number of difficulties per number of conversations (type of Sonomax used in this outcome was full block)

| Study or sub-category | Sonomax n/N | HL SmartFit n/N | RR (fixed) 95% CI | Weight % | RR (fixed) 95% CI |
|---|---|---|---|---|---|
| Wagoner 2007 | 18/73 | 20/136 | | 100.00 | 1.68 [0.95, 2.96] |

0.1 0.2 0.5 1 2 5 10
Sonomax    HL SmartFit

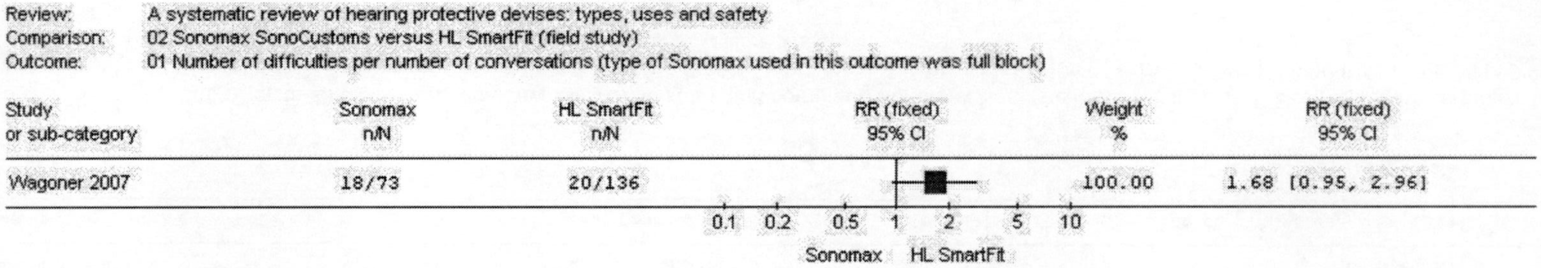

Figure 11. Representation of meta-analysis from Wagoner 2007 field study that compared Sonomax SonoCustoms versus HL SmartFit. There was no statistically significant difference between the earplugs regarding the number of difficulties per number of conversations (RR 1.68 [95% CI 0.95 to 2.96]). Note: the type of Sonomax used in this outcome was the full block.

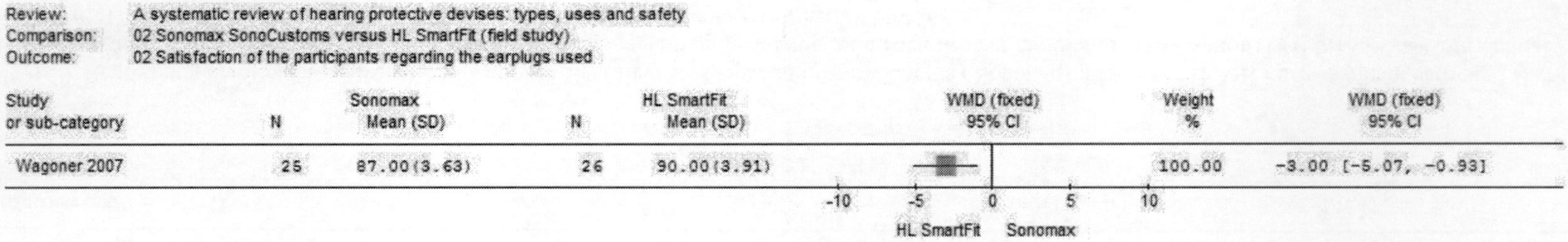

Review: A systematic review of hearing protective devises: types, uses and safety
Comparison: 02 Sonomax SonoCustoms versus HL SmartFit (field study)
Outcome: 02 Satisfaction of the participants regarding the earplugs used

| Study or sub-category | N | Sonomax Mean (SD) | N | HL SmartFit Mean (SD) | WMD (fixed) 95% CI | Weight % | WMD (fixed) 95% CI |
|---|---|---|---|---|---|---|---|
| Wagoner 2007 | 25 | 87.00 (3.63) | 26 | 90.00 (3.91) | | 100.00 | -3.00 [-5.07, -0.93] |

-10 -5 0 5 10
HL SmartFit    Sonomax

Figure 12. Representation of meta-analysis from Wagoner 2007 field study that compared Sonomax SonoCustoms versus HL SmartFit. There was a statistically significant difference favouring participants wearing HL SmartFit regarding the satisfaction of earplugs (WMD -3.00 [95% CI -5.07 to -0.93]).

(3) E-A-R Push-Ins versus HL SmartFit (field study)

Review:       A systematic review of hearing protective devises: types, uses and safety
Comparison:   03 E-A-R Push-Ins versus HL SmartFit (field study)
Outcome:      01 Number of difficulties per number of conversations

| Study or sub-category | E-A-R Push-Ins n/N | HL SmartFit n/N | RR (fixed) 95% CI | Weight % | RR (fixed) 95% CI |
|---|---|---|---|---|---|
| Wagoner 2007 | 28/89 | 20/136 | | 100.00 | 2.14 [1.29, 3.55] |
| | | | | 100.00 | |

0.1  0.2  0.5  1  2  5  10

E-A-R Push-Ins    HL SmartFit

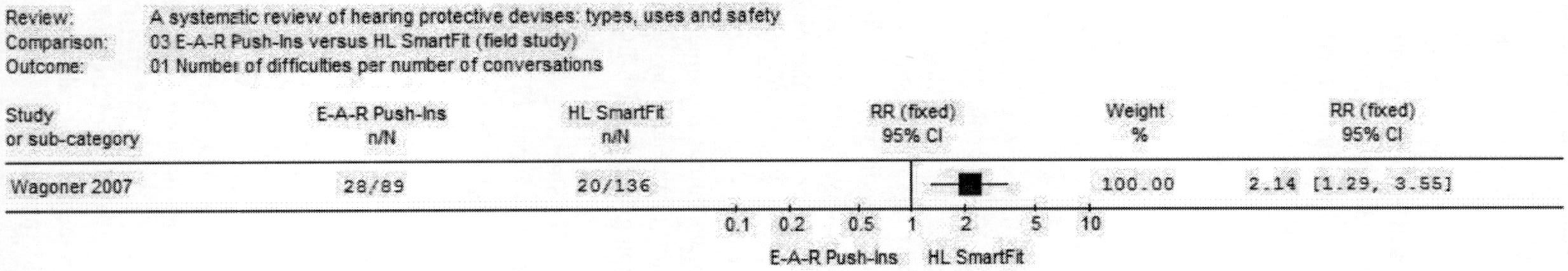

Figure 13. Representation of meta-analysis from Wagoner 2007 field study that compared E-A-R Push-Ins versus HL SmartFit. There was a statistically significant difference favouring the HL SmartFit regarding the number of difficulties per number of conversations (RR 2.14 [95% CI 1.29 to 3.55]).

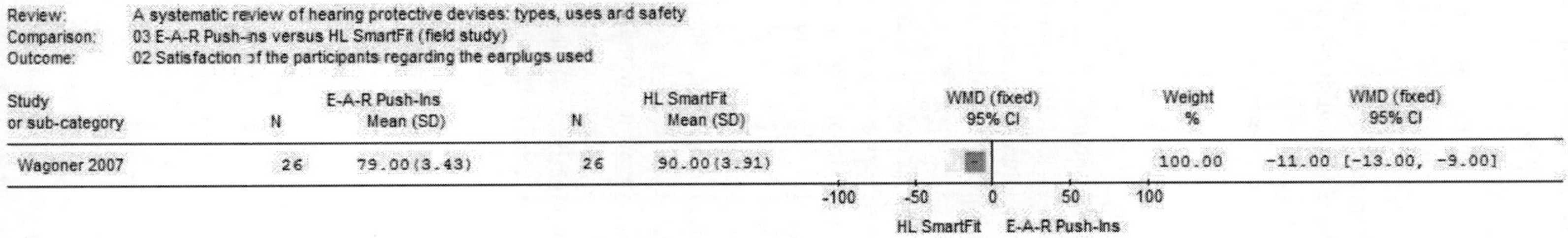

Review:       A systematic review of hearing protective devises: types, uses and safety
Comparison:   03 E-A-R Push-ins versus HL SmartFit (field study)
Outcome:      02 Satisfaction of the participants regarding the earplugs used

| Study or sub-category | E-A-R Push-Ins N | Mean (SD) | HL SmartFit N | Mean (SD) | WMD (fixed) 95% CI | Weight % | WMD (fixed) 95% CI |
|---|---|---|---|---|---|---|---|
| Wagoner 2007 | 26 | 79.00 (3.43) | 26 | 90.00 (3.91) | | 100.00 | -11.00 [-13.00, -9.00] |
| | | | | | | 100.00 | |

-100  -50  0  50  100

HL SmartFit    E-A-R Push-Ins

Figure 14. Representation of meta-analysis from Wagoner 2007 field study that compared E-A-R Push-Ins versus HL SmartFit. There was a statistically significant difference favouring participants wearing HL SmartFit regarding the satisfaction of earplugs (WMD -11.00 [95% CI -13.00 to -9.00]).

Various hearing protectors are available at the market including different materials and styles designed for specific applications and worker preferences to facilitate communication, quickly insertion and to provide a good attenuation values. It is also well know that different HPDs provide a wide range of protection levels.

To determine which hearing protector is the effectiveness device to provide workers exposure to noise levels above 80 dB(A) highest attenuation values, best communications properties, elimination of threshold shift caused by continuous noise of high intensity as well as comfort and convenience, we had decided to summarize the findings in the literature in a systematic review. The systematic reviews (a summary of research that uses explicit methods to perform a thorough literature search and critical appraisal of individual studies to identify the valid and applicable evidence) aim to reduce uncertainty in order to help to make uniform clinical decisions.

This systematic review offers up to date but limited evidence supported by two randomized controlled trials on the effectiveness of just one type of hearing protective device: earplugs. The methodological quality of the studies was very poor, even though there was a substantial risk of selection bias in both included studies due to the lack of description in the allocation concealment procedure. However, Lempert 1983 study used a valuable method to avoid contamination bias and it is often used in occupational health settings: the cluster randomization.

The two studies that we found (Wagoner 2007 and Lempert 1983) compared different types of earplugs to determine its attenuation values and speech intelligibility. It was possible to present some of the data from Wagoner 2007 study graphically, but not possible to combine the results with the other included study due to the diversity of the outcomes reported, furthermore in Lempert 1983 study the authors did not separate the data from high versus low noise exposure categories.

With regards to the number of difficulties per number of conversations outcome reported in Wagoner study, there was only a statistically significant difference favouring the participants that worn HL SmartFit compared to the other earplug E-A-R Push-Ins (Figure 13). The same applies for the outcome satisfaction self-reported by the participants which there were a statistically significant difference favouring the HL SmartFit earplug when compared to Sonomax SonoCustoms and the E-A-R Push-Ins devices (Figure 12 and 14).

Although audiometric test are the ideal way for managing a hearing loss induced by noise exposure and evaluate the worker, this is considered a long-term outcome to be studied and support the effectiveness of HPDs. Thereby, there are others methods that provide us an immediate assessment of HPD effectiveness such as perceived benefits and barriers to use of hearing protection. None included studies reported about the perceived benefits and barriers of each hearing protector. This would be important information by characterizing this population and even the information to be used for the design of further types of earplugs and earmuffs that best fit the workers exposed to noise levels above 80 dB(A).

A cross-sectional study of systematic reviews has found that the majority of Cochrane reviews highlight the absence or poor evidence around the questions on health care that has been covered by them. Around half of the reviews analysed in this study did not offer enough evidence for clinical practice, and the authors asked for further research (El Dib 2007). The same was observed in this systematic review of hearing protectors that, although it is considered the highest level of evidence in the research field, unfortunately, it does not provide us enough evidence to determine which HPD is more effective with regards attenuation values, hear communication, comfort, etc. Future researchers should focus on the first part of this chapter to allow a better design of their clinical trials and answer which HPD has highest attenuation values, best communications properties, most comfort and convenience for the workers exposed at noisy activities.

# 7. REVIEWERS' CONCLUSIONS

## 7.1. Implications for Practice

The evidence found in this review showed that the HL SmartFit earplug is more effective compared to E-A-R Push-Ins foam earplug regarding the number of difficulties per number of conversations. Furthermore, the HL SmartFit earplug is also more effective related to the satisfaction in wear the hearing protector self-reported by the participants when compared to Sonomax SonoCustoms and the E-A-R Push-Ins devices.

## 7.2. Implications for Research

More randomized controlled trials are needed with standard outcomes and interventions to make the combination of the results into a meta-analysis. To avoid the risk of contamination cluster randomised trials are preferred, proper adjustments should be made for the cluster effect and intra cluster correlation coefficients should be reported. Future trials should have standardised outcomes measures such as attenuation, speech intelligibility and audibility (hear communication) in the noise environment, worker acceptance of HPDs and the likelihood that workers will wear them consistently, hearing loss thresholds by audiometric test, costs and others. Drop-outs and loss to follow up should be reported. Future researchers should guide their clinical trials with reliable and realistic protocols to assess the real attenuation values and consider workers' beliefs, comfort and convenience.

# 8. POTENTIAL CONFLICT OF INTEREST

None known.

# REFERENCES

Abel SM, Odell P. Sound attenuation from earmuffs and earplugs in combination: maximum benefits vs. missed information. *Aviat Space Environ Med*, 2006, 77(9), 899-904.

Alaska Occupational Audiology and Health Services. Hearing Protection Devices (HPD's). Available from http://www.alaskaoccupationalaudiology.com/hearing-protection-devices. htm

Arezes, PM; Miguel, AS. Hearing protectors acceptability in noisy environments. *Annals of Occupational Hygiene*, 2002, 46(6), 531-536.

Bhattacharya, SK; Tripathi, SR; Kashyap, SK. Assessment of comfort of various hearing protection devices (HPD). *J Hum Ergol (Tokyo)*, 1993, 22(2), 163-72.

Chung, DY; Hardie, R; Gannon, RP. The performance of circumaural hearing protectors by dosimetry. *J Occup Med*, 1983, 25(9), 679-82.

Dancer, A; Grateau, P; Cabanis, A; Barnabé, G; Cagnin, G; Vaillant, T; Lafont, D. Effectiveness of earplugs in high-intensity impulse noise. *J Acoust Soc Am*, 1992, 91(3), 1677-89.

El Dib, R; Mathew, JL. Interventions to promote the wearing of hearing protection. Cochrane Database of Systematic Reviews 2009, Issue 4. Art. No.: CD005234. DOI: 10.1002/14651858.CD005234.pub3.

El Dib, RP; Atallah, NA; Andriolo, RB. Mapping the Cochrane evidence for decision-making in health care. *Journal of Evaluation in Clinical Practice*, 2007, 13(4), 689-92.

Erlandsson, B; Håkanson, H; Ivarsson, A; Nilsson, P. The difference in protection efficiency between earplugs and earmuffs. An investigation performed at a workplace. *Scand Audiol*, 1980, 9(4), 215-21.

Higgins, JPT; Green, S. (Editors). Cochrane Handbook for Systematic Reviews of Interventions 5.0.0 [updated February 2008]. The Cochrane Collaboration, 2008. Available from www.cochrane-handbook.org.

Higgins, JPT; Green, S. (Editors). Cochrane Reviewers' Handbook 4.2.5. *Assessment of study quality*. Section 4 [updated May 2005]. In: The Cochrane Library, Issue 3, 2005. Chichester, UK: John Wiley & Sons, Ltd, 2005.

Higgins, JPT; Thompson, SG; Deeks, JJ; Altman, DG. Measuring inconsistency in meta-analysis. *British Medical Journal*, 2003, 327, 555-7.

Horie, S. Improvement of occupational noise-induced temporary threshold shift by active noise control earmuff and bone conduction microphone. *Journal of Occupational Health*, 2002, 44(6), 414-420.

Ivarsson, A; Erlandsson, B; Håkanson, H; Nilsson, P. Differences in efficiency of earplugs and earmuffs measured as hearing impairments from two workshops. *Scand Audiol Suppl*, 1980, (Suppl 12), 194-9.

Jüni, P; Witschi, A; Bloch, R; Egger, M. The hazards of scoring the quality of clinical trials for meta-analysis. *The Journal of the American Medical Association*, 1999, 282(11), 1054-60.

Leigh, J; Macaskill, P; Kuosma, E; Mandryk, J. Global burden of disease and injury due to occupational factors. *Epidemiology*, 1999 Sep, 10(5), 626-31.

Lempert, BL; Edwards, RG. Field investigations of noise reduction afforded by insert-type hearing protectors. *Am Ind Hyg Assoc J*, 1983, 44(12), 894-902.

Lin, JH; Li, PC; Tang, ST; Liu, PT; Young, ST. Industrial wideband noise reduction for hearing aids using a headset with adaptive-feedback active noise cancellation. *Med Biol Eng Comput*, 2005, 43(6), 739-45.

Malchaire, J; Piette, A. A comprehensive strategy for the assessment of noise exposure and risk of hearing impairment. *Annals of Occupational Hygiene*, 1997, 41(4), 467-84.

Nakao, T; Horie, S; Tsutsui, T; Kawanami, S; Sasaki, N; Inoue, J. Earplug-type earphone with built-in microphone improves monosyllable intelligibility in noisy environments. *J Occup Health*, 2008, 50(2), 194-6.

Neitzel, R; Somers, S; Seixas, N. Variability of real-world hearing protector attenuation measurements. *Ann Occup Hyg*, 2006, 50(7), 679-91.

Ong, M; Choo, JT; Low, E. A self-controlled trial to evaluate the use of active hearing defenders in the engine rooms of operational naval vessels. *Singapore Med J*, 2004, 45(2), 75-8.

Pääkkönen, R; Lehtomäki, K; Savolainen, S. Noise attenuation of communication hearing protectors against impulses from assault rifle. *Mil Med*, 1998, 163(1), 40-3.

Pääkkönen, R; Lehtomäki, K. Protection efficiency of hearing protectors against military noise from handheld weapons and vehicles. *Noise Health*, 2005, 7(26), 11-20.

Royster, LH; Royster, JD; Cecich, TF. An evaluation of the effectiveness of three hearing protection devices at an industrial facility with a TWA of 107 dB. *J Acoust Soc Am*, 1984, 76(2), 485-97.

Royster, LH. An evaluation of the effectiveness of two different insert types of ear protection in preventing TTS in an industrial environment. *Am Ind Hyg Assoc J*, 1980, 41(3), 161-9.

Sataloff, R; Sataloff, RT. Documenting hearing conservation tests equipment's effectiveness. *Occup Health Saf*, 198, 55(2), 28-36.

Smith, CR; Wilmoth, JN; Borton, TE. Custom-molded earplug performance: a retrospective study. *Scand Audiol*, 1980, 9(2), 113-7.

Taniewski, M; Zaborski, L; Szczepański, C; Nitka, J. [Effectiveness of ear protective devices]. *Med Pr*, 1978, 29(4), 307-16.

Wagoner, L; McGlothlin, J; Chung, K; Strickland, E; Zimmerman, N; Carlson, G. Evaluation of noise attenuation and verbal communication capabilities using three ear insert hearing protection systems among airport maintenance personnel. *J Occup Environ Hyg*, 2007, 4(2), 114-22.

Wagstaff, AS; Woxen, OJ. Double hearing protection and speech intelligibility-room for improvement. *Aviat Space Environ Med*, 2001, 72(4), 400-4.

WHO - World Health Organization. The World Health Report (Chapter 4) Selected occupational risks. http://www.who.int/whr/2002/chapter4/en/index8.html 2002.

Witt B. Putting the personal back into PPE: hearing protector effectiveness. *Occupational Health & Safety*, 2007, 76(6), 90, 92, 94.

# APPENDIX 1

| Database | Search strategy for randomized clinical trials |
|---|---|
| PUBMED | (randomized controlled trial [Publication Type] OR controlled clinical trial [Publication Type] OR randomized controlled trials [MeSH Terms] OR random allocation [MeSH Terms] OR double blind method [MeSH Terms] OR single blind method [MeSH Terms] OR clinical trial [Publication Type] OR clinical trials [MeSH Terms] OR (clinical* [Text Word] AND trial* [Text Word]) OR single* [Text Word] OR double* [Text Word] OR treble* [Text Word] OR triple* [Text Word] OR placebos [MeSH Terms] OR placebo* [Text Word] OR random* [Text Word] OR research design [MeSH Terms] OR comparative study [MeSH Terms] OR evaluation studies [MeSH Terms] OR follow-up studies [MeSH Terms] OR prospective studies [MeSH Terms] OR control* [Text Word] OR prospectiv* [Text Word] OR volunteer* [Text Word]) |
| **EMBASE** | ((Randomized controlled trial) or (Controlled study) or Randomization (Double blind procedure) or (Single blind procedure) or (Clinical trial) or (clinical adj5 trial*) or (doubl* or singl* or tripl* or trebl*) or (blind* or mask*) or Placebo* or Random* or (Methodology latin square) or crossover or cross-over or (Crossover Procedure) or (Drug comparison) or (Comparative study) (comparative trial*) or (control$ or prospectiv$ or volunteer$) or (Evaluation and Follow Up) or (Prospective study)) |
| **LILACS** | (Pt randomized controlled trial) OR (Pt controlled clinical trial) OR (Mh randomized controlled trials) OR (Mh random allocation) OR (Mh double blind method) OR (Mh single blind method) AND NOT (Ct animal) AND NOT (Ct human and Ct animal) OR (Pt clinical trial) OR (Ex E05.318.760.535$) OR (Tw clin$) AND (Tw trial$) OR (Tw ensa$) OR (Tw estud$) OR (Tw experim$) OR (Tw investiga$) OR (Tw singl$) OR (Tw simple$) OR (Tw doubl$) OR (Tw doble$) OR (Tw duplo$) OR (Tw trebl$) OR (Tw trip$) AND (Tw blind$) OR (Tw cego$) OR (Tw ciego$) OR (Tw mask$) OR (Tw mascar$) OR (Mh placebos) OR (Tw placebo$) OR (Tw random$) OR (Tw randon$) OR (Tw casual$) OR (Tw acaso$) OR (Tw azar) OR (Tw aleator$) OR (Mh research design) AND NOT (Ct animal) AND NOT (Ct human and Ct animal) OR (Ct comparative study) OR (Ex E05.337$) OR (Mh follow-up studies) OR (Mh prospective studies) OR (Tw control$) OR (Tw prospectiv$) OR (Tw volunt$) OR (Tw volunteer$) AND NOT ((Ct animal) AND NOT (Ct human and Ct animal)) |

# APPENDIX 2

## EXTRACTION SHEET

ID – author, year of publication:

## Action

What will be asked to the author:

## Methods

1. Design:
2. Multicentre or Single-centre:
3. Period:
4. Sample size:
5. Generation of Allocation:
6. Allocation concealment:
7. Blinded assessment of treatment allocation:
8. Withdrawals and drop outs:
9. Intention-to-treat analysis:
10. Follow-up:

## Participants

1. N:
2. Sex:
3. Age (mean):
4. Setting:
5. Inclusion criteria:
6. Exclusion criteria:

## Intervention

1. Experimental group:
2. Control Group:

## Outcomes

1. Primary Outcome:
2. Secondary Outcome:
3. Continuous or Dichotomous:

## Notes

1. Conflict of interest:
2. Comments and notes:

In: Deafness, Hearing Loss and the Auditory System
Editors: D. Fiedler and R. Krause, pp.249-262

ISBN: 978-1-60741-259-5
©2010 Nova Science Publishers, Inc.

*Chapter 10*

# DPOAE Abnormalities after Perinatal Asphyxia

## Ze Dong Jiang[*]

Department of Paediatrics, University of Oxford, John Radcliffe Hospital,
Oxford, United Kingdom

## Abstract

Perinatal asphyxia is an important risk for acquired hearing impairment in infants and children. Selection and implementation of a proper plan to intervene in hearing impairment requires accurate information about all frequencies important for speech and language development. Thus, it is crucial to obtain detailed information about cochlear function in infants with hearing impairment. Distortion product otoacoustic emissions (DPOAEs) have been widely used to examine cochlear function in infants. Recent studies found that infants after perinatal asphyxia showed a decrease in DPOAE pass rates at most frequencies in the first few days after birth. The decrease occurred mainly between 1 and 5 kHz, particularly 1 and 2 kHz. Overall DPOAE pass rate was also decreased. These results suggest that perinatal asphyxia damages the neonatal cochlea, which occurs mainly at the frequencies 1-5 kHz, particular at 1 and 2 kHz. At 1 month the decreased DPOAE pass rates did show any improvement. It seems that the impairment detected in the first few days after birth is unlikely to improve in later neonatal period. Follow-up studies revealed that at 6 months after birth DPOAE pass rates were increased slightly at most frequencies, but were decreased slightly at some other frequencies. At 12 months infants after perinatal asphyxia still demonstrated a decrease in DPOAE pass rates at most frequencies, particularly 1 and 2 kHz. Similarly, overall DPOAE pass rates were also decreased. The same was true for the comparison of the pass rates at 12 months with those at 6 months. These longitudinal prospective studies of DPOAEs indicate that hypoxia-ischemia that is associated with perinatal asphyxia adversely affects cochlear function. The major affected frequencies are 1 and 2 kHz. At 1 year, cochlear function remains relatively poor. Therefore, cochlear function, mainly at 1 and 2 kHz, is impaired after perinatal asphyxia, which is persistent during the postnatal development, with only

---

[*] Corresponding author: Telephone: ++44 1865 221364; Telefax: ++44 1865 221366. E-mail address: zedong.jiang@paediatrics.ox.ac.uk

slightly improvement. These findings provide useful information for selecting and implementing early interventions in hearing impairment due to perinatal asphyxia.

# INTRODUCTION

Experiments in animal models showed that hypoxemia have a direct effect on the cochlea and an indirect effect by way of cardiovascular collapse and cerebral ischaemia (Sohmer et al., 1986). The effects may lead to sensory or sensorineural hearing impairment. In human infants there is a critical period extending from before birth to about possibly 3 months at which time the auditory system is particularly susceptible to the effects of asphyxia (Jiang, 1995). Infants who suffer hypoxemia or hypoxia-ischemia during the perinatal period, i.e. perinatal asphyxia, has been recognized to be at risk of acquired hearing impairment (Borg, 1997; Fahnenstich et al., 1999; Jiang, 1995,1998; Jiang et al., 2004a, Mencher and Mencher, 1999; Newton, 2001; Sano et al., 2005; Wilkinson and Jiang, 2006). Recent studies using the brainstem auditory evoked responses (BAERs) have provided further evidence that hearing impairment occurs in infants after perinatal asphyxia, although such impairment is largely temporary (Jiang et al., 2004a; Wilkinson and Jiang, 2006).

In a previous study of change in BAER threshold during the neonatal period in 92 term infants after perinatal asphyxia, we found that the threshold was elevated significantly on day 1 in these infants (Jiang et al., 2004a). The elevated threshold was decreased progressively on days 3 and 5, but was still significantly higher than in normal controls. The elevation was continuously decreased more slowly on day 10 and 15, and to a near normal level on day 30. Threshold elevation was seen in 31.7% of the babies on day 1, and 34.5% during the first 3 days. The rate of elevation was decreased progressively thereafter. On day 30, 10.6% of the subjects still had threshold elevation. It seems that hearing impairment after perinatal asphyxia is mostly temporary rather than permanent. However, permanent sensorineural hearing impairment does happen in some of the infants after perinatal asphyxia (Jiang, 1995).

Selection and implementation of a proper plan to intervene in hearing impairment, e.g. fitting a hearing aid or performing a cochlear implant, requires accurate information about the hearing impairment at all frequencies important for speech and language development. Thus, it is crucial to obtain detailed information about cochlear function in the infant or child who has hearing impairment. The BAER, which is elicited mostly by click stimuli, lacks frequency-specificity, and cannot identify which frequencies of the cochlear audiogram are affected in the cases with hearing impairment. In the last decade, otoacoustic emissions (OAEs), particularly distortion product otoacoustic emissions (DPOAEs), have been widely used to examine cochlear function (American Academy of Pediatrics, 1999; Joint Committee on Infant Hearing, 1995,2000; Salata et al., 1998).

The emissions are the result of non-linear properties of the cochlear basilar membrane, i.e., when two closely related pure tones at stimuli $f_1$ and $f_2$ are presented simultaneously, distortion products are generated with the largest occurring in the human ear at $2f_1-f_2$. The level of the retrogradely conducted sound is recorded by a probe microphone in the external auditory canal. The DP audiogram has proven useful in estimating audiometric configuration (Gaskill and Brown, 1993; Kimberley et al., 1994; Lonsbury-Martin and Martin, 1990). The frequency pattern of DPOAE amplitude reduction or absence often follows the configuration of hearing loss in the audiogram. DPOAE, which can be obtained quickly, have now become a widely used objective audiometric tool to assess infant's cochlear function and identify hearing impairment (Berg et al., 2005; Cone-Wesson et al., 2000; Gorga et al., 2000; Joint Committee on Infant Hearing, 1995,2000; Kemp and Ryan, 1993; Kemp et al., 1990; Mencher and Mencher, 1999; Norton and Stover, 1994; Noton et al., 2000a,b; Probst et al., 1991; Sininger, 1993; Sininger and Abdala, 1998; Smurzynski et al., 1993;Uziel and Piron, 1991; Vatovec et al., 2001). The emissions are absent when hearing loss due to cochlear pathology is 45 to 50 dB or greater (Sininger and Abdala, 1998). Hypoxia for a few minutes can severely inhibit OAE (Frolenkov et al., 1998; Kemp and Brown, 1984; Whitehead et al., 1992). Severe or lethal hypoxia damages cochlear function, leading to the DPOAEs disappearing at low-level stimulation (45–60 dB sound pressure level - SPL) (Rebillard et al., 1993).

Understanding of what frequencies on the cochlear audiogram are affected by perinatal asphyxia is important for early intervention of hearing impairment aimed at improving auditory-learning and later speech, language, and cognitive development. In recent years, we have studied DPOAEs across the frequencies between 0.50 and 10 kHz, shortly after birth (at term and 1 month after birth) in infants who were born with perinatal asphyxia to elucidate what frequencies in the cochlear audiogram are susceptible to perinatal asphyxia (Jiang et al., 2005). These infants were selected in an intensive care unit. All has clinical signs of hypoxia-ischemia (Levene, 2001; Levene and Evans, 2005; Volpe 2001), depressed Apgar score ($\leq$ 6 at 5 min), and umbilical cord blood pH <7.10 and/or meconium staining of the amniotic fluid. Those who had any perinatal conditions and/or problems, which can affect the central nervous system or the auditory system, were excluded. The selected infants were further followed up using DPOAEs at 6 and 12 months of age to examine longer-term functional status of the cochlea and depict a picture of changes in DPOAE and, in turn, cochlear function during the first postnatal year after perinatal asphyxia.

## RECORDING AND ANALYSIS OF DPOAES

Recording of DPOAEs were performed in a quiet room. Subjects lay supine in a cot. The left and right ears were tested separately. Prior to DPOAE recording, otoscopy was carried out using an otomicroscope (Jiang et al., 2005; Zang et al., 2008). The auditory meatus was inspected and cleaned of any wax. DPOAEs were recorded using an AudX Plus OAE system (Bio-logic Systems Co.). The acoustic stimuli to elicit DPOAEs were two pure tones ($f_1$ and $f_2$ primary tones; $f_2/f_1 = 1.22$), presented simultaneously, with the lower frequency primary tone at 65 dB SPL and the higher frequency primary tone at 55 dB SPL. Levels of the $2f_1$–$f_2$ DPOAEs and corresponding noise floor were registered as a function of $f_2$. For each subject, the $f_2$ primary tone was presented at 10 frequencies between 0.5 and 10 kHz.

Based on reliable emissions obtained from each ear of the subject, a "pass" or a "failure" for a DPOAE test was established. A DPOAE response with an amplitude at least 6 dB SPL above the noise floor at each frequency of the $f_2$ primary tone was classified as a "pass" while a response with an amplitude less than this level at each frequency was classified as a "failure" (Jiang et al., 2005). In individual subjects, a testing result that passed 6 or more of the 10 frequencies tested was classified as an "overall pass". The pass or failure rates (%) were compared between groups using the Chi-square test.

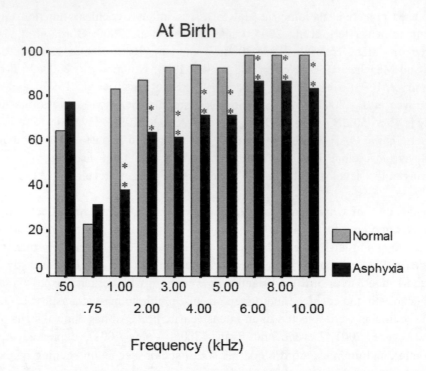

Figure 1. DPOAE pass rate (%) at different frequencies of $f_2$ primary tone in infants after perinatal asphyxia and normal control infants on days 3-5 after birth. In normal infants, the pass rates at most frequencies of the $f_2$ primary tone are very high, with a tendency that the higher the frequency, the higher is the pass rate. Across the frequencies of 1-10 kHz, DPOAE pass rates range between the highest 98.6% at 6-10 kHz and the lowest 82.9% at 1 kHz. At the lowest 0.75 and 0.50 kHz, however, the pass rate is lower (22.9% and 64.3%, respectively). Compared to the controls, the DPOAE pass rate in infants after perinatal asphyxia is much lower at most frequencies, except for the very lower frequencies 0.50 and 0.75 kHz at which the pass rate is slightly higher than in the controls. Between 1 and 10 kHz, the lower the frequency of the $f_2$ primary tone, the lower is the pass rate and the greater is the difference from the controls. "**"$P<0.01$ refers to statistical significances of the differences between the data of the infants after perinatal asphyxia and those of the controls.

## DPOAE ABNORMALITIES SHORTLY AFTER BIRTH

The first DPOAE recording was made shortly after birth (on days 3-5 after birth). DPOAE pass rates at various frequencies are plotted in Figure 1. The pass rates in infants after perinatal asphyxia were all significantly lower than in the controls across the frequency range between 1 and 10 kHz, particularly at 1-5 kHz. Overall DPOAE pass rate (83.7%) was also significantly lower than that in normal controls (95.7%).

In the normal infants DPOAE pass rate on days 3-5 after birth was decreased with the decrease in the frequency of the $f_2$ primary tone (Zang and Jiang, 2007). This trend suggests that the DPOAEs at low frequencies were more difficult to record than those at high frequencies in newborn infants, which is comparable with the finding reported by others (Lasky, 1998). In the infants after perinatal asphyxia, the DPOAE pass rates at various frequencies showed a similar trend, but the decrease was more significantly (Figure 1). It appears that the DPOAEs at low frequencies in the infants after perinatal asphyxia are even more difficult to record. At very low frequencies (0.50 and 0.75 kHz), however, DPOAE pass rates in the infants after perinatal asphyxia were slightly higher than in the normal infants. However, such a slight difference is unlikely to have any meaningful significance because at very low frequencies measurements of DPOAEs are unreliable.

The DPOAE pass rates across the frequencies between 1 and 10 kHz were very high in the normal infants. By comparison, the pass rates, particular at 1-5 kHz, were much lower in the infants after perinatal asphyxia, except at the lowest frequencies 0.50 and 0.75 kHz (Figure 1). The overall DPOAE pass rate was also lower in the infants after perinatal asphyxia. These results indicate that perinatal asphyxia depresses neonatal DPOAEs at the frequencies across 1-10 kHz, mainly 1-5 kHz.

Animal experiments in the BAER showed that fetal and neonatal threshold was elevated during and immediately following hypoxia but returned to normal shortly following the supply of normal level of oxygen (Sohmer et al., 1994a; Sohmer H, Freeman, 1991). This suggests that peripheral hearing impairment after hypoxia is reversible and the recovery occurs soon after the termination of hypoxia. Similar finding was observed in the human fetus (Sohmer et al., 1994b). Our previous study in newborn infants after hypoxia-ischaemia found that on the first days after birth BAER threshold was significantly elevated and then the elevated threshold was decreased progressively during the first month after birth (Jiang et al., 2004a). All these findings indicate that hearing impairment following perinatal asphyxia is largely transient. Earlier OAE studies revealed that hypoxia for a few minutes inhibits severely OAEs (Frolenkov et al., 1998; Kemp and Brown, 1984; Whitehead et al., 1992). Lethal hypoxia causes damage of cochlear function, leading to DPOAEs disappearing at low-level stimulation (45–60 dB SPL) (Rebillard et al., 1993). In the present study of infants after perinatal asphyxia, the recording of DPOAEs was made on days 3-5 after birth. It can be presumed that the DPOAEs had been significantly suppressed by perinatal asphyxia soon after birth. By the time at which the DPOAE recording was made, the DPOAEs were already partially or largely recovered.

In addition to perinatal asphyxia, some other problems or conditions occurring during the perinatal period may cause sensorineural hearing impairment and elevation in BAER threshold. These include hyperbilirubinaemia at serum levels requiring exchange transfusions, in utero infections, bacterial meningitis, very immaturity or very low birthweight, and ototoxic medications, etc (American Academy of Pediatrics, 1999; Borg, 1997; Fahnenstich et al., 1999; Jiang, 1995,1998; Jiang et al., 2001,2004a,b; Joint Committee on Infant Hearing, 1995; Kountakis et al., 2002; Lipkin et al., 2002; Marron et al., 1992; Mencher and Mencher, 1999; Meyer et al., 1999; Newton, 2001; Sano et al., 2005; Wilkinson and Jiang, 2006). In the present study, none of the infants who failed the DPOAE testing had any of these confounding factors. Therefore, the low DPOAE pass rates at various frequencies and the low overall DPOAE pass rate in these infants are most likely to be related to or due to perinatal asphyxia.

## DPOAE ABNORMALITIES AT ONE MONTH

The infants who suffered perinatal asphyxia were further studied with DPOAEs at 1 month after birth. Prior to recording of DPOAEs, the status of the middle ear was examined, which is critical for reliable measurement of the OAEs (Chung et al., 1993; Kemp et al, 1990; Norton and Stover, 1994; Owens et al., 1992; Plinkert et al., 1994; Sininger and Abdala, 1998). It is known that the levels and frequency extents of the DPOAEs are influenced by the middle ears retrograde transmission mechanisms (Plinkert et al., 1994; Norton and Stover 1994). With middle ear pathology, DPOAEs may not be measurable because transmission of the evoking signal into the cochlea, as well as transmission of the OAEs from the cochlea back to the ear canal, is attenuated as it travels through the dysfunctional middle ear system (Kemp et al., 1990; Owens et al., 1992). DPOAEs disappear when hearing levels exceed about 30–40 dB hearing level (HL). Therefore, normal middle ear function with a type A tympanogram (i.e. values comprised from 0.5 to 1.6 ml for the middle ear mobility and ± 50 daPa for the pressure peak) is essential for DPOAE measures. In order to examine and exclude the confounding effect of middle ear disorders on the measurement of OAEs there is a necessity to measure acoustic impedance for evaluation of middle ear status.

Due to the limitation of using conventional tympanometry and to the unreliability of the results obtained in newborn infants, acoustic impedance was not measured in the first DPOAE test, i.e. on days 3-5 after birth. However, when the subjects reached the age of 1 month after birth, impedance tympanometric measurements were conducted to detect any middle ear disorders prior to the recording of DPOAEs. The tympanometry was carried out using a standard clinical instrumentation (Grason-Stadler GSI 38 Auto Tymp, Welch Allyn Co.), with a 226 Hz probe tone that is appropriate to infants (Calandruccio et al., 2006; Prieve et al., 2008). The testing results were classified as type A (normal), B (no middle ear compliance), C (retracted tympanic membrane due to Eustachian tube dysfunction) or As (limited compliance or stiffness present) tympanogram. Any ears with an abnormal tympanogram (type B, C or As) were excluded. Only those ears that had a normal tympanogram (type A) were further studied with DPOAEs.

As shown in Figure 2, compared to those on days 3-5 after birth, DPOAE pass rates at all frequencies at 1 month tended to be decreased further. This was more significant at 1 and 2 kHz than at other frequencies. Overall DPOAE pass rate (83.8%) was the same as that on days 3-5 (83.7%). It seems that the frequency-specific hearing impairment detected on days 3-5 after birth remains or even slightly worsens at the later neonatal period.

A previous study of the BEAR revealed that at 1 month after birth 10.6% of infants after perinatal asphyxia had a threshold ≥30 dB HL (Jiang et al., 2004a). In the present study, 13 of the 80 ears with a type A tympanogram (i.e. without middle ear disorders) failed the DPOAE test at 1 month. Of the 13 ears, 7 had a BAER threshold ≥30 dB HL, suggesting sensory or sensorineural hearing impairment. The rate of hearing impairment (8.8%, 7/80 ears) is slightly lower than that in our previous BAER study (Jiang et al., 2004a), although such a direct comparison is not completely appropriate because the remaining 12 of the 92 ears (13.0%) were not included due to their type B or type As/C tympanograms. Nevertheless, even though there are some slight differences in the prevalence of peripheral hearing impairment, the results of the two studies are comparable, and suggest that around 10% of the infants after perinatal asphyxia have hearing impairment that persists for at least 1 month.

The DPOAE at 1 month in the infants after perinatal asphyxia indicates that the neonatal cochlea is impaired across the frequencies 1-10 kHz, particularly 1-5 kHz that is crucial for speech and language development. The impairment detected on days 3-5 after birth is unlikely to improve in the later neonatal period.

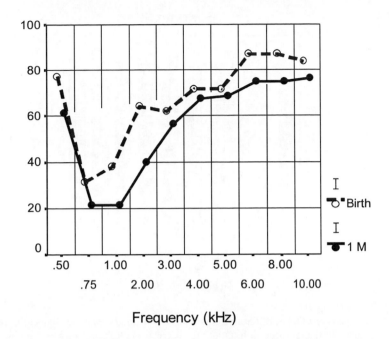

Figure 2. DPOAE pass rate (%) at different frequencies of $f_2$ primary tone in infants after perinatal asphyxia at 1 month and, for comparison, on days 3-5 after birth. The general pattern of the pass rates at different frequencies at 1 month is similar to that on days 3-5 after birth, with a clear 'dip' at the frequencies 0.75 and 1 kHz. Compared to those on days 3-5 after birth, DPOAE pass rates at one month decrease at all frequencies, and differ significantly at 0.5, 1, 2, 6 and 8 kHz. This is particularly obvious at 1 and 2 kHz.

## DPOAE ABNORMALITIES AT SIX MONTHS

Prior to the recording of DPOAEs, impedance tympanometric measurements were undertaken in all infants studied to detect any middle ear disorders. The ears with an abnormal tympanogram (type B, C or As) were all excluded from DPOAE testing. In those ears that had a normal tympanogram (type A), DPOAE pass rates, mainly at the frequencies 1-4 kHz, were lower in the infants after perinatal asphyxia, as compared with those in the normal controls (Figure 3). In the controls, almost all ears passed the DPOAE test, with an overall pass rate as high as 98.5%. In the infants after perinatal asphyxia, however, overall DPOAE pass rate is significantly lower (81.8%). Apparently, there is a certain degree of impairment in cochlear function in these infants.

The general pattern of DPOAE pass rates at various frequencies at 6 months in the infants after perinatal asphyxia was similar to that obtained at 1 month of age (Jiang et al., 2005). The same was true of overall DPOAE pass rate. However, compared to those at 1 month, DPOAE pass rates at 6 months were increased at almost all frequencies. The increase was statistically significant at 3, and 5-8 kHz. Thus, DPOAE pass rates in the infants after perinatal asphyxia has demonstrated some improvement. It seems that with time passing during the postnatal period, the cochlear impairment due to perinatal asphyxia tends to recover, but there still is a certain degree of impairment, mainly at 1-4 kHz, at 6 months of age.

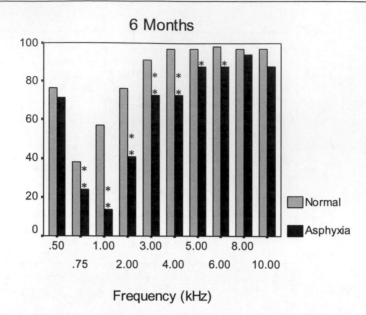

Figure 3. DPOAE pass rate (%) at different frequencies of $f_2$ primary tone in infants after perinatal asphyxia and normal infants at 6 months after birth. DPOAE pass rates at all frequencies of the $f_2$ primary tone between 1 and 10 kHz tend to be lower in infants after perinatal asphyxia than in normal controls. The pass rates at 1-6 kHz in infants after perinatal asphyxia are significantly lower than those in the normal controls, with the greatest difference at 1 and 2 kHz. "*"$P<0.05$, "**"$P<0.01$ refer to statistical significances of the differences between the data of the infants after perinatal asphyxia and those of the controls.

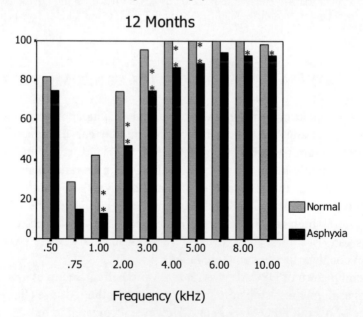

Figure 4. DPOAE pass rate (%) at different frequencies of $f_2$ primary tone in infants after perinatal asphyxia and normal infants at 12 months after birth. DPOAE pass rates at all frequencies of the $f_2$ primary tone between 1 and 10 kHz tend to be lower in infants after perinatal asphyxia than in normal controls. The pass rates at 1-10 kHz, except for 6 kHz, in infants after perinatal asphyxia are significantly lower than those in the normal controls, with the greatest difference at 1 and 2 kHz. "*"$P<0.05$, "**"$P<0.01$ refer to statistical significances of the differences between the data of the infants after perinatal asphyxia and those of the controls.

## DPOAE ABNORMALITIES AT TWELVE MONTHS

As at 1 and 6 months of age, only the wiht a type A tympanogram at 12 months were further studied with DPOAEs. The patterns of the pass rates at various frequencies of the $f_2$ primary tone at 12 months in the infants after perinatal asphyxia were similar to the pattern in the normal controls. However, the pass rates at most individual frequencies still tended to be lower (Figure 4).

Compared to those in the normal controls, DPOAE pass rates in the infants after perinatal asphyxia were decreased at all frequencies of the $f_2$ primary tone between 0.75 and 10 kHz, particularly at 1 and 2 kHz. The pass rates at all 1-10 kHz, except for 6 kHz, of the $f_2$ primary tone were significantly lower than those in the controls (Figure 4). The greatest difference occurred at the frequencies 1 and 2 kHz. Overall DPOAE pass rate in the infants after perinatal asphyxia (84.9%) was significantly lower than the rate in the controls (100.0%). These results indicate that cochlear function, particularly at 1 and 2 kHz, at 12 months after birth is relatively poor in infants after perinatal asphyxia.

## POSTNATAL DPOAE CHANGES AND COCHLEAR IMPAIRMENT

A study of development of cochlear frequency resolution in the human auditory system revealed that general shape and appearance of DPOAE suppression tuning curves (STCs) were comparable for adults and neonates, as was STC tip frequency and level (Abdala and Sininger, 1996). Statistical analyses of tuning-curve width (Q) and slope (dB/octave) failed to show any age effects. This supports the view of a similarity between adults and neonates in cochlear frequency resolution in the human auditory system. DPOAE STCs were stable, showing minimal intra- and inter-subject variability, and closely resembling and behaving like physiologic measures of tuning from the VIIIth nerve. These results suggest that cochlear tuning and related active processes are basically mature by term birth in the human auditory system, and that tuning immaturities in infants probably involve auditory-neural immaturities.

In normal term infants, DPOAEs at 10 frequencies of $f_2$ primary tone between 0.5 and 10 kHz have been studied longitudinally during the first year of life by Zang and Jiang (2007). On days 3-5 after birth there is a clear trend that the higher the frequency, the higher was DPOAE pass rate. At 6 months and 1 year, the pass rates at various frequencies in these normal infants were generally similar to those found on days 3-5. As the age was increased, the pass rate tended to be increased at most, mainly higher, frequencies, tough decreased at some lower frequencies. As a whole, during the first year of life, there are no major changes in DPOAEs or cochlear function, with only slightly age-related differences at some frequencies.

In order to depict postnatal changes in DPOAEs in the infants after perinatal asphyxia, the data of DPOAE tests obtained in these infants at different ages during the first one year of life were pooled together and plotted in Figure 5 (Jiang et al., 2005; Zang et al., 2008). Although DPOAEs were also recorded on days 3-5 after birth, these data are not included for comparison as no tympanometry was performed at that time and a possible influence of middle ear disorders in some of these infants on DPOAEs cannot be excluded. The infants born with perinatal asphyxia showed a tendency of increase in DPOAE pass rates at almost all frequencies of the $f_2$ primary tone from 1 month to 12 months, or 1 year, of age although the pass rate at 1 kHz was decreased slightly (Figure 5).

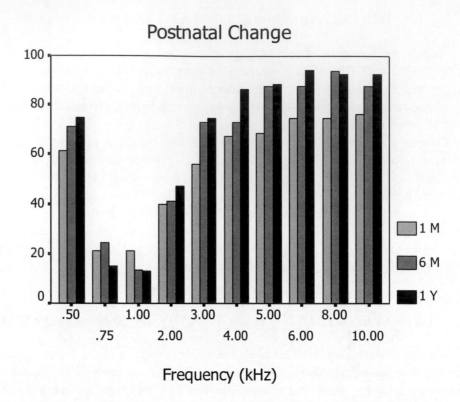

Figure 5. DPOAE pass rate (%) at different frequencies of $f_2$ primary tone in infants after perinatal asphyxia during the first year of life. As the age is increased, the pass rates tend to increase at most frequencies, except at 0.75 Hz and 1 kHz.

The general pattern of the pass rates at different frequencies at 1 year was similar to the patterns obtained at earlier ages, particularly at 6 months. There was a clear 'dip' at the frequencies 0.75 and 1 kHz. DPOAE pass rates at most frequencies tended to be increased with the increase in age. Overall DPOAE pass rate also tended to be increased with the increase in age.

In the infants after perinatal asphyxia, shortly after birth (days 3-5 after birth) DPOAE pass rates were decreased significantly across the frequencies of the $f_2$ primary tones 1 kHz to10 kHz, particularly 1 kHz to 5 kHz. Overall DPOAE pass rate was also decreased. These results suggest that the frequencies 1 kHz to 5 kHz in the cochlear audiogram are susceptible to perinatal asphyxia. A repeat DPOAE test at 1 month after birth demonstrated that DPOAE pass rates at almost all frequencies tended to be decreased further. It appears that the cochlear impairment detected shortly after birth in infants born with perinatal asphyxia is unlikely to have any significant improvement or even slightly worsens during the first month of life.

At 6 months after birth, DPOAE pass rates, mainly at the frequencies of 1 to 4 kHz, in these infants remained lower than those in the normal infants (Jiang et al., 2008). However, compared to those shortly after birth, the pass rates tended to be increased at almost all frequencies, with statistical significances at 3, 5, 6, 7 and 8 kHz. This suggests that with time passing after the first month of life, the impaired cochlear function due to the insult of perinatal asphyxia tends to recover.

At 1 year of age, the general pattern of DPOAE pass rates at various frequencies in the infants born with perinatal asphyxia was similar to that at 6 months of age (Jiang et al., 2008). DPOAE pass rates at 1 year were higher than those obtained at 6 months at most frequencies, with a statistically significant difference at 0.5 kHz. Overall DPOAE pass rate at 1 year (84.9%) was slightly greater than at 6 months (81.8%). It appears that during the second half of the first year of life the impaired cochlear function in infants born with perinatal asphyxia shows a slightly further improvement.

As a whole, at 1 year of age DPOAE pass rates at most frequencies tended to be increased when compared with those obtained at earlier ages. It appears that following the insult of perinatal asphyxia, the impairment in cochlear function improves slightly with time passing during the first postnatal year of life. By the end of the first year, there is still a certain degree of impairment.

## CONCLUSIONS

Obtaining detailed information about cochlear function in infants with hearing impairment is crucial for selecting and implementing a proper plan to intervene in the impairment. This article summarizes our longitudinal study of DPOAEs in infants after perinatal asphyxia. The results depict a picture of postnatal changes in DPOAEs and, in turn, cochlear function after perinatal asphyxia. Within the first few days after birth, cochlear function is mainly affected or impaired at 1-5 kHz, particularly 1 and 2 kHz, suggesting that hypoxia-ischemia that is associated with perinatal asphyxia adversely affects newborn cochlear function. During the postnatal development, such impairment shows only a slight improvement. By the end of the first year, cochlear function, mainly at 1 and 2 kHz, remains relatively poor. It appears that cochlear impairment attributable to perinatal hypoxia-ischemia is unlikely to completely recover. These findings contribute to the understanding of influence of perinatal asphyxia on cochlear function. The finding of persistent impairment at 1 and 2 kHz during the first year of life provides valuable information for early interventions in hearing impairment in infants after perinatal asphyxia.

## REFERENCES

Abdala, C; Sininger, YS. The development of cochlear frequency resolution in the human auditory system. *Ear Hear*, 1996, 17, 374-385.

American Academy of Pediatrics. Newborn and infant hearing loss: detection and intervention. *Pediatrics*, 1999, 103, 527-530.

Berg, AL; Spitzer, JB; Towers, HM; Bartosiewicz, C; Diamond, BE. Newborn hearing screening in the NICU: profile of failed auditory brainstem response/passed otoacoustic emission. *Pediatrics*, 2005, 116, 933-938.

Borg, E. Perinatal asphyxia, hypoxia, ischemia and hearing loss. An overview. *Scand Audiol*, 1997, 26, 77-91.

Calandruccio, L; Fitzgerald, TS; Prieve, BA. Normative multifrequency tympanometry in infants and toddlers. *J Am Acad Audiol*, 2006, 17, 470-480.

Chung, KW; White, BR; Maxon, AB. External and middle ear status related to evoked otoacoustic emission results in neonates. *Arch otolaryngol Head Neck Surg*, 1993, 119, 276-282.

Cone-Wesson, B; Vohr, BR; Sininger, YS; Widen, JE; Folsom, RC; Gorga, MP; Norton, SJ. Identification of neonatal hearing impairment: infants with hearing loss. *Ear Hear*, 2000, 21, 488-507.

Fahnenstich, H; Rabe, H; Rossi, R; Hartmann, S; Gortner, L. Neonatal screening for hearing disorders in infants at risk: incidence, risk factors, and follow-up. *Pediatrics*, 1999, 104, 900-904.

Frolenkov, GI; Belyantseva, IA; Kurc, M; Mastroianni, MA; KachaR, B. Cochlear outer hair cell electromotility can provide force for both low and high intensity distortion product otoacoustic emissions. *Hear Res*, 1998, 126, 67-74.

Gaskill, SA; Brown, AM. Comparison the level of the acoustic distortion product, $2f_1-f_2$, with behavioural threshold audiograms from normal-hearing and hearing-impaired ears. *Br J Audiol*, 1993, 27, 397-407.

Gorga, MP; Norton, SJ; Sininger, YS; Cone-Wesson, B; Folsom, RC; Vohr, BR; Widen, JE; Neely, ST. Identification of neonatal hearing impairment: distortion product otoacoustic emissions during the perinatal period. *Ear Hear.*, 2000, 21, 400-424.

Jiang, ZD. Long-term effect of perinatal and postnatal asphyxia on developing human auditory brainstem responses: peripheral hearing loss. *Int J Pediatr Otorhinolaryngol*, 1995, 33, 225-238.

Jiang, ZD. Maturation of peripheral and brainstem auditory function in the first year following perinatal asphyxia - a longitudinal study. *J Speech Lang Hear Res*, 1998, 41, 83-93.

Jiang, ZD; Brosi, DM; Wilkinson, AR. Hearing impairment in preterm very low birth weight babies at term revealed by brainstem auditory evoked responses. *Acta Paediatr*, 2001, 90, 1411-1415.

Jiang, ZD; Brosi, DM; Wang, J; Wilkinson, AR. One-third of term babies after perinatal hypoxia-ischaemia have transient hearing impairment: dynamic change in hearing threshold during the neonatal period. *Acta Paediatr*, 2004a, 93, 82-87.

Jiang, ZD; Yin, R; Shao, XM; Wilkinson, AR. Brainstem auditory impairment during the neonatal period in infants after asphyxia: dynamic changes in brainstem auditory evoked responses to clicks of different rates. *Clin Neurophysiol*, 2004b, 115, 1605-1615.

Jiang, ZD; Zheng, Z; Wilkinson, AR. Distortion product otoacoustic emissions in term infants after hypoxia-ischaemia. *Euro J Pediatr*, 2005, 164, 84-87.

Joint Committee on Infant Hearing. Position Statement: American Academy of Pediatrics. *Pediatrics*, 1995, 95, 152-156.

Joint Committee on Infant Hearing. Position statement: principles and guidelines for early hearing detection and intervention programs. *Pediatrics*, 2000, 106, 798-817.

Kemp, DT; Brown, AM. Ear canal acoustic and round window electrical correlates of $2f_1-f_2$ distortion generated in the cochlea. *Hear Res*, 1984, 13, 39-46.

Kemp, DT; Ryan, S. The use of transient evoked otoacoustic emissions in neonatal hearing screening programs. *Semin Hear*, 1993, 14, 30-43.

Kemp, DT; Ryan, S; Bray, P. A guide to the effective use of otoacoustic emissions. Ear Hear 1990, 11, 93-105.

Kimberley, BP; Hemadi, I; Lee, AM; Brown, DK. Predicting pure tone thresholds in normal and hearing-impaired ears with distortion product emission and age. *Ear Hear*, 1994, 15, 199-209.

Kountakis, SE; Skoulas, I; Phillips, D; Chang, CYJ. Risk factors for hearing loss in neonates: a prospective study. *Am J Otolaryngol*, 2002, 23, 133-137.

Lasky, RE. Distortion product otoacoustic emissions in human newborns and adults. I. Frequency effects. *J Acoust Soc Am*, 1998, 103, 981–991.

Levene, MI. The asphyxiated newborn infant. In: Levene MI; Chervenak FA; Whittle M (eds) Fetal and neonatal neurology and neurosurgery. 4th ed. Churchill-Livingstone, *Edinburgh*, 2001, 471-504.

Levene, MI; Evans, DJ. Neurological problems in the newborn: Hypoxic-ischaemic brain injury. In: Rennie, JM; editor. Roberton's Textbook of Neonatology (4th ed). Edinburgh: *Elsevier Churchill Livingstone*, 2005, 1128-1148.

Lipkin, PH; Davidson, D; Spivak, L; Straube, R; Rhines, J; Chang, CT. Neurodevelopmental and medical outcomes of persistent pulmonary hypertension in term newborns treated with nitric oxide. *J Pediatr*, 2002, 140, 306-310.

Lonsbury-Martin, BL; Martin, GK. The clinical utility of distortion-product otoacoustic emissions. *Ear Hear*, 1990, 11.144-154.

Marron, MJ; Crisafi, MA; Driscoll, JM; Jr; Wung, JT; Driscoll, YT; Fay, TH; James, LS. Hearing and neurodevelopmental outcome in survivors of persistent pulmonary hypertension of the newborn. *Pediatrics*, 1992, 90, 392-396.

Mencher, LS; Mencher, GT. Neonatal asphyxia, definitive markers and hearing loss. *Audiology*, 1999, 38, 291-295.

Meyer, C; Witte, J; Hildmann, A; Hennecke, KH; Schunck, KU; Maul, K; Franke, U; Fahnenstich, H; Rabe, H; Rossi, R; Hartmann, S; Gortner, L. Neonatal screening for hearing disorders in infants at risk: incidence, risk factors, and follow-up. *Pediatrics*, 1999, 104, 900-904.

Newton, V. Adverse perinatal conditions and the inner ear. *Semin Neonatol*, 2001, 6, 543-551.

Norton, SI; Stover, U. Otoacoustic emissions: an emerging clinical tool. In: Katz I, editor. Handbook of clinical audiology, 4th ed. Baltimore: *Williams and Wilkins*, 1994, 448-462.

Norton, SJ; Gorga, MP; Widen, JE; Folsom, RC; Sininger, Y; Cone-Wesson, B; Vohr, BR; Mascher, K; Fletcher, K. Identification of neonatal hearing impairment: evaluation of transient evoked otoacoustic emission, distortion product otoacoustic emission, and auditory brain stem response test performance. *Ear Hear*, 2000a, 21, 508-528.

Norton, SJ; Gorga, MP; Widen, JE; Folsom, RC; Sininger, Y; Cone-Wesson, B; Vohr, BR; Fletcher, KA. Identification of neonatal hearing impairment: summary and recommendations. *Ear Hear*, 2000b, 21, 529-535.

Owens, JJ; Marcy, J; McCoy, MS; Lonsbury-Martin, BL; Martin, GK. Influence of otitis media on evoked otoacoustic emissions in children. *Semin Hear*, 1992, 13, 53-66.

Plinkert, PK; Bootz, F; Vossieck, T. Influence of static middle ear pressure on transiently evoked otoacoustic emissions and distortion products. *Eur Arch Otorhinolaryngol*, 1994, 251, 95-99.

Prieve, BA; Calandruccio, L; Fitzgerald, T; Mazevski, A; Georgantas, LM. Changes in transient-evoked otoacoustic emission levels with negative tympanometric peak pressure in infants and toddlers. *Ear Hear*, 2008, 29, 533-542.

Probst, R; Lonsbury-Martin, BL; Martin, GK. A review of otoacoustic emissions. *J Acoust Soc Am*, 1991, 89, 2027-2067.

Rebillard, G; Klis, JFL; Lavigne-Rebillard, M; Devaux, P; Puel, JL; Pujol, R. Changes in $2f_1–f_2$ distortion product otoacoustic emission following alterations of cochlear metabolism. *Br J Audiol*, 1993, 27, 117–121.

Salata, JA; Jacobson, JT; Strasnick, B. Distortion product otoacoustic emissions hearing screening in high-risk newborns. *Otolaryngol Head Neck Surg*, 1998, 118, 37-43.

Sano, M; Kaga, K; Kitazumi, E; Kodama, K. Sensorineural hearing loss in patients with cerebral palsy after asphyxia and hyperbilirubinemia. *Int J Pediatr Otorhinolaryngol*, 2005, 69, 1211-1217.

Sininger, YS. Clinical applications of otoacoustic emissions. *Adv Otolaryngol Head Neck Surg*, 1993, 7, 247-269.

Sininger, YS; Abdala, C. Physiologic assessment of hearing. In: Lalwani AK; Grund KM; editors. Pediatric Otology and Neurotology. Philadelphia: *Lippicott-Raven*, 1998, 127-154.

Smurzynski, J; Jung, MD; Lafreniere, D. Distortion product and click-evoked otoacoustic emissions of preterm and full-term infants. *Ear Hear*, 1993, 14, 258-274.

Sohmer, H; Freeman, S; Gafni, M; Goitein, K. The depression of the auditory nerve-brainstem evoked response in hypoxemia - mechanism and site of effect. *Electroencephalogr Clin Neurophysiol*, 1986, 64, 334-338.

Sohmer, H; Freeman, S. Hypoxia induced hearing loss in animal models of the fetus in utero. *Hear Res*, 1991, 55, 92-97.

Sohmer, H; Freeman, S; Gafni, M; Goitein, K. The depression of the auditory nerve-brainstem evoked response in hypoxemia - mechanism and site of effect. *Electroencephalogr Clin Neurophysiol*, 1986, 64, 334-338.

Sohmer, H; Goitein, K; Freeman, S. Improvement in sensorineural auditory threshold of the guinea-pig fetus following delivery. *Hear Res*, 1994a, 73, 116-120.

Sohmer, H; Geal-Dor, M; Weinstein, D. Human fetal auditory threshold improvement during maternal oxygen respiration. *Hear Res*, 1994b, 75, 145-150.

Uziel, A; Piron, LP. Evoked otoacoustic emissions from normal newborns and babies admitted to an jntensive care baby unit. *Acta Otolaryngol*, 1991, 482 (suppl), 85-91.

Vatovec, J; Velickovic Perat, M; Smid, L; Gros, A. Otoacoustic emissions and auditory assessment in infants at risk for early brain damage. *Int J Pediatr Otorhinolaryngol.*, 2001, 58, 139-145.

Volpe, JJ. Hypoxic-ischemic encephalopathy: Clinical aspects. In: Volpe JJ, editor. Neurology of the Newborn. 4th ed. Philadelphia: *WB Saunders*, 2001, 331-394.

Whitehead, ML; Lonsbury-Martin BL; Martin, GK. Evidence for two discrete sources of $2f_1–f_2$ distortion-product otoacoustic emission in rabbit. II: Differential physiological vulnerability. *J Acoust Soc Am*, 1992, 92, 2662-2682.

Wilkinson, AR; Jiang, ZD. Brainstem auditory evoked response in neonatal neurology. *Semin Fet Neonatol Med*, 2006, 11, 444-51.

Zang, Z; Jiang, ZD. Distortion product otoacoustic emissions during the first year in term infants: a longitudinal study. *Brain Dev*, 2007, 29, 346-351.

Zang, Z; Wilkinson, AR; Jiang, ZD. Distortion product otoacoustic emissions at 6 months in term infants after perinatal hypoxia-ischaemia or with a low Apgar score. *Eur J Pediatr*, 2008, 167, 575-578.

In: Deafness, Hearing Loss and the Auditory System
Editors: D. Fiedler and R. Krause, pp.263-277

ISBN: 978-1-60741-259-5
©2010 Nova Science Publishers, Inc.

*Chapter 11*

# ROLE OF OTOACOUSTIC EMISSIONS IN HEARING LOSS EVALUATION

## *Arturo Moleti, Renata Sisto[*], Angelo Tirabasso[**] and Stefano Di Girolamo[***]*

Physics Dept., University of Roma Tor Vergata, Via della Ricerca Scientifica, Italy

## ABSTRACT

Otoacoustic Emissions (OAEs) are a promising technique for the early detection of mild hearing loss. The correlation between OAE levels and the audiometric threshold level has been well-established for transient-evoked OAEs (TEOAEs), Distortion products (DPOAEs) and stimulus-frequency OAEs (SFOAEs). Spontaneous OAEs are also correlated with minima of the audiometric threshold microstructure. The use of TEOAEs in neonatal hearing screening tests is widely accepted. The diagnostic potential of OAEs has not been fully exploited yet, partly due to intrinsic limitations (OAE responses cannot be measured at all in the profoundly hearing-impaired subjects) that permit their application only to subjects with mild or medium hearing loss levels (HL < 40-50 dB), partly because the OAE generation mechanisms are quite complex and not yet fully understood. The constant improvement of innovative acquisition and analysis techniques and the better understanding of cochlear mechanics are improving the effectiveness of OAE techniques in at least three main diagnostic fields:

(a) objective evaluation of the hearing threshold level
(b) objective evaluation of the frequency resolution of hearing (cochlear tuning)
(c) monitoring small modifications of the hearing functionality in subjects with normal-hearing or mild hearing loss.

As regards the first two applications, at the present stage, the OAE techniques can surely be considered as an important objective complement to the correspondent

---

[*] Occupational Health Dept., ISPESL, Via di Fontana Candida, 1, 00040 Monte Porzio Catone (RM), ITALY.

[**] ENT Dept., University of Roma Tor Vergata, Via della Ricerca Scientifica, 1, 00133 Roma, ITALY.

[***] ENT Dept., University of Roma Tor Vergata, Via della Ricerca Scientifica, 1, 00133 Roma, ITALY.

psychoacoustical techniques, i.e. Tonal Audiometry (TA) and the measure of the Critical Bandwidth (CB). OAE measurements can also complement the information coming from other objective techniques, such as the Auditory Brainstem Response (ABR). The third use of OAEs is very promising to monitor the hearing function of subjects exposed to noise, particularly in the case of professional exposure. Some recent studies suggest indeed that OAEs could be more sensitive than TA for this specific diagnostic task.

In this study we report a re-analysis of recently published OAE data of a population of subjects with long-term exposure to industrial noise and of another group of subjects exposed to intense noise in a discotheque, before and after exposure. The results show the potential of OAE-based tests in all the three above-mentioned tasks:

(a)  dichotomous OAE-based tests can be effective for detecting hearing loss down to sub-clinical levels (10 dB HL);
(b)  cochlear tuning can be objectively estimated from the OAE latency;
(c)  OAE levels are sensitive indicators of noise exposure in subjects with normal hearing or mild hearing loss.

# INTRODUCTION

Otoacoustic emissions (OAEs) are acoustical signals generated in the cochlea and measured in the ear canal (Probst, 1991). They are widely recognized as a by-product and a demonstration of the activity of the cochlear amplifier. They can be evoked either by acoustical or by electrical stimulation, and, in the majority of normal-hearing subjects, they can also be observed, at individual specific frequencies, without stimulation, as spontaneous emissions (SOAEs).

Clinical applications of OAEs use acoustical stimulation in the ear canal, which is obtained using ear canal probes. A standard probe consists of a miniaturized microphone and two loudspeakers, and is inserted in the ear canal using a rubber adapter, which isolates the ear canal from external noise input and fixes the probe in a stable position relative to the geometry of the ear canal cavity.

The ear canal, whose ends are closed by the tympanic membrane and by the probe, behaves like a resonant cavity. Therefore, standing waves can be sustained at its resonance frequencies, with characteristic decay times of milliseconds. The output signal detected by the probe microphone includes this spurious contribution (artifact), which must be carefully accounted for, to fully exploit the diagnostic power of OAEs.

The middle ear acts as a pressure amplifier and (more important) as an impedance adaptor, which guarantees that the input acoustic power is not reflected back due to the impedance mismatch between the air-filled (low-impedance) ear canal and the liquid-filled (high-impedance) cochlea. The transmission properties of the middle ear, both in the forward and in the backward direction, affect the OAE response. They are expressed by a transmission function matrix, which relates the pressure in the ear canal to the velocity of the stapes. Both the forward and backward transmission of the middle ear depend on the frequency of the stimulus and of the OAE (Puria, 2003). This dependence has to be taken into account in the interpretation of the spectral features of the OAE response.

The stapes vibration moves the oval window, transmitting the acoustical signal to the cochlear fluid. The acoustical stimulus propagates along the basilar membrane (BM) as a forward traveling wave of transverse BM displacement driven by differential fluid pressure. Each frequency component of the stimulus propagates longitudinally on the BM up to its own tonotopic place, whose position is related to frequency by the Greenwood's Map (Greenwood, 1990), and it is resonantly amplified and absorbed there, giving rise to frequency-specific acoustical perception. The transverse displacement amplitude reaches a sharp maximum at the resonant place, thanks to the gain (some 40 dB) of the active mechanism driven by the OHCs. The cochlear region where a large BM displacement occurs at a given frequency may become a source of OAEs of that frequency, due to partial reflection from irregularities in the BM micromechanical parameters. If a cochlear region is simultaneously excited at two different frequencies, intermodulation distortion product OAEs (DPOAEs) may be generated at frequencies that are linear combinations of the two primary frequencies. As a general rule, each OAE frequency component is generated near the correspondent tonotopic place on the BM. This is not strictly true for distortion product OAEs (DPOAEs), which can be generated by nonlinear mechanisms at places different from (but generally rather close to) that corresponding to their frequency.

Cochlear models show that significant OAE generation occurs only where the forward traveling wave is strongly amplified. Damage of the OHCs, as that produced by noise exposure, either transitory or permanent, strongly reduces the OAE level. Perturbative models of the OAE generation, based on the osculating parameter technique (e.g., Talmadge et al., 2000, Sisto and Moleti, 2008), show indeed that the cochlear reflectivity (and the consequent OAE response) is very sensitive to the amplitude of the local BM displacement, and tends to vanish rapidly as the OHC gain is reduced. As the BM displacement is also the input to our acoustical sensors (the inner ear cells, IHCs) the OAE response level is a sensitive to the hearing loss level, but only in a mild to medium hearing loss range, because severe hearing loss (above 40-50 dB HL) causes almost total OAE absence.

Due to the localization of the OAE generation, OHC damage in a limited cochlear region affects the OAE level only in the correspondent frequency range. This frequency-specificity is an important property of the OAE response.

Frequency-specificity and sensitivity to OHC damage suggested using OAEs as a fast, non-invasive, objective diagnostic tool for the detection of mild hearing loss. This task has not been fulfilled yet, although many encouraging results have been obtained. Several studies have demonstrated the correlation between OAE levels and the audiometric threshold level. In the mild hearing loss range, the evoked OAE levels are quantitatively correlated with the sensorineural HL level. Cross-section studies (e.g., Attias et al., 1995; Lucertini et al., 2002) established that frequency specific indicators based on the TEOAE and DPOAE spectral levels can effectively discriminate between populations of hearing impaired and normal hearing ears, and also between "normal hearing" populations with different levels of noise exposure.

Cross-section studies do not directly imply the possibility of developing reliable OAE diagnostic tools for evaluating the hearing threshold in a single subject. Gorga et al., (1993b), found good individual correlation between TEOAE and DPOAE levels and audiometric threshold, for HL 20 dB, but very large inter-subject variability of the OAE levels was observed. Gorga and co-workers found that both TEOAEs (Prieve et al., 1993; Gorga et al., 1993b) and DPOAEs (Gorga et al., 1993a, b, 1997) can be used for detecting hearing loss levels in the 20–30 dB HL range, using also multivariate analysis approaches (Dorn, 1999; Gorga et al., 1999, 2005; Hussain et al., 1998). Hall and Lutman (1999) compared the sensitivity of OAE techniques to that of TA, studying the individual relation between OAE levels and hearing threshold, and taking into account the different test-retest fluctuation levels. Their results show good OAE sensitivity, but large inter-subject variability.

Sisto et al. (2007) demonstrated good power for DPOAE- and TEOAE-based tests of very mild hearing impairment, down to 10 dB HL, in the 1-4 kHz range. They pointed out that part of the inter-subject fluctuations that reduce the power of OAE-based tests is due to the complexity of the OAE generation mechanisms (particularly for DPOAEs) and to the presence of SOAEs (for TEOAEs), suggesting that narrow band techniques are more vulnerable to systematic errors related to these issues. DPOAEs are generated by two different mechanisms (Shera and Guinan, 1999; Kalluri and Shera, 2001), whose interference give rise to the so-called spectral fine structure, with ample fluctuations of the response level occurring within a small fraction of an octave. As a consequence, single frequency DPOAE measurements may hit a minimum or a maximum of this fine structure, resulting in large variability of the response in subjects with similar audiometric threshold levels. The presence of two DPOAE components, one generated by nonlinear distortion and the other by linear reflection, with different phase-frequency relation, may decrease the diagnostic effectiveness of OAE tests, if not correctly taken into account. Separation of the two sources, which can be obtained by time-domain filtering, exploiting the different phase–frequency relation of the two components (Withnell et al., 2003; Long and Talmadge, 2008) could significantly improve the diagnostic power of DPOAE-based tests (Mauermann and Kollmeier, 2004, Mauermann et al., 2004).

Other studies have also shown a correlation between hearing threshold and TEOAE latency, estimated as a function of frequency by time-frequency analysis of the TEOAE responses (Sisto and Moleti, 2002; Jedrzejczak et al., 2005). Time frequency analysis techniques either based on the wavelet transform or on Matching Pursuit algorithms (Tognola et al., 1997; Jedrzejczak et al., 2004) proved indeed to be very useful for discriminating several features of the OAE response (Notaro et al., 2007). Increased latency was generally observed in hearing impaired ears, which is the opposite of what one would expect on a theoretical basis, because hearing impairment should lead to lower cochlear tuning, and shorter transmission delay. This discrepancy is explained by the fact that TEOAE latency estimates are affected by large systematic errors in hearing-impaired subjects, whose SNR may be too low, and the results of cross section analyses may easily become sensitive to arbitrary data selection choices.

Spontaneous OAEs are also correlated with the audiometric threshold structure both at the microstructure level and at mid-large scale. Indeed, SOAE frequencies coincide with minima of the threshold microstructure (Schloth, 1983), and no SOAEs are present in impaired ears, in the frequency bands where the HL level is higher than 20 dB, whereas they may be found in the same ear outside the impaired frequency range (Sisto et al., 2001). Unfortunately, SOAE presence in a given frequency band is not a necessary condition for normal hearing, so these studies have had scarce clinical implications.

Recently, the use OAEs to monitor the hearing function of subjects exposed to noise, particularly in the case of professional exposure, has been the object of interesting longitudinal studies. Some recent studies suggest indeed that OAEs could be more sensitive than TA for this specific diagnostic task. Lapsley-Miller et al. 2006, demonstrated OAE sensitivity to aircraft noise exposure, but poor correlation of the OAE levels with shifts of the audiometric threshold.

Much care is needed in the data analysis to handle OAE data with low signal-to-noise ratio (SNR), particularly in cross-section studies. Indeed, the numerical value of the measured OAE "signal" level and latency becomes largely uncertain when the SNR is of order or lower than unity. On the other hand, the simple exclusion from the analysis of the data with low SNR leads to obvious systematic errors. For example, when comparing the distributions of the OAE response of two populations of normal-hearing and hearing-impaired subjects (or exposed and non-exposed), it is not fully correct to simply exclude the OAE data with low SNR, which are expected to be more frequent in the hearing-impaired population. The simple exclusion tends to underestimate the correlation between the OAE parameters and the hearing threshold level. It can be considered therefore as a conservative approach, maybe so conservative to cancel the correlation that one is looking for. A more correct approach could be to substitute the measured response level with the noise level for all data with SNR lower than unity. This method would introduce a much smaller systematic error, always in the same conservative direction, but it requires a reliable estimate of the noise level, and cannot be applied to some important OAE parameters, such as latency. Any data selection method introduces systematic errors, the fraction of low SNR data must therefore be small to get meaningful results in cross-section studies. This observation leads to the conclusion that quantitative analysis of OAE data is limited to subjects with well-measurable OAE response, i.e., with mild to medium levels of hearing loss, depending on the sensitivity and noise level of the experimental apparatus.

## METHODS

In a first study (Sisto et al., 2007), otoacoustic emissions were measured with the ILO96 system (Otodynamics, Ltd.) in a population of 82 workers, long-term exposed (from a few years to fifteen years) to variable levels of industrial noise. Absence of middle ear pathologies and of extra-professional exposure suggested that any hearing impairment were mostly due to the exposure to industrial noise. TEOAE were measured using 80 dBpSPL click stimuli, in a 20 ms interval after the click, in the nonlinear derived mode of acquisition to suppress the linear ringing artifact. DPOAEs were measured using $L_1 = 65$, $L_2 = 55$ dB SPL stimuli, $f_2/f_1 = 1.22$, with a resolution of one third of octave. These stimulus settings are widely used in the clinical practice, because they give rise to well-measurable OAE response in subjects with mild to medium hearing loss, while maintaining sufficiently high sensitivity to the lowest levels of hearing loss, for which lower stimulus levels could be the optimal choice. No SNR-based data selection rule has been applied to these data. Statistical analyses were performed using multivariate regression and ROC curve analysis, in the R software framework.

In a second study (Nataletti et al., 2008), TEOAEs and DPOAEs were measured using the ILO292 portable system, and the same stimulus settings of the first study, in a population of 18 young normal hearing subjects, before and after exposure to high levels of noise ($L_{eq}$ of order 100dBA) in discotheques. Only the OAE data with SNR higher than unity both before and after exposure have been considered in this analysis. As stated before, this is a very conservative approach, which means that the statistical significance of the results could have been underestimated.

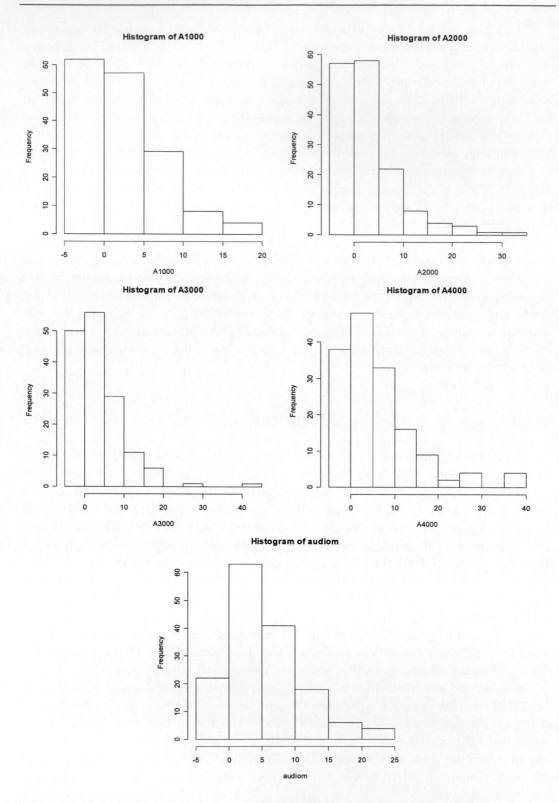

Figure 1. Statistical distributions of the hearing threshold level in four frequency bands from 1 to 4 kHz and of the average threshold (audiom) in the whole range.

Standard spectral analysis was applied to the TEOAE waveforms, as well as time-frequency analysis, based on the wavelet transform, to get estimates of the individual relation between TEOAE latency and frequency. The algorithm proposed by Moleti and Sisto (2003) and refined in Sisto and Moleti (2007) was also used to get objective cochlear tuning estimates from the TEOAE latency estimates.

# RESULTS

## A. Professional Long-term Exposure to Industrial Noise

In Figure 1 we show the histogram of the audiometric hearing threshold level in the whole population of workers, at 1, 2, 3, and 4 kHz, and of the average level in the 1-4 kHz range. The main loss is at 4 kHz, as typically observed in noise-exposed subjects, but some hearing threshold shift is observed also at lower frequencies, and the distribution of the average threshold is more regular and symmetrical.

In Figure 2 we show the ROC curve that can be obtained by straightforward application of a single variable (the DPOAE level at 4 kHz) test to discriminate between two subgroups separated according to their audiometric threshold at 4 kHz, setting the discrimination level at the standard clinical level of 20 dB. The area below the curve quantifies the predicting power of the test. A power of 88% is obtained, showing that the potential of the OAE data is large, but also that such a simple test would imply a large fraction of false alarms and/or false negatives. The use of a slightly more sophisticated approach is therefore justified.

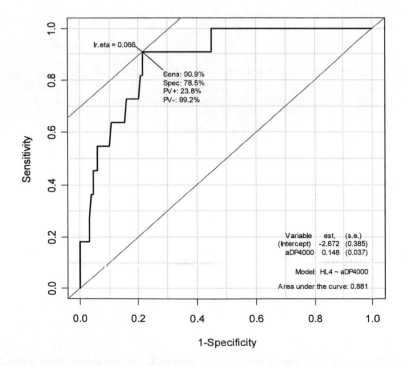

Figure 2. ROC curve obtained for a single variable test of the hearing threshold level at a single frequency (4 kHz). The discrimination hearing threshold level is 20 dB.

**Table I. DPOAE multivariate regression for the model optimized to predict the average 1-4 kHz audiometric threshold. Only the significant, used by the model, parameters are reported. The other DPOAE data were neglected in the model.**

|             | Estimate | Std. Error | t value | Pr(>|t|)       |
|-------------|----------|------------|---------|----------------|
| (Intercept) | 8.239    | 0.434      | 18.951  | < 2e-16 ***    |
| DP1200      | -0.147   | 0.049      | -2.996  | 0.003 **       |
| DP3100      | -0.286   | 0.067      | -4.277  | 3.32e-05 ***   |
| DP4000      | -0.129   | 0.054      | -2.385  | 0.018 *        |

Signif. codes: 0 '***' 0.001 '**' 0.01 '*' 0.05 '.' 0.1 ' ' 1
Residual standard error: 3.897 on 153 degrees of freedom
Multiple R-Squared: 0.4815, Adjusted R-squared: 0.4714
F-statistic: 47.36 on 3 and 153 DF, p-value: < 2.2e-16

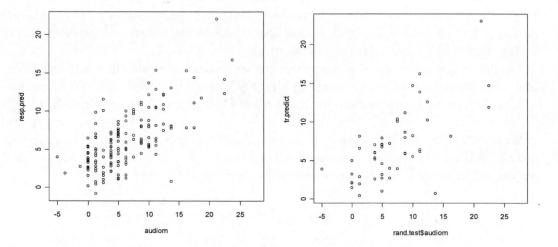

Figure 3. Multivariate regression analysis showing (a) the actual threshold versus the threshold predicted using a linear model using DPOAE levels, in a training subset of 110 ears. Three DPOAE frequency resulted significant. The relation is applied to an independent test subset of 56 ears (b).

In Table I and Figure 3a we show the results of a multivariate analysis, in which a linear regression model is optimized to get maximum correlation between the average 1-4 kHz hearing threshold level and a linear combination of the DPOAE measured levels in the same frequency range, on a randomly chosen training subset of 110 ears. The DPOAE data of frequency bands giving non significant contributions to the explanation of total variance were excluded from the regression, ending up with a three variable (the DPOAE levels at 1.2, 3.1 and 4 kHz) regression. In Figure 3b we show the result of the application of the model to the prediction of the average threshold on the remaining ears, constituting the test subset. The results are satisfactorily similar, showing that the randomly chosen training and test subsets are not statistically different from each other.

The whole population has then been divided into two audiometric subgroups, according to the average 1-4 kHz threshold level, with different choices of the average audiometric threshold level used to separate the two subgroups. By doing so, one is able to evaluate with a series of ROC curves the different power of OAE-based tests of the average hearing level, for different levels of average hearing impairment.

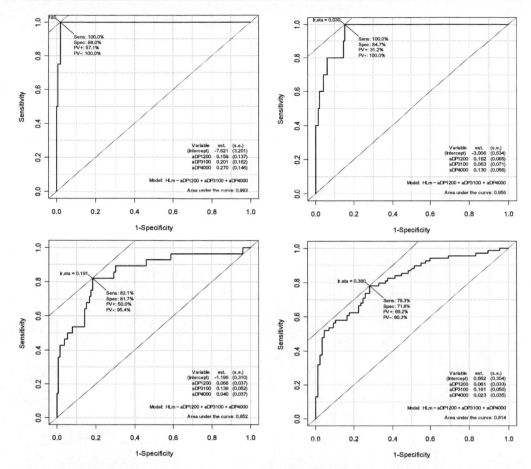

Figure 4. ROC curves of the model of Figure 3 relative to a discriminating average threshold level of 20 (top left), 15 (top right), 10 (bottom left) and 5 dB (bottom right).

In Figure 4 the ROC curves of the model of Figure 3 relative to a discriminating average 1-4 kHz threshold level between 5 and 20 dB are shown. As regards the predicting power of such tests, it can be noted that values of power well above 80% can be obtained for tests capable of discriminating threshold levels as low as 5 dB. This is an interesting result, confirming that DPOAEs can be used for diagnostic tests in a very mild hearing loss range.

Returning to the prediction of the audiometric threshold level at 4 kHz, which is an issue of clinical interest because, in most cases, noise-induced hearing loss manifests itself first at this frequency, we note that the multivariate approach can be useful also in this case to get better test performances. In this case a new model has been optimized for the prediction of the 4 kHz threshold and it turned out that including several data of DPOAE levels down to 1 kHz improved the power of the test, with respect to that of the simple single-variable test of Figure 2. In Figure 5 we show the ROC curves relative to four different choices of the audiometric discrimination level, which show that power values above 90% can be obtained down to hearing thresholds of 15 dB at 4 kHz. This result confirms the validity of using a multivariate approach also for the detection of hearing loss at a single frequency. The explanation for this result may also be related to the fine structure of DPOAEs, which introduces variability of the response at a single frequency that can be reduced by considering together DPOAE levels of different spectral regions.

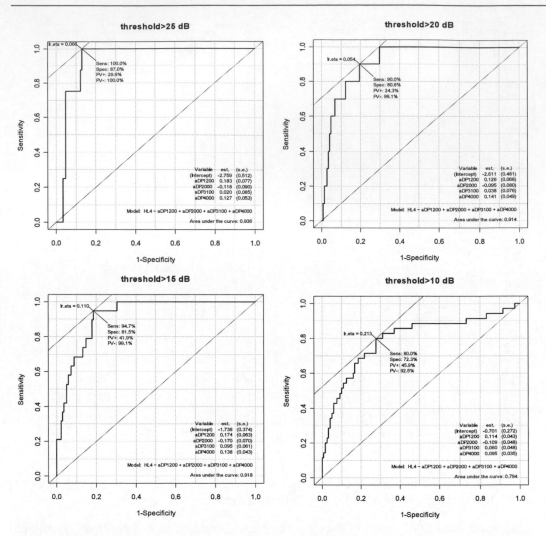

Figure 5. ROC curves for the diagnosis of the 4 kHz audiometric threshold level using a multivariate model. The four curves refer to different audiometric threshold levels used to discriminate between two audiometric subgroups.

The application of the same analysis procedures to the TEOAE response level data gives, as already noted in Sisto et al. (2007), slightly less significant results, which are not reported here, for brevity.

## B. Intense Transitory Noise Exposure in Discotheques

In Figure 6 we show the average TEOAE (top) and DPOAE (bottom) levels as measured before and after exposure to noise in the discotheque. The level change is clearly visible, and it can be compared with the size of the error bars, representing one standard error. In Table II the p-values of the t-tests are also reported, showing the statistical significance of the differences. Setting the significance threshold at $p < 0.05$, the TEOAE level differences result significant for several frequency bands and, particularly, for the global response, while for DPOAEs, the only significant result is obtained for the global response.

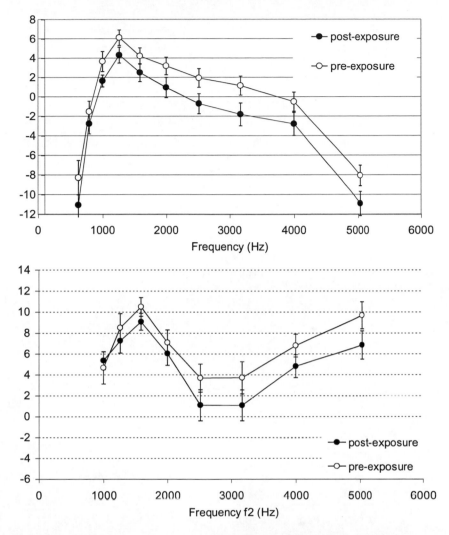

Figure 6. Average TEOAE (top) and DPOAE (bottom) levels in dB SPL as measured before and after exposure to noise in the discotheque. The statistical significance of the band and global differences are reported in Table I.

**Table II. Comparison between the pre-exposure and post-exposure TEOAE and DPOAE response levels, and statistical significance of the difference between the two distributions.**

| Frequency | 625 | 800 | 1000 | 1250 | 1600 | 2000 | 2500 | 3200 | 4000 | 5000 | Global |
|---|---|---|---|---|---|---|---|---|---|---|---|
| TE Post-exp. | -11.1 | -2.8 | 1.6 | 4.3 | 2.5 | 0.9 | -0.7 | -1.8 | -2.8 | -10.9 | 20.3 |
| TE Pre-exp. | -8.3 | -1.5 | 3.6 | 6.1 | 4.2 | 3.2 | 1.9 | 1.1 | -0.5 | -8.1 | 22.2 |
| TE p(t-test) | 0.04 | 0.15 | 0.04 | 0.08 | 0.11 | 0.06 | 0.04 | 0.03 | 0.08 | 0.07 | 0.003 |
| DP Post-exp. | - | - | 5.4 | 7.3 | 9.1 | 6.0 | 1.1 | 1.1 | 4.8 | 6.8 | 25.3 |
| DP Pre-exp. | - | - | 4.7 | 8.5 | 10.5 | 7.1 | 3.7 | 3.7 | 6.8 | 9.7 | 27.1 |
| DP p(t-test) | | | 0.35 | 0.24 | 0.12 | 0.26 | 0.10 | 0.11 | 0.10 | 0.07 | 0.02 |

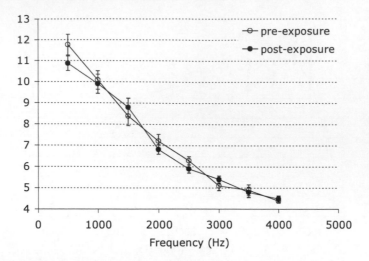

Figure 7. Average TEOAE latency (in ms) measured before and after exposure to noise in the discotheque. No statistically significant difference is obseved.

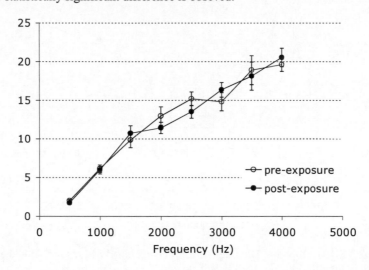

Figure 8. Average cochlear tuning derived from TEOAE latency measured before and after exposure to noise in the discotheque.

This result encourages further study about the diagnostic power of OAEs for detecting temporary hearing impairment due to intense noise exposure. It is interesting to note that TEOAEs performed better than DPOAEs for this particular diagnostic purpose, whereas for long-term noise exposure to lower noise levels the opposite has been reported (Sisto et al., 2007).

The comparison between the OAE latencies, estimated using a time-frequency wavelet technique to analyze the TEOAE waveforms, shows instead no significant difference between the latency measured before and after the exposure, as shown in Figure 7. Level measurements seem to be more effective than latency measurements for this particular diagnostic purpose.

The objective cochlear tuning estimates derived from the TEOAE latency data are shown in Figure 8. No difference is obviously found due to exposure, because the tuning estimates are directly derived from the latency data that showed no significant difference. The expected increase of tuning with frequency can be observed, even if the slope is significantly steeper than that reported by psychoacoustical studies. This steep slope suggests that the simple analytical cochlear model concepts used to predict the dependence of latency on tuning (Moleti et al., 2005; Sisto and Moleti, 2007) could overestimate the tuning dependence on frequency. This dependence, observed also by behavioral studies (Glasberg and Moore, 1990; Unoki et al., 2007), leads, by violating the scale-invariance symmetry, to the actually measured OAE latency-frequency relation, which is slower than that expected for a scale-invariant cochlea.

## CONCLUSIONS

The results reported in this study confirm the diagnostic potential of OAE-based techniques to detect hearing loss down to sub-clinical levels and that OAE levels are sensitive indicators of temporary effects of noise exposure in normal-hearing subjects. The possibility of obtaining objective estimates of cochlear tuning is also a new application of the OAE analysis. We conclude that an objective, subclinical evaluation and an accurate frequency resolution of hearing dysfunction can be obtained by a specific analysis of OAE data.

## REFERENCES

Attias, J., Furst, M., Furman, V., Reshef, I., Horowitz, G. & Bresloff, I., (1995). "Noise-induced otoacoustic emission loss with or without hearing loss," *Ear Hear.*, *16*, 612-618.

Dorn, P. A., Piskorski, P, Gorga, M. P., Neely, S. T. & Keefe, D. H. (1999). "Predicting audiometric status from distortion product otoacoustic emissions using multivariate analyses," *Ear Hear.*, *20*, 149-163.

Glasberg, B. R. & Moore, B. C. J. (1990). "Derivation of auditory filter shapes from notched-noise data," *Hear. Res.*, *47*, 103-138.

Gorga, M. P., Dierking, D. M., Johnson, T. A., Beauchaine, K. L., Garner, C. A. & Neely, S. T. (2005). "A validation and potential clinical application of multivariate analyses of distortion-product otoacoustic emission data," *Ear Hear.*, *26*, 593-607.

Gorga, M. P., Neely, S. T. & Dorn, P. A. (1999). "Distortion product otoacoustic emission test performance for a priori criteria and for multifrequency audiometric standards," *Ear Hear.*, *20*, 345-362

Gorga, M. P., Neely, S. T., Bergman, B. M., Beauchaine, K. L., Kaminski, J. R., Peters, J. & Jesteadt, W. (1993). "Otoacoustic emissions from normal-hearing and hearing impaired subjects: distortion product responses," *J. Acoust. Soc. Am.*, *93*, 2050-2060.

Gorga, M. P., Neely, S. T., Bergman, B. M., Beauchaine, K. L., Kaminski, J. R., Peters, J., Sculte, L. & Jesteadt, W. (1993). "A comparison of transient-evoked and distortion product otoacoustic emissions in normal-hearing and hearing-impaired subjects," *J. Acoust. Soc. Am.*, *94*, 2639-2648.

Gorga, M. P., Neely, S. T., Ohlrich, B., Hoover, B., Redner J. & Peters, J. (1997). "From laboratory to clinic: a large scale study of distortion product otoacoustic emissions in ears with normal hearing and ears with hearing loss," *Ear Hear.*, 18, 440-455

Hall, A. J. & Lutman, M. E. (1999). "Methods for early identification of noiseinduced hearing loss," *Audiology*, *38*, 277-280.

Hussain, D. M., Gorga, M. P., Neely, S. T., Keefe, D. H. & Peters, J. (1998). "Transient evoked otoacoustic emissions in patients with normal hearing and in patients with hearing loss," *Ear Hear.*, *19*, 434-449.

Jedrzejczak, W. W., Blinowska, K. J. & Konopka, W. (2005). "Time-frequency analysis of transiently evoked otoacoustic emissions of subjects exposed to noise," *Hear. Res*, *205*, 249-255.

Jedrzejczak, W. W., Blinowska, K. J., Konopka, W., Grzanka, A. & Durka, P. J. (2004). "Identification of otoacoustic emission components by means of adaptive approximations," *J. Acoust. Soc. Am.*, *115*, 2148-2158.

Kalluri, R. & Shera, C. A. (2001). "Distortion-product source unmixing: A test of the two-mechanism model for DPOAE generation," *J. Acoust. Soc. Am.*, *109*, 622-637.

Lapsley Miller, J. A., Marshall, L., Heller, L. M. & Hughes, L. M. (2006). "Low-level otoacoustic emissions may predict susceptibility to noise-induced hearing loss," *J. Acoust. Soc. Am.*, *120*, 280-296.

Long, G., Talmadge, C. L. & Lee, J. (2008). "Measuring distortion product otoacoustic emission using continuously sweeping primaries," *J. Acoust. Soc. Am.*, *124*, 1613-1626.

Lucertini, M., Moleti, A. & Sisto, R. (2002). "On the detection of early cochlear damage by otoacoustic emission analysis," *J. Acoust. Soc. Am.*, *111*, 972-978.

Mauermann, M. & Kollmeier, B. (2004). "Distortion product otoacoustic emission (DPOAE) input/output functions and the influence of the second DPOAE source," *J. Acoust. Soc. Am.*, *116*, 2199-2212.

Mauermann, M., Long, G. R. & Kollmeier, B. (2004). "Fine structure of hearing threshold and loudness perception," *J. Acoust. Soc. Am.*, *116*, 1066-1080.

Mauermann, M., Uppenkamp, S., van Hengel, P. W. J & Kollmeier, B. (1999). "Evidence for the distortion product frequency place as a source of distortion product otoacoustic emission (DPOAE) fine structure in humans. II. Fine structure for different shapes of cochlear hearing loss," *J. Acoust. Soc. Am.*, *106*, 3484-3491.

Moleti, A. & Sisto, R. (2003). "Objective estimates of cochlear tuning by otoacoustic emission analysis," *J. Acoust. Soc. Am.*, *113*, 423-429.

Nataletti, P., Sisto, R., Pieroni, A., Sanjust, F. & Annesi, D. (2008). "Studio pilota dell'esposizione a rumore dei frequentatori e dei lavoratori delle discoteche di Roma," Atti del 35° Convegno Nazionale AIA, Milano 11-13 giugno 2008 (in Italian).

Notaro, G., Al-Maamury, A. M., Moleti, A. & Sisto, R. (2007). "Wavelet and Matching Pursuit estimates of the transient-evoked otoacoustic emission latency," *J. Acoust. Soc. Am.*, *122*, 3576-3585.

Prieve, B. A., Gorga, M. P., Schmidt, A., Neely, S., Peters, J., Schultes, L. & Jesteadt, W. (1993). "Analysis of transient-evoked otoacoustic emissions in normal-hearing and hearing-impaired ears,". *J. Acoust. Soc. Am.*, *93*, 3308-3319.

Probst, R., Lonsbury-Martin, B. L. & Martin, G. K. (1991). "A review of otoacoustic emissions," *J. Acoust. Soc. Am.*, *89*, 2027-2067.

Puria, S. (2003). "Measurements of human middle ear forward and reverse acoustics: Implications for otoacoustic emissions," *J. Acoust. Soc. Am.*, *113*, 2773-2789.

Schloth, E. (1983). "Relation between Spectral Composition of Spontaneous Oto-acoustic Emissions and Fine-structure of Threshold in Quiet," *Acustica*, *53*, 250-256.

Shera, C. A. & Guinan, J. J. Jr. (1999). "Evoked otoacoustic emissions arise from two fundamentally different mechanisms: A taxonomy for mammalian OAEs," *J. Acoust. Soc. Am.*, *105*, 782-798.

Sisto, R. & Moleti, A. (2007). "Transient evoked otoacoustic emission latency and cochlear tuning at different stimulus levels," *J. Acoust. Soc. Am.*, *122*, 2183-2190.

Sisto, R. & Moleti, A. (2008). "Comparison between otoacoustic and auditory brainstem response latencies supports slow backward propagation of otoacoustic emissions," *J. Acoust. Soc. Am.*, *123*, 1495-1503.

Sisto, R. & Moleti, A. (2002). "On the frequency dependence of the otoacoustic emission latency in hypoacoustic and normal ears," *J. Acoust. Soc. Am.*, *111*, 297-308.

Sisto, R., Moleti, A. & Lucertini, M. (2001). "Spontaneous Otoacoustic Emissions and relaxation dynamics of long decay time OAEs in audiometrically normal and impaired subjects," *J. Acoust . Soc. Am.*, *109*, 638-647.

Talmadge, C. L., Tubis, A., Long, G. R. & Tong, C. (2000) "Modeling the combined effects of basilar membrane nonlinearity and roughness on stimulus frequency otoacoustic emission fine structure," *J. Acoust. Soc. Am.*, *108*, 2911-2932.

Tognola, G., Ravazzani, P. & Grandori, F. (1997). "Time-frequency distributions of click-evoked otoacoustic emissions," *Hear. Res.*, *106*, 112-122.

Unoki, M., Miyauchi, R. & Tan, C. T. (2007). "Estimates of tuning of auditory filter using simultaneous and forward notched-noise masking," in *Hearing – From sensory processing to perception*, B. Kollmeier, G. Klump, V. Hohmann, U. Langemann, M. Mauermann, S. Uppenkamp, & J. Verhey, (Eds.), (Springer, Berlin), 19-26.

Withnell, R. H., Shaffer, L. A. & Talmadge, C. L. (2003). "Generation of DPOAEs in the guinea pig," *Hear. Res.*, *178*, 187-195.

In: Deafness, Hearing Loss and the Auditory System
Editors: D. Fiedler and R. Krause, pp.279-289

ISBN: 978-1-60741-259-5
©2010 Nova Science Publishers, Inc.

*Chapter 12*

# SODIUM ENOXIPARIN IN THE TREATMENT OF IDIOPATHIC SUDDEN SENSORINEURAL HEARING LOSS

## *Angelo Salami, Renzo Mora, Francesco Mora, Barbara Crippa, Luca Guastini and Massimo Dellepiane*

ENT Department, University of Genoa, Italy

## ABSTRACT

The audiovestibular system can be affected by an immunological etiology; the presence of immune mediated sensorineural hearing loss (IMSNHL) as part of or in combination with other autoimmune diseases is well documented in the literature. Hearing loss can be caused by autoimmune disorders localized to the inner ear or secondary to systemic immune diseases (Cogan's syndrome, juvenile chronic arthritis, ulcerative colitis, Wegener's granulomatosis, scleroderma, pulseless disease, and SLE). A systemic autoimmune disorder can be present in fewer than one-third of cases

The clinical presentation of immune inner-ear disease is extremely variable and depends on the type of immune reaction and on the site of injury within the inner ear. IMSNHL typically presents with an idiopathic, progressive unilateral and successive bilateral rapidly progressive sensorineural hearing loss; the course of the hearing loss occurs over weeks to months and is most common in middle-aged women; it may be accompanied by tinnitus and vertigo and is almost always unilateral.

IMSNHL is still a diagnostic and therapeutic dilemma, and predicting recovery from it is very difficult. Different factors may influence a prognosis: e.g., severity of hearing loss, duration of symptoms before treatment, presence of vertigo, type of audiogram, and age of patients. The therapeutic approaches normally used for this pathological condition include the systemic and local administration of cortisone, vasoactive agents, anticoagulants, vitamin complexes, a cytotoxic agent and plasmapheresis. These drugs can be effective in reversing such hearing loss, although at the cost of occasionally severe side effects.

Currently, evaluating the importance of an autoimmune phenomenon in the genesis of inner-ear disease is difficult because the clinical and biological criteria of autoimmune deafness have not yet been well defined. A positive response to treatment is a criterion for the diagnosis of immune inner-ear disease.

This chapter aims to assess the effect of sodium enoxaparin on the recovery of hearing in patients affected by ISSNHL. Sodium enoxaparin was administered subcutaneously at a dose of 4,000 IU once a day for 10 days.

Sodium enoxaparin is a particular kind of heparin with a low molecular weight (LMWH) and is endowed with a high antithrombotic activity.

The literature does not report any therapeutic protocols for autoimmune IMSNHL treatment with sodium enoxaparin or other kinds of unfractionated heparin. Our decision to use enoxaparin was based both on the pathogenesis of this condition and on evaluation of the other classes of drugs currently used.

# INTRODUCTION

Sudden sensorineural hearing loss (SSNHL) is a symptom of cochlear injury. It is characterized by sudden onset, and it may be accompanied by vertigo and tinnitus. Many potential causes can trigger SSNHL but, despite extensive evaluation, the majority of cases elude definitive diagnosis and therefore remain idiopathic.

Hearing loss can obviously range from barely detectable to profound: *idiopathic sudden sensorineural hearing loss (ISSNHL) is defined as a sudden (<72 h) and demonstrating threshold change for the worse of at least 30 dB in at least three contiguous audiometric frequencies.* ISSNHL is almost always unilateral.

Tinnitus is usually present (>90%), and vertigo is frequent, either spontaneous (as in acute vestibular neuritis) or isolated positional vertigo [1]. Sixty-five percent of patient recover completely with or without treatment, most within 2 weeks [2].

There has been considerable speculation about viral and vascular causes, with rather more evidence for the former than the latter. Consequently, the idea that immunity might participate in the causation of inner ear disease and ISSNHL, has only recently become accepted.

In 1979, McCabe first brought the attention to a possible discrete clinical entity when he presented a series of patients with bilateral, progressive hearing loss showing improvement following treatment with corticosteroids. Since that time, autoimmunity has been proposed as a cause of other inner ear disorders, including Mèniére disease, SSNHL and acute vertigo [3-5].

Although other authors had over the years described patients with ear-related illness associated with systemic disorders, none had collected such a large series or speculated that these patients might have an organ specific illness [4,5].

Patients with ISSNHL, without obvious antecedent cause should receive a careful otologic history and examination, as well as an audiologic assessment (pure tone audiometry, otoacustic emission, auditory brainstem response, etc). The importance of pure tone audiometry and auditory brain response is well established. Otoacustic emissions (OAEs) are sometimes present (implying sparing of the outer hair cell) in ISSNHL, but is unclear whether the OAE testing is clinically useful, that is, whether the results can assist in selecting therapy. Magnetic resonance imaging with gadolinium contrast injection is only appropriate to detect a schwannomas of the cochlear nerve, when the audiologic tests highlight a possible presence [6].

In particular, when an immune-mediated sudden sensorineural hearing loss (IMSSNHL) is believed: *the importance of autoimmune phenomenon in the genesis of inner ear disease is difficult to evaluate because the clinical and biological criteria of autoimmune deafness has not yet been well defined. Individual diagnostic criteria (clinical presentation, laboratory studies and response to treatment) are non-specific but, when used in combination, can diagnose immune-mediated inner ear disease with reasonable success [7].*

Although immuno-mediated ear disease can present as the sole manifestation of a systemic autoimmune disease, many attempts have been made to develop inner ear-specific assays in order to find a diagnostic marker for isolated immune-mediated ear disease. Diverse immunological tests are used in clinical investigation and diagnosis and to form the basis for an immunological therapeutic decision: *but laboratory test appears to be positive in more than 30 to 40% of patients who otherwise fit the criteria for autoimmune disease.* One possible explanation for this is that IMSSNHL has a number of different causes, include autoimmune, viral, genetic, vascular, perhaps metabolic, etc. Another possibility is that autoimmunity exists to a variety of inner ear antigens.

*It is generally agreed that IMSSNHL should be bilateral and rapidly progressive, the involvement of the second ear may take months or even years to occur.*

IMSSNHL is a rare disorders, but the true incidence remains unknown; although patients of all the ages have been described with the disorder, the disease most commonly affects middle-aged adults. Men and women are affected at equal rates; no racial predilection has been identified.

The therapeutic approaches normally used for this pathological condition include the systemic and local administration of corticosteroids, cytoxic agents, vasoactive agents, anticoagulants, vitamin complexes, and plasmapheresis.

*Although these drugs can be effective in reversing such hearing loss, they present side effects: until now, no standard therapeutic protocol is available for the management of these conditions.*

## SODIUM ENOXAPARIN

IMSSNHL is still a diagnostic and therapeutic dilemma, and predicting recovery from it is very difficult: several factors may influence a prognosis (e.g., severity of hearing loss, duration of symptoms before treatment, presence of vertigo, type of audiogram, and age of patients).

*A positive response to treatment is a criterion for the diagnosis of immune inner ear disease, treatment guidelines are controversial but include corticosteroids, cytotoxic agents, vasoactive agents, anticoagulants, vitamin complexes and plasmapheresis* These drugs can be effective in reversing such hearing loss, although at the cost of occasionally severe side-effects [8]

*Sodium enoxaparin is a particular kind of heparin with a low molecular weight (LMWH) and endowed with a high antithrombotic activity.* Like all the other types of heparin, it belongs to the class of anticoagulants, but offers a number of clinical advantages and has therapeutic effects superior to the other types of non-fractionated heparin: this drug exerts its effects essentially on capillary blood viscosity, erythrocyte deformability, thrombocyte aggregation, antiphospholipid antibody activity and shows an anti-inflammatory action in subcutaneous administration [9,10].

*The success of unfractionated heparin with pregnancy outcomes in women with antiphospholipid antibody syndrome has our stimulated interest to implement a protocol using an anticoagulant, sodium enoxaparin, for patients with IMSSNHL [11,12].*

For these reasons, we have decided to analyze the efficacy of sodium enoxaparin in the treatment of IMSSNHL: *the aim of this chapter has been to evaluate the efficiency and applicability of sodium enoxaparin in the treatment of IMSSNHL.*

## PERSONAL EXPERIENCES

Before the treatment, all patients undergo the following instrumental examinations: blood tests, pure tone audiometry, tympanometry, otoacoustic emissions and otoacoustic products of distortion.

We perform the following blood tests: prothrombin and fibrinogen levels; erythrocyte sedimentation rate; C-reactive protein; rheumatoid factors; anti-nuclear and anti-tyroglobulin antibodies; anti double-stranded DNA antibodies; circulating immunoglobulins class G, M, A (IgG, IgM, IgA) and complement levels (CH50, C3, C4).

*No single blood immune parameter can supporter a diagnosis of immune-mediated disease: we consider the possibility of an immune-mediated disease when the patients show a modification of almost six blood immune parameters.*

Patient with ISSNHL are included if they present: an history of immunological disorder and/or an alteration of almost 6 of 12 immune blood parameters examined before the treatment; a threshold change for the worse of at least 30 dB in at least three contiguous audiometric frequencies.

**Table I. blood test result (mean value ± standard deviation) before (t=1) and at the end (t=2) of the treatment with sodium enoxaparin.**

|                                        | t=1    |      | t=2    |      |
|----------------------------------------|--------|------|--------|------|
|                                        | Mean   | ±SD  | Mean   | ±SD  |
| erythrocyte sedimentation rate (mm/hr) | 64.9   | 1.03 | 14.1   | 1.24 |
| C-reactive protein (mg/dl)             | 8.5    | 0.85 | <3.2   |      |
| rheumatoid factor (IU)                 | 281.4  | 1.76 | 189.2  | 1.68 |
| C3 complement component (mg/dl)        | 194.3  | 0.98 | 176.4  | 0.93 |
| Fibrinogen (mg/dl)                     | 313.4  | 1.89 | 313.3  | 1.01 |
| Prothrombin (seconds)                  | 98.8   | 0.83 | 98.5   | 0.71 |
| IgG (mg/dl)                            | 1855.1 | 2.03 | 1623.3 | 1.87 |
| IgM (mg/dl)                            | 286.3  | 1.21 | 234.1  | 1.08 |
| IgA (mg/dl)                            | 411.7  | 0.73 | 406.4  | 1.35 |
| C4 complement component (mg/dl)        | 48.4   | 0.53 | 37.7   | 0.57 |
| CH50 complement component (U)          | 198.8  | 1.88 | 197.4  | 1.60 |
| anti-tyroglobulin antibodies (IU/ml)   | 240.4  | 1.75 | 107.3  | 1.27 |

We don't treat patients with: a history of thrombocytopenia following heparin treatment; hemorrhagic manifestations or tendencies due to disorders of haemostasis that are not heparin-dependent or related to consumption coagulopathy; organic injuries at risk of bleeding; renal failure; acute infectious endocarditis; hemorrhagic cerebrovascular events; allergy to enoxaparin; use in the last six months of cortisone or immunosuppressive drugs; concurrent use of ticlopidine, salicylate or non steroidal anti-inflammatory drugs (NSAIDs) with sodium enoxaparin and association with platelet anti-coagulants (dipyridamole, sulfinpyrazone, etc.).

## Enoxaparin is Administered Subcutaneously at a Dose of 4,000 IU Once a Day for 10 Days

All the previous audiologic and blood tests are repeated, in each patients, at the end of the treatment.

## Until now, no Patients Experienced Side Effects

Actually, we have obtained a recovery of the hearing loss in the 84% of the patients (n=120) treated with sodium enoxaparin and affected by IMSSNHL.

In these patients, the blood test revealed: *1) a reduction and normalization of erythrocyte sedimentation rate, C-reactive protein and rheumatoid factor; 2) significant decrease of C3 and C4 complement levels; 3) decrease of the IgG and IgM plasmatic levels; 4) reduction of anti-tyroglobulin antibodies plasmatic levels.*

We found no significant differences in the others parameters. (Table 1)

## DISCUSSION

Sudden sensorineural hearing loss is one of the most controversial issues in otology. General agreement surrounds the definition of the clinical entity: unilateral sensorineural hearing loss of at least 30 dB for three consecutive frequencies on the tonal audiogram with onset within the last 3 days. However, pathogenesis and appropriate treatment remain open questions [13,14].

Several experimental studies have attempted to reproduce the mechanisms of infection, ischemic trauma, or autoimmunity leading to sudden-onset cochlear dysfunction, but extrapolation to the clinical situation is hazardous [13,14].

For at least two reasons, clinicians have had great difficulty in unraveling this clinical entity. First, exploring the inner ear directly is impossible, basically owing to the lack of any usable electrochemical data. Second, therapeutic trials are hampered because of the difficulty of recruiting a sufficiently large population within a reasonable time span [13,14].

Among the causes of sudden sensorineural hearing loss, the presence of IMSSNHL as part of or in combination with other autoimmune diseases is well documented in the literature. Hearing loss can be caused by autoimmune disorders localized to the inner ear or secondary to systemic immune diseases (Cogan's syndrome, juvenile chronic arthritis, ulcerative colitis, Wegener's granulomatosis, scleroderma, etc). A systemic autoimmune disorder can be present in fewer than one-third of cases [15-18].

Unlike other organs and tissues, the inner ear is not amenable to biopsy for expressed intent of investigating to underlying immunopathogenesis of purported autoimmune disorders affecting it. What little histopathology has been published from patients with suspected IMSSNHL shows fibrosis and/or bone deposition in the labyrinth, consistent with the late sequelae of inflammation [19,20]. Specific immune reactivity against inner ear antigens is often detected in patients with IMSSNHL, but result vary [21].

*Recent reports have shown that the inner ear does not represent an immune-privileged site but can generate a local immune response after either local or systemic immunization of antigen. These immune response are dependent on the presence of an intact endolymphatic sac.* These findings confirm the role of the endolymphatic sac in mediating immunity of the inner ear, as well as, the communication of the normal sac with circulating lymphocytes.

This provides an additional foundation for autoimmunity as an etiology in disorders involving the inner ear and demonstrates that the inner ear, although protected by systemic immunity can be damage by a local immune response.

The route of entry of the inflammatory cells into the inner ear following antigen or viral challenge of the inner ear appears predominantly to be via the spiral modiolar vein: during the inflammatory response, this vein takes on the characteristics of an activated venule and expresses intercellular adhesion molecule-1 (ICAM-1) on the endothelial cell surface that facilitates the passage of circulating immunocompetent cells into the scala tympani [22,23].

Once in the inner ear, these cells divide, release inflammatory mediators, and set in motion events that lead to cellular proliferation: shortly after entering the cochlea, hearing loss occurs [22,23].

Although these recent evidences, the pathophysiology of immune mediated disorders in the middle and inner ear is still not well understood. Multiple potential mechanisms have been identified that can result in immune-mediated ear pathology. The immune-mediated and the autoimmune pathology can affect the middle and inner ear by antibodies (Abs) against inner ear antigens and or specific immune system activation.

Although sera from patients, with immune-mediated ear pathology, contain Abs capable of immunostaining human inner ear tissues, the antigen (Ag) specificity of the autoantibodies is currently unclear. Heat shock protein 70 (HSP70) has been implicated as a possible target Ag in immune-mediated sensory-neural hearing loss (IMSNHL), but its ability to target inner ear-specific pathology is questionable in light of its expression in a variety of non inner ear tissues. Also collagen II has also been proposed as a target Ag in IMSNHL. However, the ubiquitous expression of collagen II in numerous organs makes it an improbable candidate for targeting the inner ear-specific autoimmune features prevalent in patients with "primary" IMSNHL who show no signs of additional inflammatory disorders or systemic autoimmunity [24].

Most putative autoimmune diseases are linked to T helper (Th) cells activation [24]. It is demonstrated that Th cells could be allocated to two subsets, Th1 (type 1) and Th2 (type 2), according to their cytokine production. Th1 cells activate cellular immunity by producing interleukin (IL) -2, interferon (IFN) - $\gamma$ and tumour necrosis factor (TNF) -$\beta$. Therefore, they ensure defence against viral, bacterial, fungal and protozoal infections [25].

The Th2 cells, that stimulate humoral immunity, produce IL-4, IL-5, IL-10 and IL-13. They have roles in some helminthic infections with immunoglobulin of class E (IgE) and of class G (IgG) responses and in allergic disorders [25].

It is not known clearly which factor initiate cell development as Th1 and Th2. But it was found that IL-12 and IL-4 are the two important cytokines that polarize the development of Th1 and Th2 cells inversely. The natural immune response at the beginning of an infection probably regulate the deviations in the predominance of Th1 and Th2 cells [25].

Th1 clones produces INF-γ and IL-2, but not IL-4 or IL-5. However, Th2 cells produce IL4, IL-5, IL-10 and IL-13, but they do not produce INF-γ and IL-2 cytokines [25].

Lymphokines secreted from Th1 cells activate the cellular immune system by stimulating the production of macrophages and causing B cells to produce immunoglobulin (Ig) of class M (IgM) and of class G (IgG). INF-γ and IL-2 cytokines change the Th polarization to Th1 while IL-4 changes it to Th2 [25].

The divergent effects of Th1 and Th2 cells are also seen in their association with deleterious immune reactions in humans. In particular, autoimmune disorders associated with the destruction of host tissues, such as diabetes mellitus, multiple sclerosis, or inflammatory bowel disease, predominantly involve Th1 response. By contrast, allergic disorders (e.g. seasonal rhinitis, asthma, and contact dermatitis) in which IgE, mast cells, and eosinophils play a prominent role are dominated by Th2 cells [25].

The involvement of autoreactive T cells has been particularly difficult to demonstrate primarily because of the lack of widespread availability of human inner ear antigens. Nevertheless, autoreactive T cells were first implicated in ISNHL in studies involving inhibition of leukocyte migration. Direct involvement of autoreactive T cells was confirmed by Hughes et al. (1986) who showed increased proliferative responses to human inner ear homogenate by peripheral blood mononuclear cells from ISNHL patients [26].

Recent studies showed that 25% of IMSSNHL patients have profoundly elevated concentrations of T cells capable of producing IFN-γ in recall responses to a homogenate of human inner ear antigens. These results provide evidence implicating inner ear specific IFN-γ producing proinflammatory T cells in the pathogenesis of ISNHL [3]. These T cells make only one cytokine that contributes to the overall Th1 phenotypic response (IL-2, IFN-γ, TNF-α) [26].

The clinical presentation of immune-mediated inner-ear disease can be fairly variable and may include symptoms similar to those of Ménière's syndrome or clinical conditions associated with unilateral or bilateral rapidly progressive forms of sensorineural hearing loss [15-18].

Currently, evaluating the importance of an autoimmune phenomenon in the genesis of inner-ear disease is difficult because the clinical and biological criteria of autoimmune deafness have not yet been well defined. Individual diagnostic criteria (clinical presentation, laboratory studies, and response to treatment) are nonspecific but, when used in combination, can diagnose immune-mediated inner-ear disease with reasonable success.

Immunoserological assays of patients with sudden deafness and progressive hearing losses have revealed the presence of different antibodies, leading to the assumption that immunological processes may be involved. Recent investigations have demonstrated that these patients have phospholipid antibodies that can cause venous or arterial vasculopathies [10,11].

Antiphospholipid antibodies are immunoglobulins of IgG, IgM, and IgA isotypes that target phospholipid. They are thought to induce thrombosis by binding to phospholipids on the surface of platelets and the vascular endothelium. This binding complex is characterized by decreased prostacyclin production by endothelial cells, increased thromboxane production by platelets, and decreased protein C activation, resulting in vasoconstriction [10,11].

Although refinements in laboratory tests for specific inner ear antigens are being made, non-specific laboratory indicators of inflammatory or systemic immune disease may be useful in confirming the diagnosis: for these reasons we have decided to execute the previously listed blood tests to the beginning and the end of the treatment.

*The final reduction observed in the group A of the erythrocyte sedimentation rate, C-reactive protein and rheumatoid factor confirms the anti-inflammatory action of sodium enoxaparin in subcutaneous administration. This action is highlighted by the reduction of C3 plasmatic level (its higher level observed before the treatment, shows an activation of the first part of the complement cascade and therefore a possible inflammatory cause).*

*The normalization of erythrocyte sedimentation rate, C-reactive protein and rheumatoid factor supports the combined interaction of the drug with the immune system and inflammatory mechanisms.*

*The final decrease of the IgG and IgM plasmatic levels shows the possible role of sodium enoxaparin in the antiphospholipid syndrome in patients with immune-mediated inner ear disease.*

Hearing loss accompanies some of thyroid gland diseases especially those with hypothyroidism: some authors state it correlates with autoimmune background of certain thyroid gland disturbances. According with literature our data suggest an association between the immune-mediated disease and the thyroid blood hormones level [27].

*The final reduction of anti-tyroglobulin antibodies plasmatic levels highlight the combined anti-inflammatory and immune-modulated action of the drug.*

The pathogenesis of IMSSNHL is probably multifactorial: immune mechanisms may be the primary and triggering stimuli, whereas such risk factors as hyperlipoproteinemia or lipoprotein elevation may accelerate the progression of the disease. In IMSSNHL, the hyperviscosity is determined by the development of immune complexes; such complexes are usually caused by binding of polyclonal IgG to monoclonal IgM.

*The significant reduction of C3, C4, IgG, and IgM blood levels leads to a significant improvement of capillary blood flow and to a drop in the rheumatoid factors.*

The possible side effects are slight hemorrhaging, usually due to preexisting risk factors; thrombocytopenia; sometimes serious cutaneous necrosis near the injection site; cutaneous or systemic allergy; and increased transaminase levels [28].

The blood tests, performed at the beginning of the therapy, highlighted modifications of the single immune parameters in all the patients: the hematic alterations of the immune parameters, the positive response to the treatment in the patients treated and the specific mechanisms of action of sodium enoxaparin can support a diagnosis an immune-mediated inner ear disease, in this group of patients.

At the beginning of the treatment, our data show and high incidence of high blood values of erythrocyte sedimentation rate, C-reactive protein and rheumatoid factors. The final normalization of these three parameters highlighted their importance in the diagnosis of IMSNHL.

The literature does not report any therapeutic protocols for autoimmune sensorineural hearing loss treatment with sodium enoxaparin or other kinds of unfractionated heparin. Our decision to use enoxaparin was based both on the pathogenesis of this condition and on evaluation of the other classes of drugs currently used.

## CONCLUSIONS

There are at present no uniform criteria for diagnosing immune-mediated middle and inner-ear diseases, and evidence-based diagnostic criteria and assessment tools remain a significant challenge. Individual diagnostic criteria are non-specific but, when used in combination, can diagnose immune-mediated inner-ear disease more accurately.

The diagnosis of immune-mediated middle and inner ear disorders is ascertained by the history, clinical findings, an immunologic evaluation of the patient's serum and response to immunosuppressive medication.

Different routine immunological laboratory test batteries have been recommended to evaluate patients with suspected immune-mediated middle and inner ear disorders, but these are "disease-non-specific routine immunological laboratory tests".

Diagnosis of immune-mediated sensorineural hearing loss is still based on not sufficiently diagnostic parameters as clinical impressions and laboratory tests, the existence of a typical profile patient, including clinical course, immunological changes and the response to therapy can facilitate diagnosis.

The role of tissue-specific antibodies in the disease process is poorly defined and no pathognomonic pattern of non-specific antibodies in relation to middle and inner-ear diseases have yet been shown. However, detection of circulating autoantibodies in patients with suspected immunemediated inner-ear disease remains a valid tool in establishing the diagnosis and classifying the disease.

Limited understanding of the pathogenesis of immune mediated middle and inner ear diseases has led to the adoption of "empirical" treatments with anti-inflammatory, corticosteroid and immunosuppressive agents.

We have tested sodium enoxaparin in IMSSNHL, because of that outcome, we believe it has a very important role in the therapeutic management of this disease. Avoidance of the need for monitoring anticoagulation appears to be the major advantage of this agent over unfractionated heparins.

The low number of patients suggests further studies to confirm the first data that we obtained but, as far as we are concerned, this kind of therapy appears to give encouraging results in the treatment and diagnosis of IMSSNHL.

## REFERENCES

[1]    Karlberg, M; Halmagyi, GM; Buttner, U; Yavor RA. Sudden unilateral hearing loss with simultaneous ipsilateral posterior semicircular canal benign paroxysmal positional vertigo. *Arch Otolaryngol Head Neck Surg,* 2000, 126, 1024-9.

[2]    Mattox, DE; Simmons FB. Natural history of sudden sensorineural hearing loss. *Ann Otol Rhinol Laryngol*, 1977, 86, 463-80.

[3]   McCabe, BF. Autoimmune sensorineural hearing loss. *Ann Otol Rhinol Laryngol*, 1979, 88, 585-9.

[4]   Du, X; Mora, R; Yoo, TJ. Distribution of beta-tubolin in guinea pig inner ear. *ORL J Otorhinolaryngol Relat Spec*, 2003, 65, 7-16.

[5]   Mora, R; Dellepiane, M; Mora, F; Jankowska, B. The use of recombinant tissue-type plasminogen activator for the treatment of sudden and chronic hearing loss. *International Tinnitus Journal*, 2005, 11, 181-184.

[6]   Sakashita, T; Minowa, Y; Hachikawa, K; Kubo, T; Nakai, Y Evoked otoacustic emissions from ears with idiopathic sudden deafness. *Acta Otolaryngol*, 1991, 486, 66-72.

[7]   Dornhoffer, JL; Arenberg, JG; Arenberg, IK; Shambaugh, GE Jr. Pathophysiological mechanisms in Immune Ear Disease. *Acta Otolaryngol*, 1997, 26, 30-36.

[8]   Ryan, AF; Harris, JP; Keithley, EM. Immune-mediated hearing loss: basic mechanisms and options for therapy. *Acta Otolaryngol Suppl*, 2002, 548, 38-43.

[9]   Franklin, RD; Kutteh, WH. Effects of unfractionated and low molecular weight heparin on antiphospholipid antibody binding in vitro. *Obstet Gynecol*, 2003, 101, 455-62.

[10]  Masamoto, H; Toma, T; Sakumoto, K; Kanazawa, K. Clearance of antiphospholipid antibodies in pregnancies treated with heparin. *Obstet Gynecol*, 2001, 97, 394-398.

[11]  Ermel, LD; Marshburn, PB; Kutteh, WH. Interaction of heparin with antiphospholipid antibodies (APA) from the sera of women with recurrent pregnancy loss (RPL). *Am J Reprod Immunol*, 1995, 33, 14-20.

[12]  Kutteh, WH; Wester, R; Kutteh, CC. Multiples of the median: Alternate methods for reporting antiphospholipid antibodies in women with recurrent pregnancy loss. *Obstet Gynecol*, 1994, 84, 811-815.

[13]  Ziegler, EA; Hohlweg-Majert, B; Maurer, J; Mann, WJ. Epidemiological data of patients with sudden hearing loss: A retrospective study over a period of three years. *Laryngorhinootologie*, 2003, 82, 4-8.

[14]  Berrocal, JR; Ramirez-Camacho, R. Sudden sensorineural hearing loss: Supporting the immunologic theory. *Ann Otol Rhinol Laryngol*, 2002, 111, 989-997.

[15]  Cogan, DG. Syndrome of nonsyphilitic interstitial keratitis and vestibuloauditory symptoms. *Arch Ophthalmol*, 1945, 33, 144-149.

[16]  Weber, RS; Jenkins, HA; Coker, NJ. Sensorineural hearing loss associated with ulcerative colitis. A case report. *Arch Otolaryngol*, 1984, 110, 810-812.

[17]  Leone, CA; Feghali, JG; Linthicum, FHJ. Endolymphatic sac: Possible role in autoimmune sensorineural hearing loss. *Ann Otol Rhinol Laryngol*, 1984, 93, 208-209.

[18]  Veldman, J. Immune-mediated sensorineural hearing loss. *Auris Nasus Larynx*, 1998, 25, 309-17.

[19]  Schuknecht, HF. Ear pathology in autoimmune disease. *Adv Otorhinolaryngol*, 1991, 46, 50-70.

[20]  Hoistad, DL; Schachern, PA; Paparella, MM. Autoimmune sensorineural hearing loss : a human temporal bone study. *Am J Otolaryngol*, 1998, 19, 33-9.

[21]  Soliman AM; Zanetti F. Improvements of a method for testing antibodies in sensorineural hearing loss. *Adv Otorhinolaryngol*, 1988, 39, 13-7.

[22]  Suzuki, M; Harris, JP. Expression of intercellular adhesion molecule-1 during inner ear inflammation. *Ann Otol Rhinol Laryngol*, 1995, 104, 69-75.

[23] Keithley, EM; Woolf, NK; Harris, JP. Development of morphological and physiological change in the cochlea induced by cytomegalovirus. *Laryngoscope,* 1989, 99, 409-14.

[24] Baek, MJ; Park, HM; Johnson, JM; Altuntas, CZ; Jane-wit, D; Jaini, R; Solares, CA; Thomas, DM; Ball, EJ; Robertson, NG; Morton, CC; Hughes, GB; Tuohy, VK. Increased frequencies of cochlin-Specific T Cells in patients with autoimmune sensorineural hearing loss. *The Journal of Immunology*, 2006, 177, 4203-4210.

[25] Keles, E; Godekmerdan, A; Kalidag, T; Kaygusuz, I; Yalcin, S; Alpay, C; Aral, M. Ménière's disease and allergy:allergens and cytokines. *The journal of laryngology & Otology*, 2004, 118, 688-693.

[26] Harris, JP; Sharp, PA. Inner ear autoantibodies in patients with rapidly progressive sensorineural hearing loss. *Laryngoscope*, 1990, 100, 319-25.

[27] Gawron, W; Pospiech, L; Noczynska, A; Klempous, J. Two cases of hearing loss following Hashimoto disease. *Wiad Lek*, 2002, 55, 478-82.

[28] Depasse F. & Samama M.M. (2000). Heparin-induced thrombocytopenia. *Ann Biol Clin (Paris)*, 58, 317-26.

In: Deafness, Hearing Loss and the Auditory System          ISBN: 978-1-60741-259-5
Editors: D. Fiedler and R. Krause, pp.291-300          ©2010 Nova Science Publishers, Inc.

*Chapter 13*

# MOLECULAR SCREENING OF DEAFNESS IN POPULATIONS AND PATIENTS WITH NONSYNDROMIC CONGENITAL DEAFNESS FROM THE VOLGA-URAL REGION OF RUSSIA

*Lilya U. Dzhemileva*[*], *Irina M. Khidiyatova*
*and Elza K. Khusnutdinova*

Institute of Biochemistry and Genetics Ufa Scientific Center Russian Academy of
Science, Russia, Ufa, 450054, Prospect Octyabrya 71.

## ABSTRACT

We studied the molecular basis of NSHL in the Volga-Ural region. The Volga–Ural region of Russia is of particular interest, because its ethnic populations mostly belong to the Turkic, Finno-Ugric, and Slavonic linguistic groups and have complex ethnogenesis and combine the Caucasian and Mongoloid components in various proportions. A total number of 100 patients of Tatars, Russian or mixed ethnicity and 768 population samples were analyzed by PCR-SSCP followed by direct sequencing of the *GJB2* gene. The *GJB6* gene deletion and the common non-syndromic deafness-causing mitochondrial mutations were also tested when appropriate. The 35delG mutation was predominant among patients from Volga-Ural region. Mutation 312del14 in *GJB2* gene is the second most frequent cause of non-syndromic hearing impairment in the Volgo-Ural region.

Our data testify to the founder effect and suggest an eastward distribution of 35delG, since its frequency in Finno-Ugric populations gradually decreases from Estonia to Komi. The question whether the Volga-Ural region could be one of the founder sources for the 235delC and 167delT mutations, widespread in Asia and Israel community, is open. Also, the 312del14 mutation in *GJB2* is the second most frequent cause of non-syndromic hearing impairment in the Volga-Ural region.

**Keywords:** Turkic, Finno-Ugric, and Slavonic linguistic groups, the Volga-Ural region, profound prelingual deafness, GJB2, GJB6.

---

[*] Corresponding author: +73472356088 (tel), +73472356088 (fax), e-mail Dzhemilev@anrb.ru

# INTRODUCTION

Hearing impairment is one of the most common disorders of sensorineural function and is an economically and socially important cause of human morbidity. The incidence of profound prelingual deafness is about one per 1,000 at birth and includes many known genetic and environmental causes. In most cases, hearing loss can be caused by environmental factors, including perinatal infection, acoustic or cerebral trauma affecting the cochlea, or ototoxic drugs such as aminoglycoside antibiotics [1]. It can be genetic, resulting from a mutation in a single gene (monogenic forms) or from a combination of mutations in different genes and environmental factors (multifactor forms). However, single-gene mutations can lead to hearing loss. In all these cases, hearing loss is a monogenic disorder with an autosomal dominant, autosomal recessive, X-linked, or mitochondrial mode of inheritance. These monogenic forms of hearing loss can be syndromic (characterized by hearing loss in combination with other abnormalities) or nonsyndromic (with hearing loss only) [2]. Approximately 50 percent of cases are due to monogenic forms of hearing loss; perinatal factors and infantile infections or traumas are responsible for the second half [3].

Mutations in the *GJB2* and *GJB6* genes for DFNB1 (13q12) are the most frequent cause of monogenic hearing loss, they are responsible for about half of all cases of autosomal recessive prelingual hearing loss [4].

More than 100 different mutations in *GJB2* have been identified in patients with non-syndromic deafness and a significant difference in the frequency and distribution of the mutations has been observed in different populations [http://www.iro.es/cx26deaf.html]. Most interestingly, a single *GJB2* gene mutation, 35delG, accounts for up to 70% of Northern and Southern European, as well as American, Caucasian populations, with a carrier frequency ranging from 1.3% to 2.8% [5 - 12]. Another *GJB2* gene mutation, 167delT, accounts for 40% of the pathologic alleles in the Jewish deaf population [13] and has a 4% carrier frequency among Ashkenazi Jews [14]. Both the 35delG and 167delT mutations are absent or exceptionally low in some Asian populations, in which another mutation 235delC, is the most prevalent; this mutation accounts for up to 80% of pathogenic *GJB2* alleles among Japanese [15], Koreans [16], and Chinese [17], with carrier rates ranging from 1.0% to 1.3%. Interestingly, 235delC has not been detected in South Asian populations from India, Pakistan, Bangladesh, and Sri Lanka, were W24X and W77X the *GJB2* mutations are prevalent [17, 18]. Recent investigations have shown that heterozygous mutations in *GJB2* compound with Δ(GJB6-D13S1830) GJB6 gene mutation is a subset of patients with nonsyndromic hearing loss. Δ(GJB6-D13S1830) was identified in 66% of affected individuals (originating from Spain and Cuba) carrying a *GJB2* mutation on one allele only [19].

The Volga–Ural region of Russia, which is located at the boundary between Europe and Asia, is of particular interest, because its ethnic populations mostly belong to the Turkic, Finno-Ugric, and Slavonic linguistic groups and have complex ethnogenesis and specific features of the gene pool and genetic structure; and combine the Caucasian and Mongoloid components in various proportions. To optimize the DNA diagnostics of non-syndromic recessive deafness in the Volga-Ural region of Russia, it is necessary to analyze *GJB2* and *GJB6* mutations in patients from various ethnic groups.

# MOLECULAR ASPECTS OF IN PATIENTS WITH NON-SYNDROMIC RECESSIVE DEAFNESS AND IN ETHNIC GROUPS OF THE VOLGA–URAL REGION

Here we report the results of the study based on patients presenting mainly prelingual deafness, with the mutation analysis of the *GJB2* gene and screening of the GJB6-D13S1830 deletion involved in inherited nonsyndromic sensorineural deafness. Moreover, the *GJB2* gene screening was performed in 768 unrelated control subjects of different ethnic origin.

The aim of this work was to study the 35delG, 167delT, 235delC *GJB2* gene mutations and Δ(GJB6-D13S1830) mutation frequencies in patients with non-syndromic recessive deafness and in ethnic populations of the Volga–Ural region. We report the spectrum of *GJB2* and *GJB6* mutations among 100 unrelated patients of different ethnic affiliation (Russians, n=38; Tatars, n=32; Bashkirs, n=5; mixed and other ethnicity, n=25) with non-syndromic sensorineural hearing loss in the Volga-Ural region. To be included in this study, families have to meet the following criteria: 1) hearing loss confirmed by audiologic testing; 2) hearing loss in the absence of other clinical features; 3) a pedigree structure consistent with autosomal recessive and autosomal dominant inheritance; 4) both parents with normal hearing; and 5) two or more affected family members. Pure-tone audiometry was done in a sound chamber. Assessment of age at onset, severity and pattern of hearing loss by pure-tone audiometry, tympanometry, auditory brainstem response and transient evoked otoacoustic emissions were performed according to the recommendations of the European Workgroup on Genetics of Hearing Impairment [The European Concerted Action Project on Genetic Hearing Impairment, http://hear.unife.it].

We also analyzed 240 Bashkirs of four ethnogeographic groups, 96 Tatars, 100 Chuvashes, 80 Udmurts, 80 Mordvinians, 80 Komi-Permyaks, and 92 Russians. All population DNA were sampled in the rural indigenous populations of the Volga–Ural region. 768 unrelated subjects with no familial history of hearing problems were used as controls. All DNA samples were obtained from the populations living in the Volga-Ural region. Subjects were classified by the place of the residence. All DNA samples studied were anonymized.

**Table 1. Oligonucleotides primers were used for sequencing.**

| Name of primer | DNA sequence | References |
|---|---|---|
| 35delG I | ctt ttc cag agc aaa ccg ccc | [21] |
| 35delG II | tgc tgg tgg agt gtt tgt tca c | |
| 167delT I | atg agc agg ccg act ttg tct g | This oligonucleotides are created with the help of computer program Primer select 5.05 (1999-2002) |
| 167delT II | gtg gga gat ggg gaa gta gtg a | |
| 235delC I | acg atc act act tcc cca tct c | |
| 235delC II | act agg agc gct ggc gtg gac | |
| Δ(GJB6-D13S1830) I | tat tgg ata ctt gaa tct gct g | |
| Δ(GJB6-D13S1830) II | tgc atc acc tca cat agg tta | |

**Table 2. Different mutations identified among deaf patients from the Volga-Ural region of Russia**

| Ethnic affilation | Affected subjects (n=100) | 35delG/ 35delG | 35delG/+[1] | 35delG/ 167delT | 35delG/ 235delC | 167delT/+ | 235delC/+ | 312del14/312del14 | 312del14/+ | +/+ |
|---|---|---|---|---|---|---|---|---|---|---|
| Russians | 38 | 18 | 2 | 2 | - | - | - | - | 2 | 14 |
| Tatars | 33 | 8 | 7 | 1 | 1 | 1 | 1 | 2 | - | 12 |
| Bashkirs | 5 | - | - | - | - | - | - | - | - | 5 |
| Mixed ethnicity | | | | | | | | | | |
| Russians/Tatars | 13 | 3 | 1 | 1 | - | - | - | - | 1 | 7 |
| Belarussians/Tatars | 1 | 1 | - | - | - | - | - | - | - | - |
| Russians/Chuvashes | 2 | 1 | - | - | - | - | - | - | - | 1 |
| Mordvinians/Tatars | 1 | - | 1 | - | - | - | - | - | - | - |
| Bashkirs/Tatars | 1 | - | 1 | - | - | - | - | - | - | - |
| Other ethnicity | | | | | | | | | | |
| Ukrainians | 4 | 3 | 1 | - | - | - | - | - | - | - |
| Armenians | 1 | 1 | - | - | - | - | - | - | - | - |
| Chuvashes | 1 | - | - | - | - | - | - | - | - | 1 |
| Total | 100 | 35 | 13 | 4 | 1 | 1 | 1 | 2 | 3 | 40 |

Genomic DNA was isolated from 8 ml of peripheral blood by the standard protocol [5]. The coding exons of the *GJB2* and *GJB6* genes were divided into several fragments, obtained by polymerase chain reaction (PCR) for 35delG, 167delT, 235delC and Δ(GJB6-D13S1830) mutations screening.

We performed direct sequence analyses (ABI PRISM 310 (Applied Biosystems)) to reveal other different mutations in the *GJB2* gene.

Proportion, chi-square and Fisher's exact test were used to test differences between groups. All p-values were taken to be significant at <0.05. When observed or expected values were below 5, Fisher exact test was performed.

Table 2 summarizes the mutations observed in this study. Analysis of *GJB2* gene showed four mutations, segregated with the hearing loss phenotype and genotype, in a total of 100 affected unrelated subjects.

Herein, four different frequent mutations were observed (Table 2), with mutation 35delG accounting for 44% of *GJB2* alleles. Thirteen of 53 patients (24.5%) had at least one 35delG allele and 40 (75%) were 35delG homozygous. We also identified two types of compound heterozygosis in four unrelated families: del167T/del35G (7.5 % of all 35delG homozygotes patients) and del235C/del35G (3% of all patients). This high frequency of 35delG mutation of the *GJB2* gene could be attributed to the gene drift/founder effect in a certain population. The 35delG mutation of the *GJB2* gene is responsible for deafness in 53% (20 out of 38) of the

---

[1] "+" denotes that no GJB2 gene mutations were detected

independent Russian families tested and the it is carried by 55% of the Russian alleles. Three common sequence changes 312del14, del167T and 235delC, which are pathological, were also found among deaf patients.

The 312del14 mutation of the *GJB2* gene accounts for up to 4% of pathogenic *GJB2* alleles among patients with nonsyndromic hearing impairment from The Volgo-Ural region. Segregation of the *GJB2* gene 312del14 mutation with the disease is confirmed in the families by SSCP analysis [20].

The screening of five known mitochondrial mutations (A1555G, 7445A>G, 7472insC, 7510T>C, 7511T>C) of the *12S rRNA* gene was performed in the *GJB2* negative patients who were compatible with a maternal inheritance of hearing impairment.

Screening of the (*GJB6-D13S1830*) and *12S rRNA* gene mitochondrial mutations 1555A>G, 7445A>G, 7472insC, 7510T>C, 7511T>C was negative in patients who had no *GJB2* mutations.

Specific *GJB2* mutations spectrum and different *GJB2* contributions for deafness were observed for seven main Volga-Ural ethnic groups studied (Table 3).

The genetic origin of deafness is suspected in more than half of the congenital deafness cases [6]. Despite being a heterogeneous disorder with many genes contributing to its pathology, a high proportion of autosomal recessive nonsyndromic sensorineural hearing loss (ARNSHL) has been shown to be linked to DFNB1, which codes *GJB2*, a gap junction protein, connexin 26. DFNB1 causes 20% of all childhood deafness and may have a carrier rate ranging from 0 % to 8 % in different populations [3]. A high number of sequence variations have been described in the *GJB2* gene and the associated pathogenic effects are not always clearly established. The prevalence of a number of mutations is known to be population specific, and therefore population specific testing should be a prerequisite step when molecular diagnosis is offered. Moreover, population studies are needed to determine the contribution of *GJB2* variants to deafness. 35delG *GJB2* gene mutation is particularly common, representing two-thirds of all Cx26 mutations in DFNB1 patients originating from various ethnic backgrounds [7]. In our early reports we studied the 35delG *GJB2* gene mutation frequency in patients with non-syndromic recessive deafness and in ethnic groups of the Volga–Ural region. So, we present our findings from the molecular diagnostic screening of the *GJB2* and *GJB6* genes over a four year period, together with a population-based study of *GJB2* variants.

Mutations were found in 59 of 100 (59%) NSHL patients and more frequently in familial (33.1%) than in sporadic cases (25.9%). Assortative mating can accelerate the genetic response to relaxed selection and it may have doubled the frequency of connexin deafness in developing countries during the past two centuries. In combination with positive selection, linguistic homogamy may also have accounted for the rapid fixation of the mutations required for the acquisition of speech 100,000 – 150,000 years ago [22]. This high frequency of 35delG mutation of the *GJB2* gene could be attributed to the gene drift/founder effects in a certain population. The high level of Cx26 mutations and the finding that separate populations carry other common mutations suggest that heterozygote advantage for 35delG exists or existed under certain circumstances. Given the widespread expression of the gene in many tissues, reduced expression may confer a selective advantage via a multitude of pathways, making it difficult to predict a selection mechanism [2].

Nance et al. proposed a hypothesis for the high frequency of DFNB1 in many large populations of the world, on the basis of an analysis of the proportion of noncomplementary marriages among the deaf during the 19th century, which suggested that the frequency of DFNB1 may have doubled in the United States during the past 200 years. These so-called noncomplementary marriages between individuals with the same type of recessive deafness are incapable of producing hearing offspring, and the square root of their frequency among deaf marriages provides an upper limit for the prevalence of the most common form of recessive deafness at that time. To explain the increase, they suggested that the combination of intense assortative mating and relaxed selection increased both the gene and the phenotype frequencies for DFNB1. The proposed model assumed that in previous millennia the genetic fitness of individuals with profound congenital deafness was very low and that genes for deafness were then in a mutational equilibrium. The introduction of sign language in Europe in the $17^{th}$ - $18^{th}$ centuries was a key event that dramatically improved the social and economic circumstances of the deaf, along with their genetic fitness. In many countries, schools for the deaf were established, contributing to the onset of intense linguistic homogamy, i.e., mate selection based on the ability to communicate in sign language [22].

Our findings correlate with earlier reported data concerning Russian subjects with hearing loss [23] and confirm the main contribution of the 35delG mutation in deafness among Caucasian populations [24]. Other mutations, identified in this study, 312del14, del167T and 235delC have been reported previously [3].

Sequence analysis of further 200 control chromosomes does not detect any deletion, suggesting that the 312del14 mutation is not variant of alleles in the general population and that it is the basis of the disease in the deaf families. The 312del14 mutation is believed to be pathological: first, because of it location and conservation and, second, because no change has been observed in a series of normal control. The molecular mechanism underlies pathogenesis of the *GJB2* gene 312del14 mutation, affects the cytoplasmic loop of connexin 26 and results in a premature termination of protein biosynthesis. So, 312del14 *GJB2* mutation in the intracellular loop also causes loss of intracellular transport: connexons are formed but ionic transport is deficient because of incorrect alignment of connexons or inability to form a functional gap junction between two connexons [10]. Also the 312del14 mutation in *GJB2* gene is the second most frequent cause of non-syndromic hearing impairment in the Volga-Ural region.

In parallel, we have performed a molecular epidemiology study on 768 blood samples and established the frequency of the *GJB2* variants in the Volga-Ural populations (Table 3). This study has revealed prevalence of the *GJB2* sequence variations among Volga-Ural region populations. *GJB2* gene contribution in deafness among deaf patients from the Volga-Ural region (46% all patient's alleles) is mainly defined by recessive mutation 35dellG. The 35delG frequency in Mordvinians and Russians were similar to those established for the populations of Southern Europe, including Spain (3%) [7], Greece (3.5%) [1], and Italy, and for the Estonian population, which has the highest known frequency of 35delG mutation [24]. Other ethnic groups of the Volga–Ural region were similar in 35delG frequency (0.02) to the North and Central European populations and to American Caucasians [11].

This mutation is specific for some European populations (German, French, Estonian) with an allelic frequency up to 30% among deaf patients and carrier frequency from 0% to 6% in normal populations and represents the most prevalent *GJB2* pathogenic mutation as it accounts for up to 80% of the pathogenic alleles in patients [24]. The Volga-Ural region shows a significantly higher carrier rate of the 35delG (1.4%), compared to the North-East part of Europe (0.9 % − 1/110 among 1,212 controls) and a lower carrier rate compared to other south European areas such as Spain (2.31 % − 1/43), Italy (3.45 % − 1/32) and Greece (3.54 % − 1/28) [24]. This situation has direct implications for genetic counseling as well as for the development of potential diagnostic kits.

We identified 167delT *GJB2* gene mutation in Chuvashes (2/100, 2%) and Komis (2/80, 2.5 %). Morell et al. (1998) found homozygosity for 167delT and compound heterozygosity for this mutation of *GJB2* and the 35delG mutation in Ashkenazi Jewish families with nonsyndromic recessive deafness [14]. In the Ashkenazi-Jewish population, the prevalence of heterozygosity for 167delT, which is rare in the general population, was 4.03%. The frequency of the 167delT mutation carriers (total 4.76%) predicted a prevalence of 1 deaf person among 1,765 persons, which may account for most cases of nonsyndromic recessive deafness in the Ashkenazi Jewish population. Conservation of the haplotype flanking the 167delT mutation suggested that this allele had a single origin, whereas multiple haplotypes with the 35delG mutation suggested that this site is a hotspot for recurrent mutations. So, the 167delT mutation is the second most common connexin 26 mutation described and has only been reported previously among the Ashkenazi Jews [13]. The ancestry of *GJB2* 167delT is more difficult to determine, because the shared haplotype carrying 167delT is common in the general population.

Recent studies have established that the 235delC mutation among East Asian populations was derived from a common ancestral founder. Yan (2003) stated that high frequency of the 235delC mutation in multiple East Asian populations suggested that it resulted from recurrent deletion at a mutation hotspot or was derived from a common ancestral founder [25]. Among East Asians, they observed significant linkage disequilibrium between 235delC and 5 linked polymorphic markers, suggesting that 235delC had derived from a common founder. The detection of this mutation only in East Asians, but not in Caucasians, and the small chromosomal interval of the shared haplotype suggested that it was an ancient mutation that had arisen after the divergence of Mongoloids and Caucasians. The finding that this mutation appears with a single haplotype argues against the possibility of recurrent mutation as an explanation for the high frequency of the allele. The 235delC mutation was screened in a total of 768 populations samples and detected in Mordvinians (carrier frequency is 0,012).

## CONCLUSION

Although a high heterogeneity of sequence variation was observed in patients, the 35delG mutation remains the most common pathogenic mutation in our region. Our data testify to the founder effect and suggest an eastward distribution of 35delG, since its frequency in Finno-Ugric populations gradually decreases from Estonia to Komi. The question whether the Volga-Ural region of Russia could be one of the founder sources for the 235delC and 167delT mutations, widespread in Asia and Israel community remains open. The 312del14 mutation in *GJB2* is the second most frequent cause of non-syndromic hearing impairment in the Volga-Ural region.

The high frequency of *GJB2* mutations among deaf patients, testing of *GJB2* among deaf children in the Volga-Ural region is worthwhile to provide special services at an early age. Furthermore, unnecessary invasive follow-up could be avoided, since *GJB2* mutations are not associated with syndromic hearing loss or with inner ear malformations [1].

Mutations in *GJB2* account for a large percentage of hearing loss in the Volga-Ural populations, making *GJB2* of primary importance in diagnostic and research program for understanding genetics of deafness in our region.

**Table 3. Frequency of the *GJB2* sequence variations among population of Volga-Ural region[5].**

| Population of Volga-Ural region | N | Number of chromosomes | del35G | | del167T | | del235C | |
|---|---|---|---|---|---|---|---|---|
| | | | carrier frequency | alleles frequency | carrier frequency | alleles frequency | carrier frequency | alleles frequency |
| Bashkirs | 240 | 480 | 0<br>0<br>(0-0.015) | 0<br>0<br>(0-0.007) | 0<br>0<br>(0-0.015) | 0<br>0<br>(0-0.007) | 0<br>0<br>(0-0.015) | 0<br>0<br>(0-0.007) |
| Tatars | 96 | 192 | 1<br>.010<br>(0.000264 – 0.05667) | 1<br>0.0052<br>(0.000132 – 0.02867) | 0<br>0<br>(0-0.030) | 0<br>0<br>(0-0.019) | 0<br>0<br>(0-0.030) | 0<br>0<br>(0-0.019) |
| Russians | 92 | 184 | 2<br>0.021<br>(0.002615 -0.075533) | 2<br>0.0104<br>(0.001264 – 0.03712) | 0<br>0<br>(0-0.039) | 0<br>0<br>(0-0.019) | 0<br>0<br>(0-0.039) | 0<br>0<br>(0-0.019) |
| Chuvash | 100 | 200 | 0<br>0<br>(0-0.036) | 0<br>0<br>(0-0.018) | 2<br>.020<br>(0.002431 - 0.07038) | 2<br>0.0100<br>(0.001213 – 0.03565) | 0<br>0<br>(0-0.036) | 0<br>0<br>(0-0.018) |
| Mordvinians | 80 | 160 | 5<br>0.062<br>(0.020603 -0.139857) | 5<br>0.0313<br>(0.010223 – 0.07141) | 0<br>0<br>(0 – 0.04) | 0<br>0<br>(0 – 0.022) | 1<br>.012<br>(0.000316-0.06768) | 1<br>0.0063<br>(0.00015 – 0.03432) |
| Komi | 80 | 160 | 0<br>0<br>(0 – 0.040) | 0<br>0<br>(0 – 0.022) | 2<br>.025<br>(0,003042 - 0,08740) | 2<br>0,0125<br>(0,001517 - 0,04442) | 0<br>0<br>(0 – 0.04) | 0<br>0<br>(0 – 0.022) |
| Udmurts | 80 | 160 | 3<br>.037<br>(0.007801 - 0.10570) | 3<br>0.0188<br>(0.003884 – 0.05381) | 0<br>0<br>(0 – 0.04) | 0<br>0<br>(0 – 0.022) | 0<br>0<br>(0 – 0.04) | 0<br>0<br>(0 – 0.022) |

---

[5] Number of unrelated chromosomes tested frequency (95% confidence interval)

# REFERENCES

[1]     Petersen, M; Willems, P. Non-syndromic, autosomal-recessive deafness. *Clin Genet,* 2006, 69, 371-392.

[2]     Walter, EN. The genetic of deafness. *Ment Retard,* 2003, 9, 109-119.

[3]     Rothrock, CR; Murgia, A; Sartorato, EL. et al. Connexin 26 35delG does not represent a mutational hotspot. *Hum. Genet,* 2003, 113, 18-23.

[4]     del Castillo, I; Villamar, M; Moreno-Pelayo, M. et al. A Deletion involving the connexin 30 gene in nonsyndromic hearing impairment. *NEJM* 2002, 346, 243-249.

[5]     Lucotte, G; Mercier, G. Meta-analysis of GJB2 mutation 35delG frequencies in Europe. *Genet Test,* 2001, 5, 2, 149-152.

[6]     Morton, NE. Genetic epidemiology of hearing impairment. *Ann N Y Acad Sci,* 2000, 630, 16-31.

[7]     Estivill, X; Fortina, P; Surrey, S; Rabionet, R. et al. Connexin – 26 mutations in sporadic and inherited sensorineural deafness. *Lancet,* 1998, 351, 394-398.

[8]     Goodenough, DA; Goliger, JA; Paul, DL. Connexins, connexons and intracellular communication. *Ann Rev Biochem,* 1996, 65, 475-502.

[9]     Van Camp, G; Smith, RH. [Hereditary hearing loss homepage] 2004: http://dnalab-www.uia.ac.be/dnalabhhhh/.

[10]    Bruzzone, R; White, TV; Scherer, SS; Fishbeck, KH; Paul, DL. Null mutation of connexin 32 in patients X-linked dominated Charcot-Mari-Tooth disease. *Neuron,* 1994, 135, 1253-1260.

[11]    Gasparini, P; Rabionet, R; Barbujani, G. et al. High carrier frequency of the 35delG deafness mutation in European populations. *Eur J Hum Genet,* 2000, 8, 19-23.

[12]    Green, GE; Scott, DA; McDonald, JM. et al. Carrier rates in the midwestern United States for GJB2 mutations causing inherited deafness. *JAMA,* 1999, 281, 2211-2216.

[13]    Sobe, T; Vreugde, S; Shahin, H. et al. The prevalence and expression of inherited connexin 26 mutations associated with nonsyndromic hearing loss in the Israeli population. *Hum Genet,* 2000, 106, 50-57.

[14]    Morell, RJ; Kim, HJ; Hood, LJ. et al. Mutations in the connexin 26 gene (GJB2) among Ashkenazi Jews with nonsyndromic recessive deafness. *N Engl J Med,* 1998, 339, 1500-1505.

[15]    Kudo, T; Ikeda, K; Kure, S. Novel mutations in the connexin 26 gene (GJB2) responsible for childhood deafness in the Japanese population. *Am J Med Genet,* 2000, 90, 141-145.

[16]    Park, HJ; Hahn, SH; Chun, YM. et al. Connexin26 mutations associated with nonsyndromic hearing loss. *Laryngoscope,* 2000, 110, 1535 -1538.

[17]    Dai, P ; Yu, F ; Han, B. et al. GJB2 mutation spectrum in 2,063 Chinese patients with nonsyndromic hearing impairment. *J Transl Med,* 2009, 7, 26 - 29.

[18]    Richard, S; Kelsell, DP; Sirimana, T. et al. Recurrent mutations in the deafness gene GJB2 (connexin 26) in British Asian Families. *J Med Genet,* 2001, 38, 530-533.

[19]    del Castillo, I; Villamar, M; Moreno-Pelayo, MA. et al.. A deletion involving the connexin 30 gene in nonsyndromic hearing impairment. *New Engl J Med,* 2002, 346, 243-249.

[20] Orita, M; Iwahana, H; Kanazawa, H. et al. Detection of polymorphism of human DNA by gel electrophoresis as single cell conformation polymorphism. *Proc Natl Acad Sci,* 1989, 86, 2766-2770.

[21] Kelsell, DP; Dunlop, J; Stevens, HP. et al. Connexin 26 gene mutations in hereditary non-syndromic sensorineural deafness. *Nature,* 1997, 387, 80-83.

[22] Nance, WE; Kearsey, M J. Relevance of connexin deafness (DFNB1) to human evolution. *Am J Hum Genet,* 2004, 74, 1081-1087.

[23] Anichkina, A; Kulenich, T; Zinchenko, S. et al. On the origin and frequency of the 35delG allele in GJB2-linked deafness in Europe. *Eur J Hum Genet,* 2001, 9(2),151.

[24] Gasparini, P; Rabionet, R; Barbujani, G. et al. High carrier frequency of the 35delG deafness mutation in European populations. *Genetic Analysis Consortium of GJB2 35delG. Eur J Hum Genet,* 2000, 8(1), 19-23.

[25] Yan, D; Park, HJ ; Ouyang, XM ; et al. Evidence of a founder effect for the 235delC mutation of GJB2 (connexin 26) in east Asians. *Hum Genet,* 2003, 114(1), 44-50.

[26] Morell, RJ; Kim, HJ; Hood, LJ. et al. Mutations in the connexin 26 gene (GJB2) among Ashkenazi Jews with nonsyndromic recessive deafness. *New Eng J Med,* 1998, 339, 1500-1505.

In: Deafness, Hearing Loss and the Auditory System
Editors: D. Fiedler and R. Krause, pp.301-311

ISBN: 978-1-60741-259-5
©2010 Nova Science Publishers, Inc.

*Chapter 14*

# SIGNS OF BINAURAL PROCESSING WITH BILATERAL COCHLEAR IMPLANTS IN THE CASE OF SOMEONE WITH MORE THAN 50 YEARS OF UNILATERAL DEAFNESS

*Celene McNeill[1,2*], William Noble[3,4] and Anna O'Brien[5]*

[1]Healthy Hearing & Balance Care.
[2]Macquarie University, Australia.
[3]University of New England, Australia.
[4]University of Iowa.
[5]National Acoustic Laboratories, Australia.

## ABSTRACT

A case is presented of a 70-year-old man with a profound sensorineural hearing loss in the right ear since childhood and who developed sudden severe hearing loss in the left ear at age 63. Eventually, after he received cochlear implants in both ears, he started to present behavioural auditory processing skills associated with binaural hearing, such as improved ability understanding speech in the presence of background noise, and sound localization. Responsiveness and outcomes were measured using cortical auditory evoked potentials, speech perception in noise, sound localization performance , and a self-rating questionnaire. The results suggest that even after more than 50 years of unilateral deafness it is possible to develop binaural interaction and sound localization.

## INTRODUCTION

Plasticity of the auditory brain has been of increasing interest, especially since the advent of cochlear implants. Pre-lingually deaf children have responded well to electric auditory stimulation and the earlier the intervention the more their auditory processing skills are

* Corresponding author: 1204/1 Newland St, Bondi Junction NSW, Australia 2026, E-mail: cmcneill@tpg.com.au

similar to those of normal hearing children. Adults with acquired profound hearing loss also present very good outcomes but these have been reported to correlate negatively with duration of deafness and absence of previous auditory stimulation (Tyler and Summerfield, 1996). Adults with long-term deafness have been considered less likely to develop good auditory outcomes with cochlear implantation. However, outcomes of electric stimulation in long-term deafness have not been widely explored.

The present study is of a 70 year-old male, profoundly deaf in the right ear since childhood. He had experienced the common problems associated with a unilateral hearing loss such as head shadow effects, difficulty understanding speech in noise and inability to localize sounds. At the age of 63 he developed a sudden severe sensorineural hearing loss in his left ear and a hearing aid was fitted, with limited success. Six months later he received a cochlear implant in the right ear and retained a hearing aid in the left ear. After three years he stopped wearing the hearing aid for lack of perceived benefit and received an implant in that ear. Two years following constant bilateral electric stimulation he began showing signs of binaural function.

Unilateral hearing loss is known to alter neuronal activation and binaural interactions in the auditory pathways. Khosla et al. (2003) found reduction in ipsilateral-contralateral amplitude differences for N1-P2 by measuring cortical auditory evoked potential (CAEP) in patients with profound left ear deafness. This finding indicates reorganisation in the auditory cortex in unilateral left deafness, with cortical activation increasing in the left hemisphere. In contrast, patients with unilateral right deafness have not shown evidence of reduced ipsilateral-contralateral amplitude differences. This suggests there is less compensatory plasticity increase in activation of the left hemisphere with deafness in the right ear alone.

This case study is of a 70 year-old male (P.M.) with a profound sensorineural hearing loss in the right ear since childhood and a later onset fluctuating moderate-severe sensorineural hearing loss in the left ear. The duration of profound hearing loss in the right ear was longer than 50 years and was attributed to mumps in early childhood. P.M. first became aware of his profound hearing loss in the right ear at school when he was 8 years old. In 2001 he had a sudden hearing loss in the left ear, which was diagnosed as secondary endolymphatic hydrops. Computerized tomography scans of the temporal bones revealed an asymmetry in size of the cochlear aqueducts, the left being larger than the right.

# TEST METHODS, MEASURES AND RESULTS

## Speech Perception and Auditory Evoked Potentials

P.M. was referred to the audiologist for hearing aid assessment after the episode of sudden left hearing loss, and a hearing aid was fitted in the left ear. Hearing levels in the left ear continued to fluctuate, making it difficult to programme the hearing aid. P.M. was not considered a suitable candidate for a cochlear implant, as audiological assessment showed aided speech recognition scores of 95% with his left hearing aid in free-field using CID sentences. This result was above CI candidacy guidelines at the time, which recommend aided speech scores in quiet worse than 70% as a criterion for implantation (Dowell et al., 2003). Furthermore, the right ear had not had auditory stimulation for over 50 years, which was considered a contra-indication for implantation. In spite of this it was agreed that an implant in the right ear would be attempted, as there was "nothing to lose".

P.M's CAEP with the CI in the right ear and hearing aid in the left ear were recorded using a high frequency stimulus 6 months and 9 months after implantation to follow his cortical responses. The stimulus was selected based on previous evidence for robust cortical responses to 4 kHz tone bursts in adult CI users (Kelly et al., 2005). Changes were also expected for cortical responses in this frequency region based on previous evidence for high frequency cortical reorganisation in humans with acquired hearing loss (e.g. Dietrich et al., 2001; Thai-Van et al., 2003). The results 6 months following cochlear implantation showed auditory responses elicited via a CI even after more than 50 years of unilateral auditory deprivation. Changes in speech scores over time and differences in performance comparing left hearing aid, right implant and bimodal stimulation also reflected the CAEP results.

Speech test performance became very poor in the left ear after implantation of the right ear, but the hearing loss was fluctuating at this time and more difficult speech material was used for post-CI testing. Despite this, at nine months post-CI the CUNY speech scores indicated that bimodal listening was superior to the CI alone.

Eighteen months after implantation P.M. reported great satisfaction with the implant. He was using bimodal stimulation (CI in the right ear and hearing aid in the left ear) but reported that he was relying mostly on the CI. He was back at work and reporting significant improvement in hearing ability.

The difference in bimodal listening compared to CI or hearing aid alone was evident in the cortical responses at six and nine months post-CI (Figure 1 and 2). These show a binaural interaction effect, with different cortical responses in the bimodal condition than with either device alone. Hearing in the left ear continued to deteriorate. Speech scores with the hearing aid alone deteriorated to 20% using BKB/A in quiet, in spite of hearing aid optimisation. P.M. started to rely more and more on the right CI alone for hearing and communication. After three years of attempted bimodal hearing, and the left ear having deteriorated so greatly, P.M. had his left ear implanted in 2005.

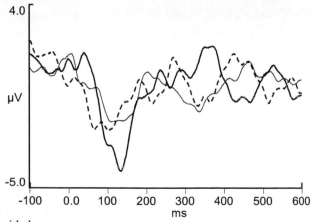

Thicker line: hearing aid alone,
Dashed line: CI alone
Thinner line: bimodal

Figure 1. CAEP 6 months post-CI.

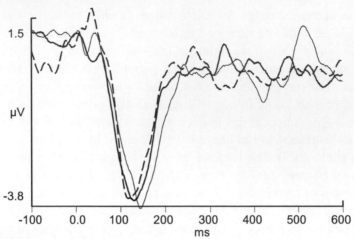

Thicker line: hearing aid alone
Dashed line: CI alone
Thinner line: bimodal

Figure 2. CAEP at 9 months post-CI.

Twelve months after receiving the second implant P.M. scored 90% with bilateral implants for BKB/A sentences presented at 65 dB SPL in babble noise at +10 dB signal-to-noise ratio.

CAEP with bilateral implants was attempted but waveforms resulted in a large artefact so that it was not possible to objectively determine whether a cortical response was present. This illustrates one of the problems of CAEP recordings in bilateral CI users (McNeill et al, 2009). The artefact usually occurs when the speech processor is activated and lasts at least as long as the duration of the stimulus (Gilley et al, 2005). Distribution of the artefact on the scalp varies according to type of CI and mode of stimulation, and although it can occur with unilateral CIs it is more prominent with bilateral stimulation. CAEP has the potential to be a fast and reliable tool for CI assessment but there are still some limitations that need to be overcome in order to make it more clinically useful. While further research is undertaken regarding the use of CAEP with bilateral CI, performance and subjective measures are relied on to assess responsiveness and outcomes.

## Auditory Localization

### Background

A primitive function of the binaural auditory system is enabling listeners to tell the whereabouts of audible events in the environment — basic to safe and effective orientation. This hearing function relies on detection and discrimination of interaural differences that vary with the location of audible events relative to the listener's position; referred to as spatial hearing (Blauert, 1983) or auditory localization (Mills, 1972). For human listeners, sounds occurring at points away from the body's midline, and containing energy up to about 1200 Hz, can be spatially distinguished on the basis of differences in phase relations between the two ears. As energy in a signal extends higher in frequency, becoming more complex, the head casts an increasingly marked acoustic shadow, which in turn yields detectable interaural differences in the overall level of the signal at any position away from the body's midline.

Cochlear implants do not allow reliable detection of low-frequency phase differences, but the shadowing effect of the head is a biophysical given, hence people with bilateral implants should be able to detect the whereabouts of complex sounds on the basis of interaural level differences. Studies confirm that bilateral CI users are indeed able to localize such sounds (Dunn et al., 2008; Litovsky et al., 2004; van Hoesel & Tyler, 2003).

### Test procedure

Localization was tested in a medium-sized anechoic chamber using a circular array (1.7-meter radius) of 20 loudspeakers at 18° intervals in the horizontal plane. P.M. sat in the centre of the array, the seat adjusted to align his interaural axis with the loudspeakers at 90° and 270° azimuth. Loudspeakers were masked with a curtain of optically opaque acoustically transparent material printed with progressively numbered marks at 10° intervals. The listener's task was to identify the number judged closest to the source, on each trial, by reference to the numbers on the curtain or a map of the loudspeaker layout. On an initial set of trials, the listener kept his head stationary during each trial, while fixating a point at 0°. In a repeat test session the same procedure was used, followed by groups of trials in which he was free to move his head.

Various signals were used in groups of 40 trials, with random presentation (each loudspeaker activated twice), and sound level at 65 dB, but jittered at random through ±3 dB. Tests were conducted under conditions of both bilateral and unilateral CI listening.

### Results

*Initial test (head stationary):* Various narrowband and broadband signals were employed in different groups of trials, as well as a speech signal (BKB/A sentence spoken by a male). Figures 3a-c show scatterplots of source-response relations listening to the speech signal with both CIs, under right CI only, and left only. When listening with only the right CI activated, as indicated in Figure 3a, all the sounds were heard as located around the rightward (90°) loudspeaker; and all were heard as coming from around the leftward (270°) loudspeaker when only the left CI was activated (Figure 3b). In the bilateral condition (Figure 3c) all signals were correctly lateralized — there are no errors across the midline. The data also show that P.M. discriminated to a certain extent among sources within the left and right hemifields, but that he attributed some rearward signals to somewhat "mirror-image" locations in front. His performance with the noise signals (only tested bilaterally) was similar to that shown in Figure 3c.

*Repeat test (head stationary then mobile):* On a second visit, testing was repeated under bilateral CI conditions using broadband noise, with the further condition added of allowing P.M. to move his head/torso while the sound was activated. A longer (2-sec.) as well as shorter (0.9-sec.) duration signal was also employed. Under stationary listening for both durations, and under mobile listening for the shorter signal the outcome was essentially the same as that shown in Figure 3c. Under mobile listening with a 2-sec. signal, there were signs that the front-rear signals were resolved to their correct regions (Figure 4).

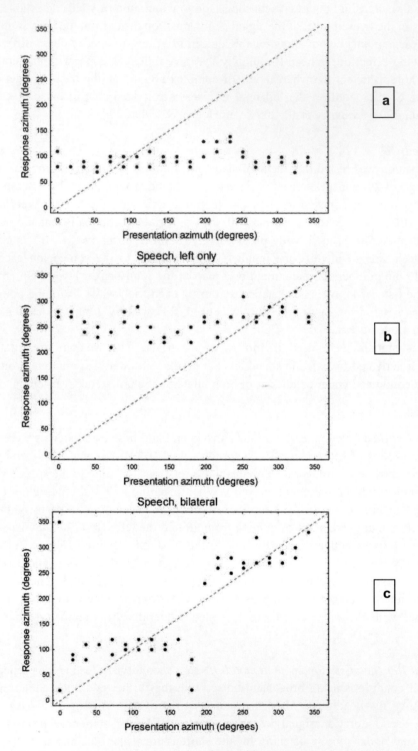

Figure 3. Localization response patterns for male speech with a) right CI only, b) left CI only and c) bilateral CIs.

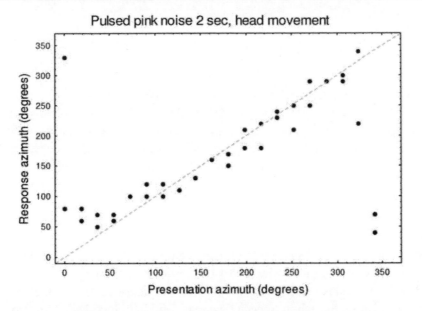

Figure 4. Localisation response pattern for 2 second broadband stimulus, head mobile.

**Table 1. P.M.'s self-ratings on ten SSQ subscales compared with the averages of 36 bilateral CI patients; right-hand column shows SSQ benefit (from second implant) scores. [In square brackets next to P.M.'s SSQ scores are scores of a case of unilateral deafness.]**

| SSQ Subscales<br>*Speech* | P.M.<br>(n = 1) | CI+CI<br>(n = 36) | P.M. benefit scores |
|---|---|---|---|
| Speech in quiet | 9.5 [7.5] | 8.1<br>(1.3) | +5.0 |
| Speech in noise | 6.5 [6.0] | 5.7<br>(1.9) | +4.0 |
| Speech in speech contexts | 8.3 [8.3] | 5.3<br>(2.2) | +3.8 |
| Multiple speech-stream processing and switching | 6.0 [4.2] | 4.1<br>(2.2) | +2.0 |
| *Spatial* | | | |
| Localization | 7.2 [0] | 5.8<br>(2.3) | +4.2 |
| Distance and Movement | 6.8 [0.5] | 5.7<br>(1.9) | +3.6 |
| *Quality* | | | |
| Sound quality and naturalness | 5.8 [9.4] | 6.9<br>(2.0) | +4.0 |
| Identification of sound and objects | 5.6 [9.4] | 6.6<br>(2.1) | +3.6 |
| Segregation of sounds | 8.7 [2.7] | 6.0<br>(2.2) | +4.3 |
| Listening effort[*] | 5.0 [2.0] | 6.1<br>(1.8) | +4.0 |

## Self-rating

### Background

Various measures have been devised to assess people's self-ratings of their abilities in the domain of hearing disabilities; a recent one is the *Speech, Spatial and Qualities of Hearing* scale (SSQ: Gatehouse & Noble, 2004). This scale was developed to cover as broad as possible a range of hearing functions and experiences, with particular attention to capacities that implicate the binaural system, including spatial hearing. The SSQ has been applied in the case of people with one versus two CIs (Noble et al., 2008; Summerfield et al., 2006), and revealed evident self-rated advantage for spatial hearing in the case of the bilateral CI profile. Thus, it is appropriate to apply the SSQ in the present case.

### Test procedure

The SSQ comprises 49 items in three main sections, addressing speech hearing, spatial hearing and other qualities of hearing. Most of the items comprising these sections can be aggregated as 10 subscales that have been labelled (Gatehouse & Akeroyd, 2006) Speech in Quiet, Speech in Noise, Speech in Speech Contexts, Multiple Speech-Stream Processing and Switching, Localization, Distance and Movement, Sound Quality and Naturalness, Identification of Sound and Objects, Segregation of Sounds, and Listening Effort. Each item is accompanied by a 0-10 scoring ruler such that zero represents complete inability with respect to the item in question, and 10 represents perfect ability.

A paper-pencil version of the SSQ was mailed to P.M, which he completed and returned. Shortly thereafter, a new version of the SSQ was sent to him with the request he complete that. This new version — SSQ(B) — is currently under development for use as a benefit measure. Respondents are asked to rate each item on a −5-to-+5 scoring ruler in terms of whether their abilities and experiences are much worse (-5), unchanged (0) or much better (+5) as a consequence of whatever intervention has been undertaken. In the case of P.M. the intervention of interest was the acquisition of a second CI. It was fully recognized (and explained to P.M.) that applying the SSQ(B) in his case was purely exploratory, given that he had been using two implants for three years, and thus may not be able to rate his abilities and experiences now against those he remembered from three years previously, when he had a CI in the right ear and a hearing aid in the left. P.M. nonetheless felt able to respond to the SSQ(B).

## RESULTS

In Table 1 are the self-ratings of P.M. on the ten subscales of the SSQ, and, for comparison, the averages (SD's in brackets) of 36 bilateral CI cases from the University of Iowa Hospital (Noble et al., 2008). P.M. rates his abilities in the speech and spatial domains higher than the Iowa sample, although it can be noted from the standard deviation values that his ratings are within the Iowa range. There is also a measure of similarity between this case and the Iowa sample in the relative ranking of the subscales (P.M.'s Speech in Noise rating might be seen as aberrant in this respect, and we return to that in the Discussion). By contrast, the ratings on three of the four qualities subscales are lower than the Iowa sample. In square brackets alongside P.M.'s SSQ subscale scores are the scores of a case of right ear unilateral deafness. This case can be seen as an approximation to how P.M. might have rated his abilities and experiences while his left ear was functioning normally. We return to the comparisons with the Iowa sample and this other individual case in the Discussion section.

On the SSQ(B) P.M. rates his abilities/experience as consistently improved under bilateral compared with unilateral listening, but not uniformly across subscales. This outcome is in agreement with the Iowa data, when unilateral and bilateral patients' scores are compared (Noble et al., 2008). That said, we reiterate that the findings using the SSQ(B) can only be regarded as indicative given the length of time since P.M. listened with only one CI.

# DISCUSSION AND CONCLUSIONS

## Performance Data

The speech test data demonstrate that P.M. is functioning almost at a normal hearing level when listening to a purely auditory signal in background noise. This highly proficient performance is echoed in his self-ratings. It can be assumed, from the CAEP observations in his earlier (bimodal) profile, that the bilateral CI condition is enabling binaural processing of speech.

The localization performance data from the initial test session, with immobile listening, demonstrate the evident contrast between unilateral and bilateral listening. There are no reliable cues to direction with only one CI activated and the sensation experienced would lead to attribution to a source more or less in line with the activated side. By contrast, interaural level differences become available with two devices active, leading to accurate lateralization and a degree of azimuthal discrimination. Because of the geometry of interaural differences it is not straightforward to distinguish sources at "mirror-image" positions behind and in front of the interaural axis. The repeat session confirmed the latter outcome for stationary listening. The condition in which the listener was free to move during signal presentation showed some resolution of front/back reversals, especially when the signal is 2-sec. rather than 1-sec. Such resolution is feasible because the change of interaural differences under head movement is in one direction when a sound is in the front hemifield, and in the opposite direction when the sound is in a "mirror-image" location to the rear.

## Self-rating Data

The particular history of the present case, namely, most of his life with normal hearing in one ear, makes comparison with typical CI patients difficult to predict. At interview, P.M. reported a lifelong involvement in stage acting and singing, which could explain his particularly high self-ratings for speech understanding. We also note a strong influence of visual input in speech understanding: On an item of the SSQ asking how he gets on when not all conversation members are in sight P.M. gave a very low rating (which pulls down his speech-in-noise average score). He also observed that he was quite conscious of the reduction in quality and identifiability of sounds since becoming reliant solely on electric stimulation (and was aware of the livelier quality of what he hears on the side that was more recently normal). These features may account for the lower Qualities ratings than found in the Iowa sample.

It is instructive to note the sharp contrasts in Spatial and certain Qualities ratings between P.M. and the case of unilateral deafness. In the latter case Spatial hearing is rated as non-existent, but naturalness and identifiability are rated very highly. These contrasts are telling as regards the substantial benefit for spatial hearing provided by bilateral implantation, whilst also indicating the loss of quality that flows from the limited patterning available by this means of connection to the audible world. Nonetheless it confirms that the provision of bilateral auditory information, despite degraded signal quality and the age of the brain, can enable cortical plasticity to take place and auditory processing skills to develop.

## References

Blauert, J. (1983). *Spatial hearing*. Cambridge, Mass.: MIT Press.

Dietrich, V., Nieschalk, M., Stoll, W., Rajan, R. & Pantev, C. (2001). Cortical reorganization in patients with high frequency cochlear hearing loss. *Hearing Research, 158,* 95-101.

Dowell, R., Hollow, R. & Winton, L. (2003). Changing selection criteria for cochlear implants – the Melbourne experience. Cochlear N95506 ISSI.

Dunn, C. C., Tyler, R. S., Oakley, S., Gantz, B. J. & Noble, W. (2008). Comparison of speech recognition and localization performance in bilateral and unilateral cochlear implant users matched on duration of deafness and age at implantation. *Ear & Hearing, 29(3),* 352-359.

Gatehouse, S. & Akeroyd, M. (2006). Two-eared listening in dynamic situations. *International Journal of Audiology, 45(Supplement 1),* S120-S124.

Gatehouse, S. & Noble, W. (2004). The Speech, Spatial and Qualities of Hearing Scale (SSQ). *International Journal of Audiology, 43(1),* 85-99.

Gilley, P. M., Sharma, A., Finley, C. C., Panch, A. S., Martin, K. & Dorman, M. (2005). Minimization of cochlear implant stimulus artefact in cortical auditory evoked potentials. *Clinical Neurophysiology, 116,* 648-657.

Kelly, A. S., Purdy, S. C. & Thorne, P. R. (2005). Electrophysiological and speech perception measures of auditory processing in experienced adult cochlear implant users. *Clinical Neurophysiology, 116,* 1235-1246.

Khosla, D., Ponton, C. W., Eggermont, J. J., Kwong, B., Dort, M. & Vasama, J. P. (2003). Differential ear effects of profound unilateral deafness on the adult human central auditory system. *Journal of the Association for Research in Otolaryngology, 4,* 235-249.

Litovsky, R. Y., Parkinson, A., Arcaroli, J., Peters, R., Lake, J., Johnstone, P., et al. (2004). Bilateral cochlear implants in adults and children. *Archives of Otolaryngology, Head and Neck Surgery, 130,* 648-655.

McNeill, C., Sharma, M. & Purdy, S. C. (2009). Are cortical auditory evoked potentials useful in the clinical assessment of adults with cochlear implants? *Cochlear Implants International, 10,* 78-84.

Mills, A. W. (1972). Auditory localization. In J. V. Tobias (Ed.), *Foundations of modern auditory theory (Vol. II,* 303-348). New York: Academic Press.

Noble, W., Tyler, R. S., Dunn, C. & Bhullar, N. (2008). Unilateral and bilateral cochlear implants and the implant-plus-hearing aid profile: Comparing self-assessed and measured abilities. *International Journal of Audiology*, *47*, 505-514.

Summerfield, A. Q., Barton, G. R., Toner, J., McAnallen, C., Proops, D., Harries, C., et al. (2006). Self-reported benefits from successive bilateral cochlear implantation in post-lingually deafened adults: randomised controlled trial. *International Journal of Audiology*, *45*, S99-S107.

Thai-Van, H., Micheyl, C., Moore, B. C. J. & Collet, L. (2003). Enhanced frequency discrimination near the hearing loss cut-off: a consequence of central auditory plasticity induced by cochlear damage? *Brain*, *126*, 2235-2245.

Tyler, R. S. & Summerfield, A. Q. (1996). Cochlear implantation: Relationships with research on auditory deprivation and acclimatization. *Ear & Hearing*, *17(3)*, 38S-50S.

van Hoesel, R. J. & Tyler, R. S. (2003). Speech perception, localization, and lateralization with bilateral cochlear implants. *Journal of the Acoustical Society of America*, *113(3)*, 1617-1630.

In: Deafness, Hearing Loss and the Auditory System
Editors: D. Fiedler and R. Krause, pp.313-322

ISBN: 978-1-60741-259-5
©2010 Nova Science Publishers, Inc.

*Chapter 15*

# CISPLATIN OTOTOXICITY: A KEY FOR THE UNDERSTANDING OF THE INNER EAR PATHOLOGY

## *José Ramón García-Berrocal*[*], *Rafael Ramírez-Camacho,*
## *José Ángel González-García and Rodrigo Martínez-Monedero*

Servicio de Otorrinolaringología. Hospital Universitario Puerta de Hierro.
Universidad Autónoma de Madrid, Spain

## ABSTRACT

Ototoxicity is defined as the tendency of certain therapeutic agents to cause functional impairment and cellular degeneration of the inner ear and of the eighth cranial nerve. Cisplatin (cis-diamminedichloroplatinum II; CDDP) is the first generation platinum-containing antitumoral drug known to be effective against a variety of solid tumors. Ototoxicity has been observed in up to 36% of patients receiving cisplatin. Risk factors for cisplatin ototoxicity include renal insufficiency, co-administration with aminoglycosides and/or radiation therapy, and increased cumulative doses. Monitoring for ototoxicity should be individualized: an audiogram (high frequencies and ultrahigh frequencies) should be obtained at the onset of therapy, before each successive dose, and with the onset of symptoms. Second generation platinum derived drugs have been developed in order to minimize the toxic effect on the inner ear.

Only 1% of intracellular platinum (Pt) is bound to nuclear DNA with the great majority of the drug available to interact with other cellular targets. The quantification of Pt inside the inner ear by quadrupole inductively coupled plasma mass spectrometry (ICP-MS) has shown the presence of Pt-biomolecules in nuclear, cytosolic and mitochondrial fractions. The Pt-biomolecules binding could play a role in ototoxicity since the complexes were different depending on the drug and represents a future outlook in the management of cisplatin ototoxiciy.

Although classically the most prominent change seen in the cochlea after cisplatin administration consists of loss of outer hair cells (OHCs), new directions in the research allowed us to provide a main role to the supporting cells (Deiter's cells) since they appeared more sensitive than outer hair cells.

[*] Corresponding author: E-mail: jrgarciab@yahoo.com

*In vitro* and *in vivo* experiments have shown that apoptotic cell death is the primary mechanism of cisplatin antitumoral action. A novel investigation has shown that cisplatin induces apoptosis in hair cells, supporting cells, spiral ganglion cells, stria vascularis cells and spiral ligament fibrocytes by the activation of caspases, evoking an intrinsic pathway of pro-apoptotic signalling. This innovative idea has facilitated the development of several strategies to prevent oxidative stress-induced apoptosis of inner ear cells that have been exposed to cisplatin. However, the loss of the population of some type of inner ear cells could be irreversible, and then it would be necessary to replace these cells. The conversion of inner ear stem cells to sensory neurons and the search of a possible common pathway of inner ear damage need to be explored and they will lead the future trends in inner ear research.

**Keywords:** Cisplatin, ototoxicity, hearing loss, apoptosis, caspases, inner ear, outer hair cells, supporting cells, ICP-MS, stem cells.

# INTRODUCTION

Ototoxicity is defined as the tendency of certain therapeutic agents to cause functional impairment and cellular degeneration of the inner ear and of the eighth cranial nerve. Cisplatin (cis-diamminedichloroplatinum II; CDDP) is still one of the cornerstone in the treatment of epithelial malignancies. Unfortunately, cisplatin damages, indiscriminately, tumour and normal cells. Thus, severe side effects arise from the lesion of various cell types in peripheral nerves, renal tubules, bone marrow and gastrointestinal tract. Ototoxicity has been observed in up to 36% of patients receiving cisplatin [1]. Cisplatin-induced ototoxicity is characterized by a cumulative, dose-related sensorineural hearing loss and tinnitus and less frequently by vestibular impairment [2,3]. Hearing loss is progressive, irreversible, bilateral and it usually affects high frequencies first and may gradually spread to lower frequencies [4]. Risk factors for cisplatin ototoxicity include renal insufficiency, co-administration with aminoglycosides and/or radiation therapy, and increased cumulative doses. Monitoring for ototoxicity should be individualized: an audiogram (high frequencies and ultrahigh frequencies) should be obtained at the onset of therapy, before each successive dose, and with the onset of symptoms. Second generation platinum derived drugs have comparable antitumor spectrum to cisplatin, they present several side effects such as myelosuppression but they induces less nephrotoxicity and ototoxicity than CDDP.

Although the ototoxic effect of cisplatin has been extensively studied, the cellular mechanisms by which cisplatin induce degeneration of the organ of Corti remains elusive. Furthermore, the cellular sites of cisplatin uptake and accumulation in the cochlea have not yet been properly identified. It is commonly accepted that binding of cisplatin to DNA results in the formation of cisplatin-DNA adducts, which produce severe distortions in the DNA double helix. This antineoplastic effect is mediated by the platination of nucleophilic centers in DNA bases, leading to intra- or inter-strand cross-linking of the bases, to abnormal base pairing or to DNA strand breakage. Cisplatin-DNA adducts may damage outer hair cells, stria vascularis, spiral ligament and spiral ganglion cells leading to ototoxicity.

## CISPLATIN OTOTOXICITY: A REAPPRAISAL OF THE CLASSIC THEORY

Although classically the most prominent change seen in the cochlea after cisplatin administration consists of loss of outer hair cells (OHCs), new directions in the research allowed us to provide a main role to the supporting cells (**Deiter's cells**) since they appeared more sensitive than outer hair cells. Supporting cells (**Deiter's cells**) appeared more sensitive than outer hair cells and the alteration of the supporting cell ultrastructure preceded detectable changes in outer hair cells [5] (**Figure 1**). Recent studies suggest that the toxic drug initially affects the supporting cells (Deiters and Hensen cells) that help to maintain the metabolic homeostasis of outer and inner hair cells, which experience structural and functional lesions when there is an impairment of their metabolism-regulating cells [5,6]. This hypothesis may justify the increase in hearing loss in animals with a long-term survival after cisplatin injection. This alteration correlates with the degeneration of the cytoplasm of the Hensen cells that was observed prior to the destruction of inner hair cells. This finding could support the theory that the exhaustion of hair cells is influenced by damage to supporting cells and suggest an active role of supporting cells in the maintenance of hair cell function and structure. Supporting cells may provide the necessary metabolic and electrolytic conditions ($K^+$ active exchange) for hair cells mechanical and bioelectrical function.

## CELLULAR ACTION: CISPLATIN INDUCES AN INTRINSIC APOPTOTIC PATHWAY INSIDE THE INNER EAR

*In vitro* and *in vivo* experiments have shown that apoptotic cell death is the primary mechanism of cisplatin toxicity [7]. In the cochlea, cisplatin has been shown to induce apoptosis in hair cells, supporting cells, spiral ganglion cells and stria vascularis cells [8] by means of activation of caspases evoking an intrinsic pathway of pro-apoptotic signalling [9] (**Figure 2**), up-regulation of the pro-apoptotic tumor suppressor gene p53, a significant increase in bax-positive cells, a decrease in bcl-2-positive cells and the release of cytochrome c [10-12]. A high accumulation of Pt-DNA adducts has been observed in the nuclei of marginal cells of the stria vascularis but not in OHCs which have been discussed as the main target of cisplatin-induced cell damage [13]. The excessive DNA platination in the marginal cells represents the earliest event in short-term cisplatin ototoxicity triggering their functional impairment and apoptotic destruction. Marginal cell damage may lead to an impaired uptake of $K^+$ from the intra-strial space as well as an impairment $K^+$ secretion into the endolymph with subsequent dysfunction and loss of hair cells. The impairment of $K^+$ recycling process that is essential to the endocochlear potential is a known toxic effect of cisplatin induced by apoptosis of type I spiral ligament fibrocytes [14] and by the direct apoptotic effect of cisplatin on the stria vascularis, responsible for the decreased cellular $Na^+$, $K^+$ ATPase and $Ca^{2+}$ ATPase activities [15]. Morphologically, edema formation in the stria vascularis was followed by severe atrophy after CDDP treatment. The majority of marginal cells affected by CDDP exhibited expression of cleaved caspase-3 indicating that caspases are involved in the process of apoptotic cell death after CDDP treatment. However, they showed expression of cleaved caspase-9 indicating that apoptosis was started by permeabilization of mitochondrial membranes.

Studies on morphologic cell changes after cisplatin injection have shown the presence of blebs in diverse regions of the apical region such as kinocilium and other marginal areas in IHC and OHC [16] (**Figure 3**). Blebs were first recognized as a hallmark of apoptosis. Thus, blebs form within 30 minutes after exposure to cisplatin administration, coinciding with channel-mediated $K^+$ and $Cl^-$ loss during "apoptotic volume decrease" (AVD) preceding mitochondrial cytochrome C release and caspase-3 activation [17]. During apoptosis caspase-3 cleaves the Rho-kinase I (ROCK I), leading to a deregulated activity of this kinase and consequently to bleb formation [18]. These morphological findings, together with the severe hearing loss found in these animals, suggest that these blebs are a manifestation of apoptosis.

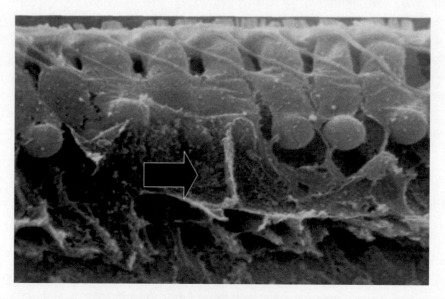

Figure 1. Organ of Corti of a guinea pig after CDDP injection showing degeneration of Deiters cells (black arrow) with outer hair cells preservation (scanning microscopy; x1500).

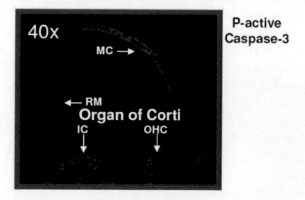

Figure 2. Immunostaining of active caspase-3 in the nuclei of inner ear cells from rats 7 days after a single dose of cisplatin (5mg/kg). MC, marginal cells of stria vascularis; RM Reissner's membrane; OHC, outer hair cells; IC, interdental cells of the spiral limbus. Magnification 400x.

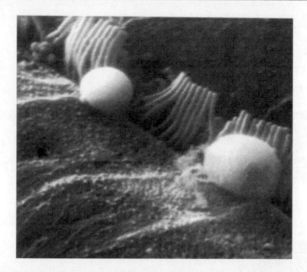

Figure 3. Scanning micrograph of the organ of Corti of a Hartley guinea pig after cisplatin treatment (5mg/kg) showing blebs emerging from the basal body of the cuticular plate in inner hair cells (x5500).

## ROLE OF PLATINUM-BIOMOLECULES AND INTRACELLULAR PLATINUM CONCENTRATION IN OTOTOXICITY

Only 1% of intracellular platinum (Pt) is bound to nuclear DNA with the great majority of the drug available to interact with other cellular targets. The quantification of Pt inside the inner ear by quadrupole inductively coupled plasma mass spectrometry (ICP-MS) has shown the presence of Pt-biomolecules in nuclear, cytosolic and mitochondrial fractions. By means of this technique, we have found a 10-fold higher deposition of Pt in inner ear than in brain, and the Pt clearance rate is faster in brain [19]. The inner ear and brain are in anatomical proximity with a common embryological origin (ectoderm) and a common vascularization. These different concentrations detected in Pt in inner ear and in brain suggest that Pt has a higher histological affinity for the structures of the organ of Corti. A revision of the proteins that are present in the inner ear but not in the brain was reported by Thalman et al [20, 21], who describes the organ of Corti proteins (OCPs), OCP1, OCP2 and oncomodulin, among others. OCP1 and OCP2 are restricted to the supporting cells of the organ of Corti and adjacent epithelia. This distribution coincides with the boundaries of the epithelial gap junction system of the cochlea, as defined by staining for connexin 26. OCP2 is diffusely distributed within the cytoplasm of the supporting cells, but is apparently absent from the nucleus [20]. Cochlear gap junction system may assist with removal of the excess $K^+$ from the hair cells and with its recirculation-via the spiral ligament-by the stria vascularis. The endolymphatic potential causes a massive $K^+$ current through the hair cells and it needs an acidification of the endolymph. The presence of an acidification system in cells bordering the scala media with a distribution similar to OCP2 suggests the role of OCP2 in pH homeostasis mechanisms [6]. Recently, the binding of Pt to biomolecules with molecular weights of 12 kDa and 25-65 kDa for inner ear samples has been demonstrated in rats after cisplatin injection [22, 23] (**Figure 4**).

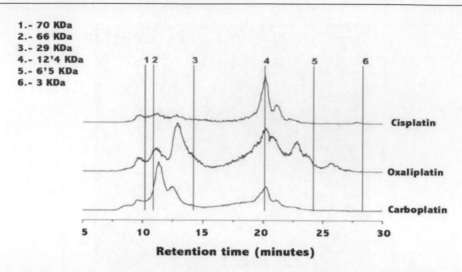

Figure 4. Chromatograms of inner ear cytosol from rats treated with cisplatin, oxaliplatin or carboplatin performed by size exclusion inductively coupled plasma mass spectrometry (SEC-ICP-MS). Molecular weight calibration markers: 1-70 kDa, 2- 66 kDa, 3- 29 kDa, 4- 12.4 kDa, 5- 6.5 kDa and 6- 3 kDa.

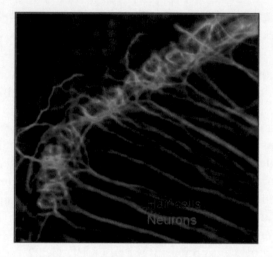

Figure 5. In vitro culture of an organ of Corti explant from a newborn mouse. The hair cells (shown in red) and the innervation of the auditory neurons (shown in green) are damaged usually in the hearing loss in humans. The regeneration of these cells and their innervation is a major goal in the search of a new therapy for the hearing loss.

The Pt-biomolecules binding could play a role in ototoxicity since the complexes were different depending on the drug and represents a future outlook in the management of cisplatin ototoxiciy.

## THERAPY STRATEGIES

Cisplatin may directly lead to the generation of reactive oxygen species (ROS) or may induce the release of reactive oxygen molecules normally sequestered within mitochondria that may trigger several mechanisms of apoptosis. ROS-mediated damage could occur as a consequence of antioxidant depletion and increased lipid peroxidation in the cochlea of rats [24]. Thus, several strategies have been suggested to prevent oxidative stress-induced apoptosis of OHCs that have been exposed to cisplatin: prevention of the formation of ROS either by binding the toxin or reversing the toxin's binding, inhibition of the lipid peroxidation, addition of exogenous free-radical scavengers and antioxidant enzymes, inhibitors of caspases and gene therapy (to upregulate antiapoptotic gene products such as Bcl-2) [12, 25]. Likewise, the administration of antioxidants could stimulate endogenous mechanisms (heat shock proteins, glutathione, adenosine A1 receptors, heme-oxygenase-1, kidney injury molecule) to prevent oxidative stress caused by cisplatin. However, protective therapy should preserve the antineoplastic efficacy of cisplatin. Unfortunately, once loss of hair or ganglion cells has been established, an irreversible hearing loss can be expected.

In mammals the sensorineural hearing loss is irreversible; underlying this loss of auditory function is the inability to replace inner ear cells by cell division and by differentiation from endogenous cells in the inner ear epithelia.

The advances in stem cell research are a new approach to inner ear regeneration in mammals. A major advance in the prospects for the use of stem cells for the replacement of inner ear cells came with the recent discovery that hair cells could be generated in vivo from embryonic stem cells, from adult inner ear stem cells and from neural stem cells [26-28}.

Loss of stem cells postnatally in the cochlea may correlate with the loss of regenerative capacity and may limit our ability to stimulate regeneration [29-31].

It may be possible to replace inner ear cells that have degenerated with the transplantation of cells that restore auditory function. In this way, the spiral ganglion neurons obtained from the cochlea of a newborn mouse reinnervated hair cells in a toxin-treated organ of Corti and expressed synaptic vesicle markers at points of contact with hair cells [32}. These findings suggest that it may be possible to replace degenerated neurons by grafting new cells into the organ of Corti.

If we use in the cell therapy stem cells as a source of transplanted cells, we can control the cell fate decisions that determine the phenotype. We can differentiate these stem cells to sensory neurons that can be grafted to the inner ear [33].

A distant future therapy for the hearing loss might be a combination of stem cell, gene therapy and drug treatment in conjunction with technical devices.

## CONCLUSION

Cisplatin is still the first-line treatment for some neoplastic entities. Its main adverse effects are ototoxicity, nephrotoxicity, bone marrow toxicity, gastrointestinal toxicity, liver toxicity and peripheral nervous system toxicity. Most of these adverse effects can be prevented and treated but inner ear damage is one of the most common reasons to discontinue chemotherapy with Pt-based compounds.

Cisplatin induces apoptosis in hair cells, supporting cells, spiral ganglion cells, stria vascularis cells and spiral ligament fibrocytes by the activation of caspases, evoking an intrinsic pathway of pro-apoptotic signalling. Several strategies have been suggested to prevent oxidative stress-induced apoptosis of OHCs that have been exposed to cisplatin. The stimulation of endogenous mechanisms to prevent oxidative stress could support the administration of antioxidants.

However, loss of hair and/or ganglion cells caused by cisplatin will induce an irreversible hearing loss. The differentiation of inner ear stem cells and the search of a possible common pathway of inner ear damage need to be explored and they will lead the future trends in inner ear research.

# REFERENCES

[1] Nagy, JL; Adelstein, DJ; Newman, CW; Rybicki, LA; Rice, TW; Lavertu, P. Cisplatin ototoxicity: the importance of baseline audiometry. *Am J Clin Oncol*, 1999, 28, 305-308.

[2] Schaefer, SD; Wright, CG; Post, JD; Frenkel, EP. Cis-platinum vestibular toxicity. *Cancer*, 1981, 47, 857-859.

[3] Anniko, M; Sobin, A. Cisplatin: evaluation of its ototoxic potential. *Am J Otolaryngol*, 1986, 7, 276-293.

[4] Waters, GS; Ahmad, M; Katsarkas, A; Stanimir, G; McKay, J. Ototoxicity due to cis-diamminedichloroplatinum in the treatment of ovarian cancer: influence of dosage and schedule of administration. *Ear Hear*, 1991, 12, 91-102.

[5] Ramírez-Camacho, R; García Berrocal, JR; Buján, J; Martin-Marero, A; Trinidad, A. Supporting cells as a target of cisplatin-induced inner ear damage: therapeutic implications. *Laryngoscope*, 2004, 114, 533-537.

[6] Ramírez-Camacho, R; García-Berrocal, JR; Trinidad, A; González-García, JA; Verdaguer, JM; Ibáñez, A; Rodríguez, A; Sanz, R. Central role of supporting cells in cochlear homeostasis and pathology. *Med Hypotheses*, 2006, 67, 550-555.

[7] Boulikas, T; Vougiouka, M. Cisplatin and platinum drugs at the molecular level. *Oncol Rep*, 2003, 10, 1663-1682.

[8] Alam, SA ; Ikeda, K ; Oshima, T ; Suzuki, M ; Kawase, T ; Kikuchi, T ; Takasaka, T. Cisplatin-induced apoptotic cell death in Mongolian gerbil cochlea. *Hear Res*, 2000, 141, 28-38.

[9] García-Berrocal, JR; Nevado, J; Ramírez-Camacho, R; Sanz, R; González-García, JA; Sánchez-Rodríguez, C; Cantos, B; España, P; Verdaguer, JM; Trinidad Cabezas, A. Antitumoral drug cisplatin induces an intrinsic apoptotic pathway inside the inner ear. *British J Pharmacol*, 2007, 116, 779-784.

[10] Devarajan, P; Savoca, M; Castaneda, MP; Parks, MS; Esteban-Cruciani, N; Kalinec, G; Kalinec, F. Cisplatin-induced apoptosis in auditory cells: role of death receptor and mitochondrial pathways. *Hear Res*, 2002, 174, 45-54.

[11] Zhang, M; Liu, W; Ding, D; Salvi, R. Pifithrin-alpha suppressers p53 and protects cochlear and vestibular hair cells from cisplatin-induced apoptosis. *Neuroscience*, 2003, 120, 191-205.

[12] Rybak, LP; Whitworth, CA; Mukherjea, D; Ramkumar, V. Mechanism of cisplatin-induced ototoxicity and prevention. *Hear Res*, 2007, 226, 157-167.

[13]  Thomas, JP; Lautermann, J; Liedert, B; Seller, F; Thomale, J. High accumulation of platinum-DNA adducts in strial marginal cells of the cochlea is an early event in cisplatin but not in carboplatin ototoxicity. *Mol Pharmacol*, 2006, 70, 23-29.

[14]  Liang, F; Schulte, BA; Qu, C; Hu, W; Shen, Z. Inhibition of the calcium and voltage-dependent big conductance potassium channel ameliorates cisplatin-induced apoptosis in spiral ligament fibrocytes of the cochlea. *Neuroscience*, 2005, 135, 263-271.

[15]  Cheng, PW; Liu, SH; Hsu, CJ; Lin-Shiau, SY. Correlation of increased activities of $Na^+$, $K^+$ ATPase and $Ca^{2+}$ ATPase with the reversal of cisplatin ototoxicity induced by D-methionine in guinea pigs. *Hear Res*, 2005, 205, 102-109.

[16]  Ramírez-Camacho, R; García-Berrocal, JR; Trinidad, A; Verdaguer, JM; Nevado, J. Blebs in inner and outer hair cells: a pathophysiological hypothesis. *J Laryngol Otol*, 2008, 10, 1-5.

[17]  Okada, Y; Maeno, E; Shimizu, T; Dezaki, K; Wang, J; Morishima, S. Receptor-mediated control of regulatory volume decrease (RVD) and apoptotic volume decrease (AVD). *J Physiol*, 2001, 532, 3-16.

[18]  Coleman, ML; Sahai, EA; Yeo, M; Bosch, M; Dewar, A; Olson, MF. Membrane blebbing during apoptosis results from caspase-mediated activation of ROCK I. *Nat Cell Biol*, 2001, 3, 339-346.

[19]  Ramírez-Camacho, R; Esteban-Fernández, D; Verdaguer, JM; Gómez Gómez, MM; Trinidad, A; García-Berrocal, JR; Palacios Corvillo, MA. Cisplatin-induced hearing loss does not correlate with intracellular platinum concentration. *Acta Otolaryngol*, 2008, 128, 505-509.

[20]  Thalmann, R; Henzl, MT; Thalmann, I. Specific proteins of the organ of Corti. *Acta Otolaryngol*, 1997, 117, 265-268.

[21]  Thalmann, R; Henzl, MT; Killick, R; Ignatova, EG; Thalmann, I. Toward an understanding of cochlear homeostasis: the impact of location and the role of OCP1 and OCP2. *Acta Otolaryngol*, 2003, 123, 203-208.

[22]  Esteban-Fernandez, D; Gómez-Gómez, MM; Cañas, B; Verdaguer, JM; Ramírez, R; Palacios, MA. Speciation analysis of platinum antitumoral drugs in impacted tissues. *Talanta*, 2007, 72, 768-773.

[23]  Esteban Fernández, D; Verdaguer, JM; Ramírez-Camacho, R; Palacios, MA; Gómez-Gómez, MM. Accumulation, fractionation and analysis of platinum in toxicologically affected tissues after cisplatin, oxaliplatin and carboplatin administration. *J Anal Toxicol*, 2008, 32, 1-7.

[24]  Rybak, LP; Husain, K; Whitworth, C; Somani, SM. Dose dependent protection by lipoic acid against cisplatin-induced ototoxicity in rats: antioxidant defense system. *Toxicol Sciences*, 1999, 47, 195-202.

[25]  Lopez-Gonzalez, MA; Guerrero, JM; Rojas, F; Delgado, F. Ototoxicity caused by cisplatin is ameliorated by melatonin and other antioxidants. *J Pineal Res*, 2000, 28, 73-80.

[26]  Li, H; Liu, H; Heller, S. Pluripotent stem cells from the adult mouse inner ear. *Nat Med.*, 2003, 9, 1293-9.

[27]  Li, H; Roblin, G; Liu, H; Heller, S. Generation of hair cells by stepwise differentiation of embryonic stem cells. *Proc Natl Acad Sci*, USA, 100, 13495-500.

[28]  Tateya, I. Fate of neural stem cells grafted into injured inner ears of mice. *Neuroreport*, 14, 1677-81.

[29]  Oshima, K; Grimm, CM; Corrales, CE; Senn, P; Martinez Monedero, R; Geleoc, GS; et al. Differential distribution of stem cells in the auditory and vestibular organs of the inner ear. *J Assoc Res Otolaryngol.*, 2007, 8, 18-31.

[30]  Martinez-Monedero, R; Edge, AS. Stem cells for the replacement of inner ear neurons and hair cells. *Int J Dev Biol.*, 2007, 51, 655-61.

[31]  Martinez-Monedero, R; Oshima, K; Heller, S; Edge, AS. The potential role of endogenous stem cells in regeneration of the inner ear. *Hear Res.*, 2007 May, 227, 48-52.

[32]  Martinez-Monedero, R; Corrales, CE; Cuajungco, MP; Heller, S; Edge, AS. Reinnervation of hair cells by auditory neurons after selective removal of spiral ganglion neurons. *J Neurobiol.*, 2006, 66, 319-31.

[33]  Martinez-Monedero, R; Yi, E; Oshima, K; Glowatzki, E; Edge, AS. Differentiation of inner ear stem cells to functional sensory neurons. *Dev Neurobiol.*, 2008 Apr, 68, 669-84.

In: Deafness, Hearing Loss and the Auditory System       ISBN: 978-1-60741-259-5
Editors: D. Fiedler and R. Krause, pp.323-332       ©2010 Nova Science Publishers, Inc.

*Chapter 16*

# MODELING THE PERCEPTUAL MASKING PROPERTIES OF THE HUMAN AUDITORY SYSTEM USING NEURAL NETWORKS

## *Hossein L. Najafi*[*]

Department of Computer Science, University of Wisconsin, River Falls,
River Falls, Wisconsin, USA

## ABSTRACT

Modeling of the perceptual masking properties of the Human Auditory System is investigated. An artificial neural network is trained to model the perceptual masking map of the human auditory system. Successful application of the model to data hiding is demonstrated.

**Keywords**: Neural Networks, Perceptual Map, Perceptual Coding, Back Propagation, Data Hiding.

## I. INTRODUCTION

The human auditory system is known to have physiological mechanisms to differentiate and mask noise-like data when presented relative to tone-like signals such as music and speech [1] [2]. This masking mechanism is known to be caused by the action of the cochlea of the ear and is a phenomenon in which one sound interferes with our perception of another sound [3]. For this masking phenomenon to take place, the two signals must have certain spectral and temporal properties relative to each other. Figure 1 (borrowed from John G. BEERENDS [4]) demonstrates a schematic representation of the frequency-domain, the time-domain and the time-frequency-domain of the masking pattern of a sinusoidal tone.

---
[*] Corresponding author: email: hossein.najafi@uwrf.edu.

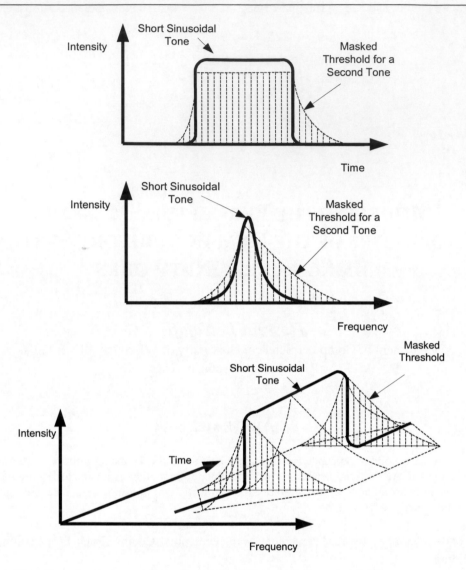

Figure 1. Time-Domain, Frequency Domain and Time-Frequency Domain Masking

Note that the cochlea is capable of performing both frequency and temporal masking. Frequency masking occurs when two signals that are close in frequency are played at the same time. In this case, one sound simply vanishes in the presence of the other sound. Temporal masking occurs when a one signal is played immediately before or after another one. In both cases one signal has the potential to mask the other. Post-masking refers to the effect of masking after a strong sound, and can be in effect up to about 200 ms. When a sound is masked by something that appears after it, it is called pre-masking. Pre-masking is relatively shorter and may last up to about 20 ms [5].

Many examples of modeling perceptual masking properties [6] [7] and perceptual measuring techniques [8] [9] [10] [11] [12] [13] [14] [15] [16] [17] are presented in the literature. The majority of these works focus on hand-crafting mathematical models of the cochlea and its signal processing capabilities. Such models are often too general and do not focus on the complete Auditory System's masking ability. Other models can only predict certain aspects of auditory sensation and do not offer a comprehensive masking model of the cochlea. In addition, to compute the masking thresholds using these models, a series of transformations (Fourier Transforms, Scale Conversions, matrix multiplications, etc.) must be performed on the signal. Such signal transformations are computationally expensive and hence not attractive for real-time applications. Mourjopoulos et al. [18] trained a neural network using the mathematical masking models to improve the computation complexity of the process. In this way, the network was trained to be an efficient representation of the corresponding hand-crafted mathematical model. However, the trained network, at best, can perform as well as the corresponding mathematical model.

In this paper we present a unique approach to modeling the perceptual masking map of the human auditory system using a back-propagation neural network [19] [20] [21]. Quality of the model is verified by its ability to inject imperceptible data into an audio stream.

## II. PROPOSED SOLUTION

The main objective of the work presented here is to build a computational model of the perceptual masking map of the human auditory system. To accomplish this, an artificial neural network was trained using the back-propagation algorithm. The first step in training a neural network is to create a feature vector set from which training and test sets can be produced. To accomplish this, real audio signals off of a reference tape were used. To improve the generalization capability of the network, the reference tape was composed of a variety of audio signals such as news clips, clips from movies, music clips, etc. The data sets were generated through interactive experiments, as described next, and were generated in such a way to represent the masking ability of the human auditory system.

As depicted in Figure 2, the audio signals from the tape are first decomposed into a set of $k$ corresponding audio bands $A_b = \{A_{b1}, A_{b2}, ..., A_{bk}\}$, using a bank of band-pass filters. The resulting band activities are then presented to an Activity Generator subsystem. The Activity Generator subsystem produces activity levels, $A_{bL}=\{A_{b1L}, A_{b2L}, ..., A_{bkL}\}$, and activity durations, $A_{bD}=\{A_{b1D}, A_{b2D}, ..., A_{bkD}\}$ of the audio bands. The Minimum Activity Detector Subsystem monitors the bands for an absolute minimum signal activity level and duration before any kind of masking is possible. When minimum signal activity is detected, the Random Data Generator subsystem is flagged to generate a data vector, $D(P_i)$. The data signal, $D(P_i)$, is then generated using one of the predefined parameter vectors $P_i = [P_{Li}, P_{Di}, P_{Ti}, P_{Bi}]$, randomly selected from the parameter set $P = \{P1, P2, ... , Pn\}$. Here, $P_L$ is the Level Parameter and identifies initial magnitude of $D$, $P_D$ is the Duration Parameter and identifies length of $D$, $P_T$ is the Decay Rate Parameter and identifies the rate at which $P_L$ is decayed during data transmission, and $P_B$ identifies a pair of neighboring bands to be used for data transmission. The data injection subsystem then injects the randomly generated data signal, with the specified magnitude, duration and decay rate into a pair of neighboring bands, identified by $P_B$, using (FSK) across the bands[1]. The resulting audio stream is then produced to a user who is given two seconds to respond if the data was heard by pressing a button on the keyboard. This user response is recorded as perceptual masking flag, $f$.

---

[1] Although the data infusion can be performed via different mechanisms, for the purpose of this study Frequency Shift Keying (FSK) across a pair of neighboring bands was used.

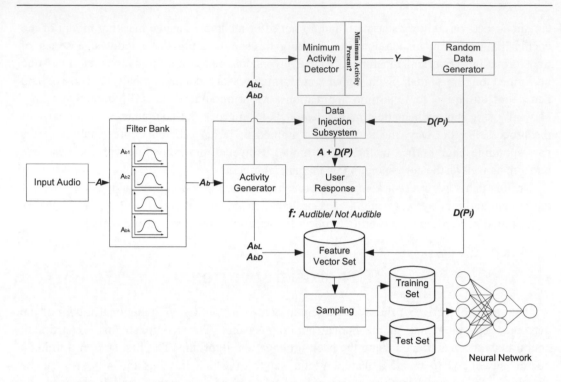

Figure 2. Training and Test Data Generation System

Data generated in this manner is then used to produce the feature vectors. Each feature vector is represented by $V = A_{bL} + A_{bD} + P_i + f$, where $A_{bL}$ is the activity level vector, $A_{bD}$ is the activity duration vector, $P_i$ is the data parameter vector used, and $f$ is the perceptual masking flag produced by the user.

The feature vector set, $V$, is then randomly sampled into a training set and a test set. These sets are then used to train and test a neural network using the standard back-propagation algorithm with momentum and adaptive learning rate. The number of hidden units is experimentally selected to produce best generalization. The trained neural network produced in this manner is then considered to be the computation model of the perceptual masking map of the human auditory system, and will be referred to as the Perceptual Masking Model (**PMM**) for the rest of this paper.

Note that, without affecting the merit of the proposed approach (i.e., Transmitting data at the Perceptual Entropy Envelope limit), other classification methods such as Projection Pursuit Regression [22], Radial Basis Functions [23], or Support Vector Machine [24] [25], can be used in place of the back-propagation neural network.

## III. APPLICATION OF THE MODEL TO DATA HIDING

Quality of the Perceptual Masking Model described in the previous section is examined by its ability to hide data in an audio stream. The model is used to monitor an audio stream for "opportunities" to infuse data signals into the stream such that the infused signals are masked according to the Perceptual Entropy Envelope of the audio signal. The model is also used to help identify and recover data signals that were injected into the channel from the corresponding audio stream. This section provides an overview of the data infusion and recovery subsystems.

## A. Data Infusion Subsystem

The data infusion subsystem uses a bank of PMMs, each representing a specific set of data parameters, for monitoring the audio channel for data transmission opportunities. To accomplish this, the input audio signal is first processed through the same Activity Detector used for generating the training and test sets. The outputs of the activity detector, $A_{bL}$ and $A_{bD}$ are then fed into the PMMs in the bank (See Figure 3). In addition to the band activity, each PMM also receives one of the predefined set of data parameters, $P_i$. Each PMM will generate its output activation value ($\alpha$) between zero and one. This value is a measure of the probability of hiding the data if transmitted with the corresponding parameters. Perceptual Masking Models with output activation values greater than threshold ($\tau$) are considered active. The threshold value $\tau$ was experimentally selected to provide maximum data capacity while keeping the perceptual quality of the audio signal intact. Active PMMs compete for data transmission. Data parameters associated with the active PMM that has the greatest output activation will be used to transmit the data. If no PMM is active, then no transmission will take place. Otherwise, the data infusion subsystem will use the data parameter $P_i$, associated with the selected active Perceptual Masking Model, $pmm_i$, to insert the data into the audio stream. Data will be inserted into the bands identified by $P_{Bi}$ at initial level specified by $P_{Li}$, with a duration specified by $P_{Di}$, and its magnitude is decayed according to $P_{Ti}$.

In this manner, the PMM bank controls the transmission frequency of the data signal, the level at which the data signal is transmitted and the timing of transmission of the data signal. Under the control of the this system, the data infusion subsystem will then combine a narrowband FSK data signal with the audio signal at the frequency, level and duration determined by the PMM bank such that the data signal has a high probability of being masked by the audio signal.

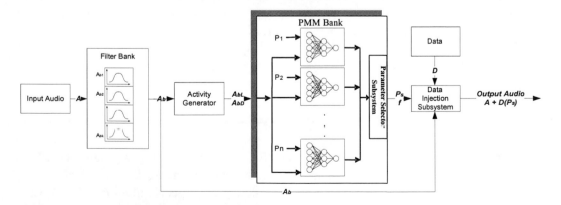

Figure 3. Data Infusion Subsystem

This process is summarized in Figure 3 with the **Parameter Selector Subsystem** implementing the following algorithm:

Given a set of Perceptual Masking Models, $PMM = \{pmm_1, pmm_2, \ldots pmm_n\}$, where $pmm_i$ is associated with the data parameters $P_i$, and where each Perceptual Masking Model, $pmm_i$ has an output activation $\alpha_i$ that represents the probability of successful transmission, if the data vector is transmitted with the data parameters $P_i$.

1.  Identify a subset of Active Perceptual Masking Models, $APMM = \{apmm_1, apmm_2, \ldots, apmm_k\}$ such that $\alpha_i > \tau$, where $\tau$ is a predefined threshold and selected experimentally to maximize data hiding capacity, while keeping the perceptual quality of audio signal intact.
2.  If $APMM$ is empty (i.e., there is no active PMM), set Inject Data Flag $f$ to **false**. No data will be transmitted.
3.  Otherwise, set Inject Data Flag $f$ to **true** and from the set $APMM$, identify the $apmm_s$ such that

$$\mathbf{apmm_s} = \underset{apmm_i}{\mathrm{argmax}}(\alpha_i).$$

4.  Output the Inject Data Flag $f$ and the data parameters, $P_s$ associated with the selected Active Perceptual Masking Model $apmm_s$.

Note that the proposed algorithm, has the same order of computational complexity as the method proposed by Mourjopoulos et al. [18].

## B. Data Extraction Subsystem

The data extraction subsystem (see Figure 4) utilizes the same PMM bank used by the data infusion subsystem. The received audio signal is decomposed and processed through the PMM bank in the same manner as at the transmitting end. The output of the parameter selector, $f$ and $P_s$ will be used to identify the location in the audio stream where a data signal with parameters $P_s$ is hiding. If the Inject Data Flag $f$ is **true**, then the corresponding parameters $P_s$ identify the FSK bands and the level, duration and decay rate of the data signal. Given this information, an FSK decoder will then retrieve the data signal from the audio stream.

## IV. SIMULATION RESULTS

Feasibility of the proposed solution was investigated by using a small number of frequency bands. The transmission bands were fixed, and the network was trained to only identify the masking level, data duration and data decay rate. Specifically, four MPEG bands centered at approximately 2.2K, 2.55K, 2.95K and 3.5K were used. The two center bands (2.55K and 2.95K) were used as the FSK transmission bands with the center at about 2.77K. Forty sets of data parameters representing combination of five data levels, four decay rates and two data durations were used. Data levels, were set at 32 dB from full scale and worked down by 3 dB. Decay rates were at 0.74 dB, 0.58 dB, 0.46 dB, and 0.36 dB per sample. Data durations where set at 24 and 32 data bits.

The Data Generation System depicted in Figure 2 was used by a group of listeners to generate the training and test data. Listeners were asked to play an audio file composed of a variety of audio signals such as news clips, clips from movies, music clips, etc. The audio stream also contained data with one of the forty random parameters. The listeners were asked to press a button on the keyboard if and when they heard an audio anomaly. If the button was pushed within two seconds of a data transmission, that data transmission was marked as audible. Activities in each sub-band (i.e., level and duration of activities), the parameters used for the data signals and the corresponding audible flag produced by the user were then stored in a data file.

The data produced by the Data Generation System was then randomly sampled into a training set and a test set. These sets were used to train and test a 3-layer feed-forward neural network using the back-propagation learning algorithm, with momentum and adaptive learning rate. To help identify a system with best generalization capability, a number of networks with different hidden layer size were trained and tested, and the network with the best performance was selected for data insertion and extraction.

In specific, the number of hidden units was increased from 2 to 10. Each network was then trained and tested using 40 different training and test sets. The performance of each network was measured in terms of its True Positive (*TP*), False Positive (*FP*), True Negative (*TN*), and False Negative (*FN*) Classification Rates.

The following observations were considered in selecting the best performing network:

- Networks with larger *TP* will have higher transmission rates
- Networks with larger *FP* will have higher audible distortions
- Networks with larger *FN* will have higher missed opportunities
- Networks with larger *TN* will have higher perceptual quality.

Using these observations, the best performing network was identified to have the maximum True Positive classification accuracy (i.e. highest insertion rate) and minimum ratio of False Positive to True Positive (i.e., relative lowest audible distortion) as formalized by the following function, *g*:

$$g = \frac{TP/(TP + FP + FN + TN)}{FP/TP} = \frac{TP^2}{FP*(TP + FP + FN + TN)}$$

Table 1 shows the average values of *g* as a function of the number of hidden units. Note that the network architecture that employed 3 hidden units give the best average performance (i.e., *g* is maximum).

Among the 40 networks trained with 3 hidden units, the network that gave the best performance was then selected and used for data insertion and extraction. This network had a *g* value of 4.41 and its Classification Rates are listed in Table 2.

Note that FP is only 2%, indicating that data inserted by best performing network will be very inaudible. Also, note that TP+TN is over 60%, indicating that the network is transmitting at close to the limits of the Perceptual Entropy Envelope. However, the FN of 36% indicates that there are missed opportunities and offers room for improving the rate of insertion.

This best performing network was then used as part of the data infusion and data extraction subsystems. The network bank was composed of forty versions of this network with each having their data parameter inputs set equal to one of the forty parameters used in this experiment. The data insertion threshold, $\tau$, was varied from 0.5 to 0.9 and it was identified that a value of 0.7 would lead to maximum data insertion capacity, while preserving perceptual quality of the audio signal.

The ultimate quality of the system was tested using a new audio file. Users were asked to listen to two audio files, one with and one without the infused data. They were then asked to identify which one contained the data. Results showed that users could not clearly identify the tape with the data. Approximately 50% of the time they identified the tape with the data correctly, and the other 50% of the time they incorrectly identified the tape with no data on it.

The quality of the data retrieval was tested in terms of the number of infused data vectors that could successfully be retrieved. This test was conducted in a lossless environment. Results indicated that all data transmissions could be retrieved successfully.

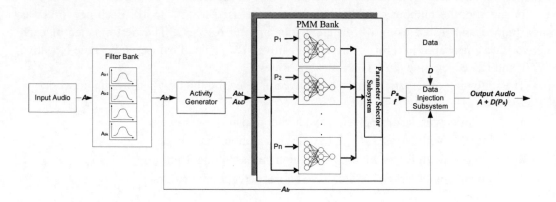

Figure 4. Data Extraction Subsystem

### Table 1. Values of $g$ as a Function of Number of Hidden Units

|   | Number of Hidden Units | | | | | | | | |
|---|------|------|------|------|------|------|------|------|------|
|   | 2    | 3    | 4    | 5    | 6    | 7    | 8    | 9    | 10   |
| g | 1.51 | 2.02 | 1.74 | 1.97 | 1.81 | 1.61 | 1.84 | 1.78 | 1.56 |

### Table 2. Best network's performance on an independent test set

| Best Network Performance | | | |
|------|------|------|------|
| TNR  | FNR  | FPR  | TPR  |
| 34%  | 36%  | 2%   | 28%  |

# CONCLUSIONS

A system that employed Artificial Neural Networks to model the masking properties of the Human Auditory System was presented. Quality of the model was examined by its application to the audio data hiding problem. Experimental results demonstrated good capacity, transparency, and robustness of the model.

# REFERENCES

[1] Hellman, R. *Asymmetry of Maksing Between Noise and Tone, Perception and Psychophysics*, Vol. 11 (3), 241-246, 1972.

[2] Schroeder, MR; Atal, BS; Hall, JL. *Optimizing Digital Speech Coder by Exploiting Masking Properties of the Human Ear,* Journal of Acoustic Society, Am. 66 (6), 1647-1652, 1979.

[3] Moore, BCJ. *An Introduction to the Psychology of Hearing.*, London, England: Academic Press, 3$^{rd}$ Edn., 1989.

[4] Beerends, JG; Stemerdink, JA. A Perceptual Audio Quality Measure Based on a Psychoacoustic Sound Representation., *Journal of Audio Engineering*, Vol. 40, No. 12, 1992.

[5] Lincoln, B. "An experimental high fidelity perceptual audio coder," March 1998, Project in MUS420 Win97

[6] Bauer, FL. *Decrypted Secrets – Methods and Maxims of Cryptology.*, Berlin, Heidelberg, Germany: Springer-Verlag, 1997, ISBN 3-540-60418-9.

[7] Nicchiotti, G; Ottaviano. E. *Non-Invertible Statistical Wavelet Watermarking*, EUSIPCO'98,- Ninth European Signal Processing Conference, September 8-11. 1998. pp. 2289-2292.

[8] Cox, IJ; Miller, ML. *A Review Of Watermarking And The Importance Of Perceptual Modeling. Proceedings of Electronic Imaging*, 1997.

[9] Nikolaidis, N; Pitas, I. *Robust Image Watermarking In The Spatial Domain. Signal Processing*, vol. 66, no. 3, pp. 385-403, May 1998, ISSN 0165-1684, European Association for Signal Processing (EURASIP).

[10] Karjalainen, M. *A New Auditory Model For The Evaluation Of Sound Quality Of Audio Systems*, in Proc. ICASSP, 1985, 608-611.

[11] Fielder, LD. *Evaluation Of The Audible Distortion And Noise Produced By Digital Audio Converters, J. Audio Eng. Soc.*, vol. 35, July-August 1987, 517-535.

[12] Seitzer, D; Brandenburg, KH; Kappust, R; Eberlein, E; Gerhäuser, H; Krägerloh, S; Schott, H. *Dsp Based Real Time Implementation Of An Advanced Analysis Tool For Audio Channels*, In Proc. ICASSP, 89, 2057-2060.

[13] Herre, J; Eberlein, E. Schott, H. Brandenburg, K. *Advanced Audio Measurement System Using Psychoacoustic Properties*, presented at the 92$^{nd}$ Convention of Audio Engineering Society, *J. Audio Eng. Soc.* (Abstracts), vol. 40, May 1992, p. 447.

[14] Paillard, B; Mabilleau, P; Morisette, S; Soumagne, J. *PERCEVAL: Perceptual Evaluation Of The Quality Audio Signals, J. Audio Eng. Soc.,* vol. 40, *January-February*, 1992, 21-31.

[15]  Hamza Özer, Bülent Sankur, Nasir Memon, *An SVD-Based Audio Watermarking Technique*, MM-SEC'05, New York, New York, 2005.

[16]  Al-Khassaweneh, M; Aviyente, S. *Robust Watermarking On The Joint Spatial-Spectral Domain*, in Proceedings of IEEE DSP Workshop, August, 2004.

[17]  Maria Calagna, Luigi V. Mancini, Huiping Guo, Sus hil Jajodia, *A Robust Watermarking System based on SVD Compression*, ACM SAC'06, April 23-27 2006, Dijon, France

[18]  Mourjopoulos, J; Tsoukalas, D. *Neural Network Mapping To Subjective Spectra Of Music Sounds*, , *J. Audio Eng. Soc.*, vol. 40, no. 4, April, 1992, 253-259.

[19]  Rumelhart, DE; Hinton, GE; Williams, RJ. *Learning Internal Representation by Error Propagation*, Parallel Distributed Processing, Chapter 8, MIT Press, 1986.

[20]  Werbos, PJ. *Beyond Regression: New Tools for Prediction and Analysis in the Behavioral Sciences*, Ph.D. Thesis. Harward University, Cambridge, MA, 1974.

[21]  Reed, RD; Marks II, RJ. *Neural Smithing – Supervised Learning In Feedforward Artificial Neural Networks*. MIT press, 1999.

[22]  Friedman, JH; Stuetzle, W. Projection Pursuit Regression, *Journal of the American Statistical Association*, Vol 76, 817-823., 1981.

[23]  Maruyama, M; Girosi, F; Poggio, T. *A Connection Between GRBF and MLP*, Artificial Intelligence Memo 1291, *Massachusetts Institute of Technology.*, 1991.

[24]  Vapnik, VN. *The Nature of Statistical Learning Theory*, Springer, 1995.

[25]  Schölkopf, B; Burges, C; Smola, A. (ed.), *Advances in Kernel Methods - Support Vector Learning*, MIT Press, 1999.

In: Deafness, Hearing Loss and the Auditory System    ISBN: 978-1-60741-259-5
Editor: D. Fiedler and R. Krause, pp. 333-372    © 2010 Nova Science Publishers, Inc.

*Chapter 17*

# PERCEPTUAL FEATURES FOR ROBUST SPEECH RECOGNITION

*Serajul Haque and Roberto Togneri*
School of Electrical, Electronic and Computer Engineering
University of Western Australia

## Abstract

Automatic speech recognition (ASR) broadly encompasses the recognition of human
speech by a machine or by some artificial intelligence. The recognition process should be
robust, that is, it should accurately recognise the spoken word in the presence of speaker
variabilities, word perplexities, and speech corrupted by noise which are introduced during
transmission and in the communication channels itself. Research in the past several decades
has produced speech processing techniques like the short-time Fourier transform (STFT),
the linear prediction (LP) and autoregressive (AR) methods, and the mel-frequency cepstral
coefficients (MFCC), which have contributed significantly to robust speech recognition.
The ability of the human auditory system to recognize speech in adverse and noisy
conditions has motivated speech researchers to include features of human perception
in speech recognition systems. Particularly in the early 1980s, several computational
models of the auditory periphery based on physiological measurements of the response on
individual fibres of the auditory nerve were proposed [1],[2],[3]. These "cochlear models"
only provided marginal improvements at higher computational costs when applied to
speech recognition. As a result, a decline in the interest in auditory models was observed
until computing resources were able to meet the intensive computational requirements of
such models. In recent years, there has been a resurgence in perceptual speech processing
after research provided evidence that it may lead to improved recognition performances
[12],[13],[14].

This chapter describes several psychoacoustic properties of the peripheral auditory system applied to a speech recognition front-end. Dynamic behaviour of the auditory nerves
are incorporated in speech parametrization utilizing temporal processing, so that time domain information as appropriate time constants are incorporated in speech parameterization.
A simplified method of synaptic adaptation as determined by psychoacoustic observations
in an auditory nerve is described. It utilizes a high pass infinite impulse response (IIR)

temporal filter to enhance the signal onsets and the subsequent dynamic and the steady-state characteristics [15],[16]. Speech features are extracted in the temporal mode utilizing a zero-crossing algorithm [5]. The two-tone suppression as observed in the non-linear response of the basilar membrane is described in a zero-crossing auditory front-end using a temporal companding strategy [18],[17]. This may introduce asymmetric gain control without degrading the spectral contrast. The word recognitions are evaluated by continuous density hidden Markov models and are shown to provide improvements over conventional parameterizations in clean and noise conditions. Some of these perceptual algorithms may also benefit people with sensorineural hearing loss and may be implemented in hearing aids and cochlear implants for the hearing impaired through VLSI implementations [18].

# 1   Introduction

Speech processing may be categorized into two main branches: speech production/synthesis and speech perception/recognition. Automatic speech recognition (ASR) has emerged in recent years as one of the most important research areas in the field of speech science and technology. ASR broadly encompasses the recognition of human speech by a machine or by some artificial intelligence. It may form the basis of a man-machine interface for human-computer interactions. One of the main functions of an ASR system is to transform speech produced by a speech production mechanism such as human voice captured by a microphone, a telephone, or some other transducer to a text sequence, usually in terms of a sequence of words. Other important applications of ASR are in document preparations and dictations, automated dialog systems over media such as telephones and radio links, device controls through voice activation, voice "finger-printing" for identification and forensic applications, database access and web enabling via voice, and many more.

The acoustic speech signals are transmitted to the receiver through some communication medium. The ASR system should accurately and robustly recognise the spoken word after it has passed through the communication channel. However, in spite of focused research in this field for the past several decades, robust and reliable speech recognition has not been achieved [13],[20],[21]. Several factors contribute to this degradation. The speech may be corrupted by external noise during the transmission process. The recognition process may fail due to speaker variabilities, that is, due to the variable speed, style, accent of the spoken word. The channel itself may introduce distortions by the convolutive noise added by the channel impulse response. A word may be misrecognised due to the context, perplexity and multiple meanings such as in the English language.

Research in speech technology in the past several decades has produced significant advances in ASR. Speech signals are pseudo-periodic with substantial random components, the statistical properties of which vary significantly over time. The short-time Fourier transform (STFT) method of speech processing [25] produces a series of feature vectors at a rate sufficient to capture the rapid instantaneous transitions in the spoken word within a short duration over which the statistical properties are reasonably stationary. This has contributed significantly to robust speech recognition. The linear prediction (LP) and autoregressive (AR) method of speech analysis utilizes the speech production process to determine the parameters of the vocal tract [22]. AR modeling yields the allpole spectrum of the speech waveform, from which the frequencies and bandwidths of the individual resonances corresponding to the formant positions of the vocal tract may be obtained. Another significant improvement was the cepstral method of speech processing introduced by Bogert *et al.* [23] in 1963, which provided reduction of feature dimensionality and decorrelation of the vocal tract excitation and the glottal waveform. Traditionally, speech enhancement methods using spectral subtraction have been employed to improve performance in noisy conditions.

The recognition problem is one of determining the most probable word spoken, and usually done by template matching with a predetermined database of sound representation. Since speech has numerous variabilities which are usually unpredictable, it is possible to model speech as a context dependent random process and then use statistical tools to analyze it. As a result, speech recognition has primarily focussed on statistical methods. The most popular and effective statistical template matching is based on a set of hidden Markov models (HMM). It utilizes statistical modeling and a grammar rule to select the highest probability of some hidden or unobservable parameters of the speech from a sequence of observation feature vectors. The Markov chain rule is one of the most widely used models describing class dependence which has contributed substantially to robust speech recognition.

In recent years, the superb ability of the human auditory system to recognise spoken words under extreme conditions has motivated researchers to include processing features of human auditory system and perceptual features in the automatic speech recognition process. In the early 1980s, several computational models of the auditory periphery, based on physiological measurements of the response on individual fibres of the auditory nerve, were proposed [1],[2],[3],[4]. These were generally referred to as "cochlear models". The primary objective of such models was speech processing for auditory research [4], hearing aids [5], cochlear implants [6], and to a lesser extent, for automatic speech recognition. While comparatively little is known about the neural mechanisms of the central auditory processing stages, much more is known about the peripheral auditory system, which encompasses first stages of auditory processing. These models of the peripheral auditory system usually include a perceptual filterbank corresponding to the critical bands of human hearing, a non-linear rectification process, automatic gain control to compress the dynamic range that can be coded into the auditory nerve, synapse processing consisting of short-term synaptic adaptation, and lateral suppression. The initial process in a peripheral auditory system enhances some perceptual information in the speech signal which assists the higher auditory system in the proper identification of the speech segments [1]. Some of these perceptual features enhance the speech segments, others suppress it to increase spectral contrasts or to suppress sources of stationary noise. It was shown that such approaches tend to provide robustness and recognition accuracy with a degree of improvement over conventional speech parameterizations either in clean conditions or in environment mismatch and noisy conditions [7], [8].

However, one disadvantage with cochlear models was the higher computation cost involved with such processing. Moreover, the use of perceptual features resulted only in marginal improvements in many cases when applied to speech recognition [2],[9],[10] and in specific cases even degraded ASR performance [11]. As a result, a decline in the interest in auditory models was observed until computing resources were able to meet the intensive computational requirements of such models. In recent years there has been a resurgence in perceptual processing of speech for speech recognition after research provided evidence that such processing may lead to improved performance [2],[13],[14],[40],[47].

Based on the progress in understanding auditory processing mechanisms, several aspects of sound processing in the auditory periphery are modeled and simulated in common front ends for ASR systems. For example, the transformation of speech vectors to spectral magnitudes emphasizes the role of the basilar membrane (BM) as a spectral analyzer. The filterbank decomposition techniques and the use of mel or Bark scales (critical bands) simulates the tonotopic processing in the BM [27]. Static compression with log or cube-root functions, and spectral smoothing are consistent with the perceptual features of auditory compression [28]. The spectrum is pre-emphasized to implement the functionalities of the outer and the middle ear, that is, the unequal sensitivity of human hearing at different frequencies corresponding to the equal loudness curves of perception [1]. In the filterbank analysis, the progressively higher bandwidths at higher frequencies give poorer frequency resolution which simulates the loss of synchrony and the ability of the auditory system to phase lock at higher frequencies. RASTA processing has some relation to the models of forward temporal masking [29].

Auditory perception is a psychoacoustic process in which the mapping between the acoustic speech and the human perception is non-linear. Because of this, an analytic treatment of auditory processing in the inner ear is often intractable, and relies substantially on experimental methods [30]. A distinction should be made between the two processes of psychoacoustic perception, which is a dynamic process, and speech recognition, which is primarily a static process. A comparison between a conventional and the perceptual speech recognition process is shown in Fig. 1. Auditory models for ASR integrate some of the dynamic features of psychoacoustic phenomena related to speech perception with the static speech features. On the other hand, conventional speech processing for ASR usually ignores the detailed effects of psychoacoustic perception. The primary objective of this project is to identify the perceptual features which are relevant and useful for the improvement of ASR performance in clean and noisy conditions.

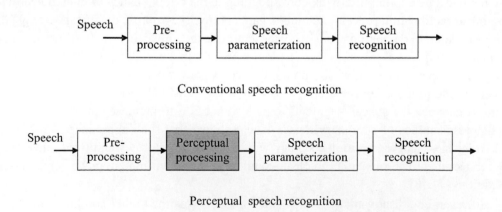

Figure 1: Comparison between the conventional and the perceptual speech recognition process.

In this chapter, the performance of two perceptual properties of the peripheral auditory system, synaptic adaptation and two-tone suppression are investigated for their roles in automatic speech recognition in clean conditions and in additive noise environment. The chapter is arranged as follows. Section 2 gives an overview of some methodologies of auditory processing related to automatic speech speech recognition. In section 3, a simplified synaptic adaptation model is developed in a zero-crossing auditory model used as a speech recognition front-end. It is shown that rapid adaptation can be implemented in temporal processing of speech, not otherwise implementable in the spectral domain. In section 4, the two-tone suppression is investigated and a method of introducing the two-tone suppression in a zero-crossing auditory front-end using temporal companding is described. This is followed in section 5 by an overall discussion and conclusion drawn from the experiments.

## 2 Some Methodologies of Perceptual Speech Recognition

In our study, we have particularly emphasized on three methodologies. Firstly, we have adopted temporal processing of speech, utilizing time-domain filters, rather than processing in the spectral domain. The temporal-place representation of auditory processing is much less affected by background noise than the rate-place representation [31]. There are several other advantages of processing in the time-domain. Auditory functions are usually dynamic in nature with substantial transient properties, which, unlike steady-state emissions, can not be fully characterized by the spectrum, although short-time Fourier transform processing may alleviate this to some extent. This is primarily because, by their very nature, transients are time-varying or non-stationary signals [32]. In many cases, the fine temporal structures and time variations are removed by the spectral feature extraction methods in the log spectral domain [14]. Recursive filtering which can simulate many of the psychophysical behaviors of human perception, is better implemented in the time domain than in the spectral domain because of the aliasing problem and the requirement of inverting an infinite dimensional Fourier transform. Time-varying cues are also useful in identifying CV (consonant followed by a vowel sound) transitions [25].

Secondly, we have chosen a temporal auditory model using a zero-crossing algorithm for implementations. The conventional features used for speech recognition, e.g., the MFCC and the PLP, mainly extract the spectral properties of the signal, and lacks in temporal information. it is well known that this deficiency in the MFCCs, and almost all other features conventionally used for speech recognition, are somewhat inadequate for the recognition of rapidly changing events such as the bursts in plosives. Moreover, formant transitions, a key aspect in the perception of speech, are also implemented inadequately in the MFCC. This is, however, compensated by the delta-delta coefficients in the MFCC, which again increase the dimensionality of the feature vectors. Using spectro-temporal features, similar to those found in the primary auditory cortex, should overcome the above mentioned problems. One method of spectro-temporal speech parameterization is the zero-crossing algorithm for speech processing, such as in the the zero-crossing peak amplitudes (ZCPA) auditory model proposed by Kim *et al.* [13]. It is based on the principle that any stimulus periodicity in the filter subband can be extracted from the zero-crossing intervals, the inverse of which shows up as a dominant frequency corresponding to the formant peaks within that subband. This is known as the dominant frequency principle [33]. The dominant frequency in a subband has more power than others, which makes the zero-crossing algorithm more robust in noisy environments. Moreover, the zero-crossing analysis is amenable to simple transformations instead of complex transformations between the time and the frequency domains such as in the spectral processing.

Thirdly, for the feature extraction process, larger time windows and filters with appropriate time constants consistent with human perception are utilized. Since time domain processing is based on extracting frequency information from periodicity, it generally utilizes larger window lengths than the short-time FFT methods. Auditory models do not make strong assumptions of quasi-stationarity. This is consistent with human auditory functions which have longer integration times with higher time constants. For example, forward masking may last up to 200 ms [14]. However, STFT processing of speech using a filter-bank approach (e.g. MFCC) is based on smaller stationary window lengths of 20-25 ms. Too short a window length produces a poor spectral representation of the speech, which usually degrades in noise condition, and is also sensitive to temporal effects of voicing. Performances at higher SNRs decrease with decreasing window lengths [25]. This has motivated several researchers to emphasize time interval processing with longer time constants for integration into the speech recognition systems [34],[35].

## 3    Speech Recognition with Synaptic Adaptation

Synaptic adaptation is a dynamic mechanism of the human auditory system. In response to tone bursts, a single auditory-nerve fibre exhibits an increased neural discharge in the initial 15 ms at the signal onset. This decays monotonically in time, reaching a steady-level within about 50 ms. This decrease in response rate, referred to as "synaptic adaptation", has been determined by physiological experiments and from responses to pure tones [37],[38]. In this section, we demonstrate a method of introducing synaptic adaptation as observed in the peripheral auditory system for automatic speech recognition. The adaptation process is implemented in a ZCPA auditory model in the temporal domain and evaluated by a HMM recognizer. We first analyse the process of synaptic adaptation in the auditory system, followed by an analysis of the zero-crossing algorithm. This is followed by an implementation method of a simplified adaptation scheme in the ZCPA auditory model using an infinite impulse response (IIR) filter. At the end, the results are presented demonstrating the benefit of the scheme both analytically and quantitatively as percentage improvements in recognition performance.

### 3.1    The Synaptic Aadaptation Process

The synaptic adaptation process is shown in Fig. 2 as a post-stimulus time histogram (PSTH) for an afferent nerve fibre. Initially, there is a surge in the response at the beginning of the stimulus which gradually decays to a steady-state response. The decay consists of an initial rapid phase with a time constant of 3 ms (rapid synaptic adaptation). It is followed by a slower exponential decay with a time constant of about 40 ms (short-term synaptic adaptation). It is observed from the figure that in the absence of the stimulus the auditory nerve fibre produces spikes at a small but discernable rate. This is called the spontaneous rate. When the tone is removed, the spike rate decreases to slightly lower than the spontaneous rate for a short time before resuming its normal rate. The synaptic adaptation process

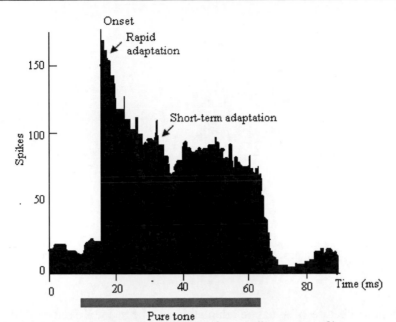

Figure 2: Poststimulus time histogram (PSTH) of an auditory nerve fibre to a pure tone burst showing the rapid and short-term synaptic adaptation (adopted from [36]).

indicates that the auditory nerve is more responsive to changes than to steady inputs. The rate of fall from the onset transient down to the synaptic adaptation level is independent of the intensity of the tone signal level [37].

Synaptic adaptation in the AN results primarily from the release of transmitter substances (neurotransmitters) from the hair cells into the synaptic cleft at the beginning of a signal onset, and the subsequent transmitter depletion of $Ca^{2+}$ in the voltage-sensitive $Ca^{2+}$ channels [39],[14]. After the release of neurotransmitters by the hair cells, the voltage-sensitive $Ca^{2+}$ channels located close to the synapses at the basal part of these cells open upon depolarization of the cell membrane. This process fills up the "readily releasable pool" (RRP). The cleft is filled up at a rate that is proportional to the concentration gradient of the transmitter across the membrane. Some transmitter within the cleft is lost which gives rise to the slow depletion of the neurotransmitters in the cleft. Some flow back through the cell membrane for recycling (reuptake) and are reprocessed to fill up the RRP. At the beginning of an acoustic stimulus, plenty of vesicles are available to fuse, causing a strong initial AN response. Subsequently, as the RRP is refilled at a lower rate than the initial vesicle fusion rate due to the loss in the cleft, the RRP depletes with time. Auditory nerve activity is, thus, depressed shortly after the stimulus onset and during sustained stimuli, producing the synaptic adaptation effect. This process is shown in Fig. 3.

Synaptic adaptation accentuates signal onsets by following a high initial discharge rate. A rapid synaptic adaptation component enhances voicing, and short-term synaptic adaptation is found to improve the immunity of the system to stationary noise [20]. This principle is used in RASTA processing of speech and shown to improve the robustness of the system [29]. However, the main difference is that RASTA processing is a bandpass modulation filtering operating on the logarithmic spectrum, which completely suppresses dc modulations, whereas the auditory nerve shows a sustained discharge rate to steady-state stimuli.

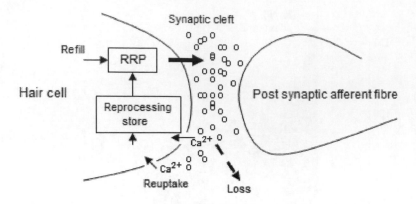

Figure 3: Synaptic adaptation process in the synapses between the inner hair cells and an auditory nerve.

The perceptual feature of synaptic adaptation has been employed in ASR by several researchers. Cohen [8] implemented an ASR front-end utilizing a Bark-scaled filterbank in which a compressive power law transformation was applied to the output of each filter approximating loudness scaling. A reservoir-type synaptic adaptation was used to model the neural discharge rate. It was shown that the error rates and decoding times in a word recognition task were substantially lower with the auditory model than with a mel filterbank implementation (3.9% vs. 6.3%).

The generalized synchrony detector (GSD) model proposed by Seneff [1] incorporated an IHC-synaptic processing stage which consisted of a saturating half-wave rectification, short-term synaptic adaptation, synchrony suppression at higher frequencies and rapid synaptic adaptation, as observed from psychophysical measurements. Jankowski [40] designed a speech recognizer using Seneff's GSD auditory model and compared the word error rates with a conventional mel filterbank using isolated words and a HMM recognizer. The GSD front-end produced better recognition performance results than the mel filterbank.

Strope *et al.* [12] described a dynamic model with a logarithmic synaptic adaptation stage based on forward masking data. The adaptation mechanism implemented was a modified form of the automatic gain control (AGC), which added an exponentially adapting linear offset to the logarithmic intensity. It showed improvements in robustness to background noise when used as a front-end for DTW and HMM based recognitions. Holmberg *et al.* [14] incorporated a simplified model of synaptic adaptation for ASR into the MFCC feature parametrization as a competitive strategy to RASTA and the cepstrum mean subtraction (CMS). A first-order infinite impulse response (IIR) high-pass filter was used to represent the decaying exponential effects of the rapid and the short-term synaptic adaptation. Evaluated with Aurora 2 database and a HMM recognizer, it showed improved ASR performance compared to the baseline MFCC, and MFCC in combination with RASTA and CMS processing. In contrast, we have proposed a time-domain approach to the adaptation and demonstrated a method of implementation in a auditory model of the human peripheral auditory system used as an ASR front-end. To demonstrate the implementation, we first introduce the zero-crossing algorithm for speech processing.

## 3.2   The Zero-crossing Analysis

For a real-valued zero mean stationary Gaussian random process $Z_t, t \in T$ for all $t_1, \ldots, t_N \in T$, the number of zero-crossings $D$, can be defined in terms of a clipped process $M_t$ for discrete time $t$ as

$$D = \sum_{t=1}^{N} (M_t - M_{t-1})^2, \qquad 0 \leq D \leq N - 1 \tag{1}$$

where

$$M_t = \begin{cases} 1 & \text{if} \quad Z_t \geq 0 \\ 0 & \text{if} \quad Z_t < 0 \end{cases}$$

for $t=1,\ldots,N$. If we define $\mu=E\{Z_t\}$ as the mean vector ($E\{.\}$ denotes the expected value), and $\gamma_k$ as the covariance matrix as a function of the lag $k$ such that

$$\begin{aligned} \gamma_k &= \text{Cov}(Z_t(k)) \\ &= E\{(Z_t - \mu)(Z_{t+k} - \mu)\}. \end{aligned} \tag{2}$$

To make the covariance invariant to scaling, it is usually useful to normalize $\gamma_k$ with respect to $\gamma_0$, and define the normalized parameter $\rho_k$ such that we can express

$$\rho_k = \frac{\gamma_k}{\gamma_0} \qquad k = 0, \pm 1, \ldots. \tag{3}$$

Using the Wiener-Khintchin theorem, a relationship between the covariance matrix $\gamma_k$ and its spectral representation may be obtained. Koopmans [41] has shown that using the Wiener-Khintchin theorem, it is possible to define a monotone increasing function, $F(\omega)$, ($\omega$ being the angular frequency with a maximum value of $\pi$), such that

$$\gamma_k = \int_{-\pi}^{\pi} \cos(k\omega) dF(\omega) \tag{4}$$

where $F(\omega)$ is the spectral distribution function (cumulative) of $Z_t$. The function $Z_t$ must satisfy the convergence property, that is, it must be square integrable,

$$\int_{-\infty}^{\infty} dt \mid Z(t) \mid^2 < \infty \tag{5}$$

If we substitute for $k=1$ in Eqn. (3), then we may write

$$\begin{aligned} \rho_1 &= \frac{\gamma_1}{\gamma_0} \\ &= \frac{\int_{-\pi}^{\pi} \cos(\omega) dF(\omega)}{\int_{-\pi}^{\pi} dF(\omega)}. \end{aligned} \tag{6}$$

The expected value of the zero-crossings count, $D$, of the Gaussian $Z_t$, $t \in T$, with zero mean is related to its spectral representation [33] by

$$\cos\left(\frac{\pi E\{D\}}{(N-1)}\right) = \frac{\int_0^\pi \cos(\omega)dF(\omega)}{\int_0^\pi dF(\omega)} \tag{7}$$

where

$$F(\xi) = \int_{-\pi}^\pi f(\xi)d\xi \tag{8}$$

is a spectral distribution function (cumulative) and $f(\xi)$, $\pi \leq \xi \leq \pi$, is the spectral density of $Z_t$. Eqn. (7) shows that $\pi E\{D\}/(N-1)$ which is the normalized expected zero-crossing rate of the random process, $Z_t$, may be represented in terms of the angular (weighted) spectral content of $Z_t$. Therefore, within a subband, if a certain frequency, $\omega_0$, becomes dominant, that is, has more power (weights) than in other bands, then it is seen from Eqn. (7)

$$\frac{\pi E\{D\}}{(N-1)} \approx \omega_0 \tag{9}$$

which states that this frequency may be represented by a corresponding average zero-crossing rate. This is referred to as the dominant frequency principle [33]. A dominant frequency in a subband has more power than others, which makes the zero-crossing algorithms more robust in noisy conditions [13]. The resolution of the subband dominant frequency estimates decreases rapidly at higher frequencies. One method to circumvent this is by up-sampling the high frequency subband signals using frequency-dependent interpolation factors [21].

## 3.3   The ZCPA Auditory Model

An auditory model based on the zero-crossing algorithm is the zero-crossing with peak amplitudes (ZCPA) proposed by Kim *et al.* [13]. It is based on the dominant frequency principle and duplicates the functions of the peripheral auditory system in some details. It is an enhancement of the ensemble interval histogram (EIH) model proposed by Ghitza [2], where it replaces the multiple levels of the EIH with a single zero level to extract the speech features from the zero-crossings. Fig. 4 shows the schematic of the ZCPA temporal auditory model used as an ASR front-end. Digitized speech is input to a bank of bandpass filters with frequency characteristics closely resembling the human frequency response along the length of the basilar membrane. It utilizes a zero-crossing detector in each channel to estimate the dominant frequencies within a filterbank channel. Each speech frame is represented by a frequency histogram obtained from the inverse of the time interval between two successive upward going zero-crossings in the filter channel outputs. The intensity is measured by a peak detector from the peak amplitudes between each zero-crossing interval. In this experiment, a computationally efficient version of the ZCPA with fewer number of filters to reduce the computational cost and suitable for hardware realization was implemented.

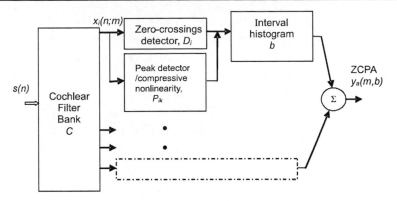

Figure 4: The ZCPA auditory model used as an ASR front-end utilizing a zero-crossing detector and a peak detector for feature extraction.

An ensemble interval histogram is constructed by summing the histograms of all the frames. An expression of the ZCPA histogram output may be obtained as follows. If we denote $m_s(n)$ the clean message speech signal which is corrupted with bandlimited white Gaussian noise, $\varphi(n)$, with a rectangular power spectrum of bandwidth, $W$, then the noisy speech $s(n) = m_s(n) + \varphi(n)$ is given by

$$s(n) = \sum_{l=0}^{M-1} A_l \cos(\omega_l n + \theta_l) + A_\varphi \varphi(n), \qquad l = 0, 1, \dots, M-1 \qquad (10)$$

where the message speech $m_s(n) = \sum_{l=0}^{M-1} A_l \cos(\omega_l n + \theta_l)$, $l \in M$ contains $M$ frequency components each with a phase $\theta_l$ within the signal, and $A_l$ and $A_\varphi$ are the signal and noise amplitudes, respectively. If the input noisy signal, $s(n)$, is filtered by a bank of bandpass cochlear filters with bandwidth, $B_i$, where $i = 1, \dots, C$ corresponds to the number of channels in the filterbank, then the output at the $i$-th bandpass filter may be expressed in discrete form as

$$x_i(n) = A_i \cos(\omega_i n + \theta_i) + A_\varphi \varphi(n). \qquad (11)$$

If $w(n)$ is a window of finite length, then the value of $x_i(n)$ at the frame index $m$ is given by $x_i(n; m) = x_i(n) w_i(m-n)$, $i = 1, \dots, C$, where $C$ is the number of filter channels.

Let $D_i$ be the number of upward-going zero-crossings at the $i$-th filter in a windowed frame $x_i(n; m)$ and $P_{ik}$ is the peak amplitude between the $k$-th and the $(k+1)$-th zero-crossing in $x_i(n; m)$. Then the output $y(m, b)$ at time $m$ is given in [13] as

$$y(m, b) = \sum_{i=1}^{C} \sum_{k=1}^{D_i-1} \log(P_{ik} + 1)\delta_{bj_k}, \qquad 1 \le b < R \qquad (12)$$

where $R$ is the number of frequency bins, $b$ is the frequency bin index and $\delta_{bj}$ is the Kronecker delta, such that

$$\delta_{bj_k} = \begin{cases} 1 & \text{if } b = j_k \\ 0 & \text{elsewhere.} \end{cases}$$

The frequency histogram is constructed by processing each channel output sequentially and counting all upward-going zero crossings within that channel. For each zero-crossing count, the index of frequency bin $j_k$ is computed by taking the inverse of the time interval between the $k$-th and $(k+1)$-th zero-crossings, for $k$=1,...,$D_i$-1. For each $k$ within a frame, the value of the frequency histogram at the frequency bin, $j_k$, is increased by logarithm of the peak value within that zero-crossing interval, $P_{ik}$. The interval histogram for all frames are combined to form the ensemble interval histogram output, $y_a(m, b)$.

In the filter subbands, the derivative windows from which zero-crossing counts are obtained are made proportional to the inverse of the channel centre frequencies. Accordingly, the zero-crossing intervals are collected over a derivative window length of 10/$f_i$ for lower frequencies and 60/$f_i$ for higher frequencies, where $f_i$ is the filter centre frequency for the $i$-th filter [21]. For example, for a $f_i$ (which is the same as CF) of 125 Hz, the derivative window length would be 80 ms, whereas for a $f_i$ of 2000 Hz, the derivative window length would be 30 ms.

In the ZCPA, a synchronous neural firing ("spike") is simulated as the upward going zero-crossing event of the input stimulus. In the temporal-rate representation of the auditory nerve coding, the auditory nerve activity occurs in synchrony with the stimulus periods. At low characteristic frequencies (CFs) the dominant frequencies are resolved with high precision and the neural discharges of the auditory nerve fibres are phase locked to the dominant frequencies, which represent the formant positions. However, at the higher CFs the frequency resolution is poor due to the wider bandwidths, and the phase-locking of the discharges is greatly reduced. In such case, the instantaneous rate of firing conveys temporal information with fine time resolution [2].

An expression for the variance of the zero-crossing perturbation in the zero-crossing detector may be obtained following the method in [13]. Considering $D$, the number of zero-crossings, as a random variable, then the variance of the time interval perturbation (TIP) between two adjacent zero-crossings of a noisy signal, $s(t)$, corrupted by white noise, $\varphi(t)$, is given in [13] as

$$\sigma_l^2 = \frac{2A_\varphi^2 B_l/W}{(\omega_l A_l)^2} \qquad (13)$$

where $B_l$ is the bandwidth of the cochlear filter corresponding to the frequency component $l$, $l \in M$, at which the variance is measured, $A_l$ and $A_\varphi$ are signal and noise amplitudes, respectively, and $W$ is the rectangular power spectrum bandwidth of the white Gaussian noise, $\varphi(t)$. From Eqn. (13), it is seen that the zero-crossing variance, $\sigma_l^2$, at a frequency component $l$, is inversely proportional to that frequency $\omega_l$ in the input speech.

## 3.4   Synaptic Adaptation in the ZCPA Auditory Model

In this section we present a method of introducing adaptation effects in the ZCPA auditory model used as an ASR front-end. Our approach is similar to the one used by Holmberg *et al.* [14] for introducing adaptation in the MFCC parameterization, but with two significant differences. Firstly, it operates in the time domain utilizing temporal processing in a zero-crossing auditory model, which is in contrast to the spectral domain implementation in [14]. Specifically, rapid synaptic adaptation, which enhances the temporal fine structure of speech signals, cannot be implemented in the spectral domain because this fine temporal structure is removed by the spectral feature extraction process [14].

Secondly, our implementation of the auditory model consisted of simple FIR filters as cochlear filters, with only 16 filters in the filterbank for computational efficiency. Moreover, The base ZCPA auditory model does not provide any synaptic processing as observed in the mammalian auditory system through which dynamic or transient properties of speech are emphasized. The proposed method extends the capabilities of the base model by implementing synaptic temporal adaptation in it. Therefore, it is expected that the ASR performance may be improved by such integrations in the feature extraction process.

Forward temporal masking can be viewed as a consequence of auditory synaptic adaptation. Particularly, recovery from synaptic adaptation may be responsible for temporal (forward) masking observed in psychoacoustic experiments [12],[42]. Ghulam *et al.* [26] combined forward and backward masking with the pitch synchronous ZCPA, which was half-wave rectified and center clipped. The addition of masking effects was found to improve recognition rates. Our approach differs from this method in that we do not utilize a half-wave rectification, because it introduces substantial higher order harmonics of the formant frequencies [1], which degrades the formant detection, and hence the ASR performance. Moreover, the mean is also raised from the zero value, and mean values higher than the zero level result in higher sensitivity in the estimated intervals and frequencies for the ZCPA [13]. Substituting Eqn. (9) for the dominant frequency into Eqn. (13), we obtain a relation of the zero-crossing variance, $\sigma_l^2$, in terms of the zero-crossings, $D_l$, for the frequency component $l$ as

$$\sigma_l^2 = \frac{2A_\varphi^2 B_l / W (N-1)^2}{\pi^2 E\{D_l\}^2 A_l^2}.$$ (14)

From Eqn. (14), it is seen that the variance of the zero-crossing perturbations is reduced more for higher zero-crossing rates corresponding to the high frequency components than for the lower frequency components. Moreover, the variance also depends inversely on the signal amplitude $A_l$. A high-pass filter may be used to further enhance the high frequency components in speech and to take the advantage of the variance reduction property of the ZCPA. A reduction in variance of the zero-crossing perturbation may improve speech recognition by increasing the precision of the unbiased estimates of the HMM model parameters that can be obtained by an iterative algorithm such as the the expectation maximization (EM). In the case of noisy speech the covariance matrices are always decorrelated so that the diagonal elements are the individual variances of the random process.

If $\theta$ is the true value and $\hat{\theta}_N$ is an estimate of the parameter of a random variable, where $N$ is the number of observations, then for an unbiased estimate, $\theta = E\{\hat{\theta}_N\}$. In order for the estimate of a HMM parameter to converge to its true value, it is necessary that the variance of the estimates go to zero as the number of observations go to infinity

$$\lim_{N \to \infty} \text{Var}\{\hat{\theta}_N\} = \lim_{N \to \infty} E\{|\hat{\theta}_N - E\{\hat{\theta}_N\}|^2 = 0$$ (15)

For an unbiased estimate of $\theta$, it is shown using the Tchebycheff inequality [43] that for any sufficiently small $\epsilon > 0$,

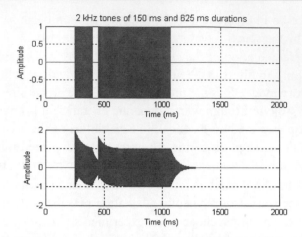

Figure 5: Rapid and short-term synaptic adaptation effects to a 2 kHz tone bursts of 150 and 625 ms durations with a time constant $\tau$=40 ms using the transfer function $H_a(z)$ (from [17])

$$\Pr\{|\hat{\theta}_N - \theta| \geq \epsilon\} \leq \frac{\text{Var}\{\hat{\theta}_N\}}{\epsilon^2} \tag{16}$$

Therefore, if the variance is sufficiently small, then the probability that the difference between the true value and the estimated value is greater than $\epsilon$ will also be smaller.

Based on the above analysis, a simplified adaption scheme suitable for ASR applications is presented. We define the first order high-pass infinite impulse response (IIR) filter function as

$$H_a(z) = \frac{10\tau f_r(1 - z^{-1})}{(10\tau f_r + 0.05) + (10\tau f_r - 0.05)z^{-1}} \tag{17}$$

where $\tau$ is the synaptic adaptation time constant in seconds and $f_r$ is the frame rate equal to 100 Hz [17]. Fig. 5 shows the transient effects of the rapid and the short-term synaptic adaptation implemented using Eqn. (17) with a time constant $\tau$=40 ms to a 2 kHz tone of 625 ms duration preceded by a tone of 150 ms may be observed. Particularly, the initial onset at the beginning of the tone and the gradual decay due to the adaptation process depending on the filter time constant can be observed in the figure.

Further in Fig. 5, effects similar to forward masking are also observed, e.g., the first tone burst is reduced in magnitude due to the presence of the second tone burst following it when the time duration separating the two tones is less than the time constant of the filter. It has been reported that forward (post-masking) and simultaneous masking can last up to 200 ms, whereas backward masking (pre-masking) are of much shorter duration, typically 10-30 ms [14]. Longer time constants are important for speech processing which may give better recognition performance. The best time constant for ASR lies between 200 and 300 ms [14]. A time constant of 250 ms was used in all our experiments utilizing temporal synaptic adaptation with a cutoff frequency of 0.636 Hz which is well below the modulation spectrum of 1-16 Hz. The modulation frequencies are regarded important for speech intelligibility [29] and the cutoff of 0.636 Hz of the high-pass filter would not interfere with the modulation frequencies. The synaptic adaptation filtering was implemented by summing the high-pass synaptic adaptation filter output with the original FIR filter output for each channel of the filterbank.

One particular issue that needs to be considered is that whether the frame sizes of 40-120 ms and the frame rates 10 ms used in auditory models, being much smaller than the adaptation time constant of 250 ms, are able to capture the effects of adaptation and the forward masking in the speech signal. The conventional frame sizes are even smaller, typically in the range of 20-25 ms. In the case of forward masking which may last upto 200 ms, the masking effect in a particular frame may depend on the statistics of the previous frames [44]. However, for the temporal synaptic adaptation used in ASR, we did not consider the effects of the previous frames, since the main objective of the adaptation process is to enhance the speech onsets, which occur within the initial 15 ms of the input stimulus. This effect may be extracted from a reasonable frame size of 80 ms which have been employed in our experiments. Moreover, the effect of synaptic adaptation on onsets is more prominent than the forward masking effect across the frames, since speech perception is more sensitive to rapid variations and dynamic changes than to the steady-state characteristics.

In the HMM a state corresponds to an acoustically stable region or a number of continuous number of frames with stationary observation vectors. Onset region detection techniques based on a hidden Markov model (HMM) utilize localization of onset regions as temporal sequences within a frame which are then combined together for speech recognition process using the HMM. Frames containing onsets regions in the speech can be detected directly from the state transition sequence in the HMM. Moreover, by using a frame advance of 10 ms a frame-based method can still capture some of the rapid synaptic adaptation effects, depending on the time alignment of the frame with respect to the onset time. In conventional feature extraction by spectral methods, detection of CVC transitions in speech which are typically dynamic in nature similar to synaptic adaptation, follow a similar detection procedure by the frame-based method. However, in the MFCC, these dynamic effects are captured more efficiently by incorporating delta-delta features.

Fig. 6 shows the post-stimulus time histogram (PSTH) obtained from the ZCPA auditory model with an IIR adaptation filter given by Eqn. (17) but with a time constant $\tau$=40 ms. The input was a 1 kHz tone of 50 ms duration. The PSTH was taken with 70 presentations of the input and collected in 400 bins with 0.2 ms bin-width. It is observed that at the signal onset, there is a rapid increase in the histogram count, followed by a rapid decrease (due to the rapid synaptic adaptation) within about 3 ms (pointer 'A'). This is followed by a more gradual and slower decay giving rise to short-term synaptic adaptation (pointer 'B') and a nearly constant steady-state response. It is observed in Fig. 6 that effects similar to the rapid synaptic adaptation may be implemented in temporal processing of speech such as in the ZCPA, not otherwise possible in spectral implementation. The Figs. 5 and 6 have been implemented with pure tone bursts to demonstrate the effects of synaptic adaptation using Eqn. (17). Speech signals are, however, more complex and the time constant of 40 ms may not be appropriate for speech recognition purposes.

Westerman et al. [38] measured the time constants in the Mongolian Gerbil to be a few milliseconds for rapid synaptic adaptation and roughly 40-60 ms for short-term synaptic adaptation. Spoor et al. [45] found that synaptic adaptation time constants in humans might differ considerably from values measured in animals. He estimated that human time

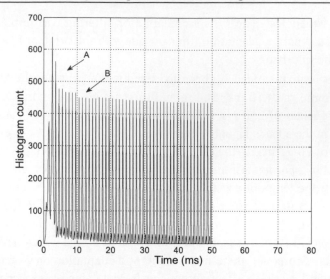

Figure 6: Post Stimulus Time Histogram (PSTH) obtained from the ZCPA showing the effects of rapid synaptic adaptation (pointer 'A') and short-term synaptic adaptation (pointer 'B'). The PSTH was obtained with a synaptic adaptation filter with a time constant $\tau=40$ ms and was taken with 70 presentations of a 1 kHz tone input of 50 ms duration in 400 bins with a bin width of 0.2 ms.

constants for recovery from synaptic adaptation are about a factor of four longer compared to gerbil data. It has been reported that forward (post-masking) and simultaneous masking can last up to 200 ms whereas backward masking (pre-masking) are of much shorter duration, typically 10-30 ms [46]. This was verified by Holmberg *et al.* by a series of experiments using Aurora 2 and 3 speech corpus and evaluating word error rates for a range of synaptic adaptation time constants. It was found that for the case of clean training with Wiener filtering, the best time constant is 80 ms, but for the case with adaptation and multi-condition training, it was found that the best time constant lies between 200 ms and 300 ms. Therefore, a synaptic adaptation time constant of 240 ms was chosen by Holmberg *et al.* in the experimentations. This time constant is also motivated by the notion that higher levels in the auditory pathway, with presumably longer adaptation time constants than the auditory nerve, contribute to the temporal processing of speech. The 240-ms time constant is consistent with other auditory models that have been used as ASR front ends [47] and with the high-pass corner frequency employed in RASTA [29] processing. Motivated by these experimental results, we have chosen a time constant of 250 ms as the adaptation time constant in all our experiments for temporal synaptic adaptation. This time constant gives a cutoff frequency of 0.636 Hz which is well below the modulation spectrum of 1-16 Hz. The modulation frequencies are regarded important for speech intelligibility [29] and the cutoff of 0.636 Hz of the high-pass filter would not interfere with the modulation frequencies. The synaptic adaptation filtering was implemented by summing the high-pass synaptic adaptation filter output with the original FIR filter output for each channel of the filterbank.

Fig. 7 shows the ZCPA with the simplified synaptic adaptation used as a preprocessing front-end. The synaptic adaptation as implemented in Eqn. (17) was introduced in each filter channel with a time constant $\tau=250$ ms. The input speech was first normalized between

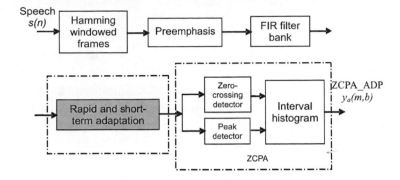

Figure 7: The ZCPA auditory model with the synaptic adaptation (ZCPA_ADP) processed on a frame data of 80 ms.

$\pm 1$ to reduce the effects of loudness. Normalization also improves noise performance by enhancing spectral contrast. Speech frames were pre-emphasized to model the outer and the middle ear functionalities that approximate the unequal sensitivity of human hearing at different frequencies. A pre-emphasis coefficient of -0.97 was used. It was then processed by a bank of 16 finite impulse response (FIR) filters of order 70 with the CFs uniformly spaced on the equivalent rectangular bandwidth (ERB) scale [48] between 10-3500 Hz.

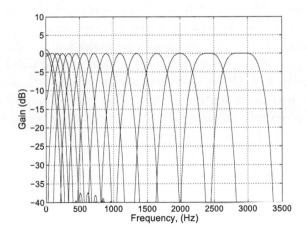

Figure 8: Frequency response of the perceptual FIR filterbank consisting of 16 FIR filters each of order 70 with the centre frequencies of each channel spaced at the ERB scale.

The frequency response of the perceptual FIR filterbank is shown in Fig. 8. Our choice of FIR filters for the filterbank was motivated by the fact that FIR filters consistently performed better than carefully designed cochlear filters when applied in ASR applications [13]. In most applications, real-time operations through hardware implementation is often the main goal. All digital signal processors (DSPs) available have architectures in powers of two, $2^n$, where $n$ is the number of available bits. This is particularly suited to FIR filtering in hardware. Moreover, FIR filters are always stable, have exactly linear phase, and are simple to implement. However, FIR filters of particularly higher orders may also introduce substantial lag or time delay. Since the outputs are extracted as frequency histogram counts, the time delay effects on the output are not considered [13].

To reduce computational time, we implemented the simplified model with fewer number of filters with some optimization of the parameters and feature extraction algorithm. However, fewer number of filters result in greater frequency overlap of adjacent frequency channels, particularly at higher frequencies due to wider bandwidths. This would result in a lower frequency resolution and an additional effect of loss of synchrony at higher frequencies. However, both of these effects are consistent with perceptual properties of the inner ear and the cochlea. This is also supported by the observation that decreasing the number of electrodes in cochlear implant patients have little or no effects on speech intelligibility [24]. Gajic *et al.* [21] made a study of the ASR performance obtained by several different choices of filter bandwidths and number of histogram bins and has quantified the results. It was observed that the choice of filter bandwidths had a significant influence on the ASR performance, while it was not very sensitive to the particular choice of the number of histogram bins. However, the influence of increased number of filters was tested by evaluating features based on 16 and 20 filters, and no significant performance difference was observed [21].

In the ZCPA, the width of the derivative windows in units of time over which the features are extracted are functions of the centre frequencies of the filterbank. In temporal processing it is usually required to use large window sizes especially for lower frequency channels to capture about 10 periods of the signal for the accumulation of temporal information [21]. Although longer time windows give better parameter estimates, the window size should not be too large to violate the stationarity assumption in the short-term processing method. Considering these, the largest window size was limited to 80 ms corresponding to the lowest frequency channel. In each filter output, inverse of zero-crossing intervals were collected in 26 frequency bins uniformly spaced between 10-4000 Hz on the ERB scale. The interval histogram was weighted by the logarithm of the peak value within two successive zero-crossings. Frame data was processed at a frame rate of 10 ms. The histogram was normalized between 0 and +1 with respect to the maximum value. Normalising the histogram produces two effects. Firstly, it limits the dynamic range of the histogram and secondly, the compression due to normalising reduces the effects of any biasing in the histogram. Thirteen cepstra were generated and retained from each speech frame.

Figs. 9 (a) and (b) show the spectrogram of the 35-th frame for the male CV utterance /ba/ without adaption and with temporal synaptic adaptation with $\tau$=250 ms, respectively [17]. The processing started at the 35th frame of the whole utterance /ba/ and ended after the processing of that frame. A single frame was taken to study the time-frequency characteristics within this frame for greater resolution and for comparison for the two cases with synaptic adaptation and without synaptic adaptation. It is assumed that the steady-state vowel /a/ and the corresponding formants are captured in this frame in addition to the high frequency speech segments in that frame. It is observed in (b) that the high frequency segments are enhanced by the application of the temporal synaptic adaptation strategy. However, the low frequency formants are not affected.

Fig. 10 shows a spectrogram-like (narrowband) time-frequency plots of the point pro-

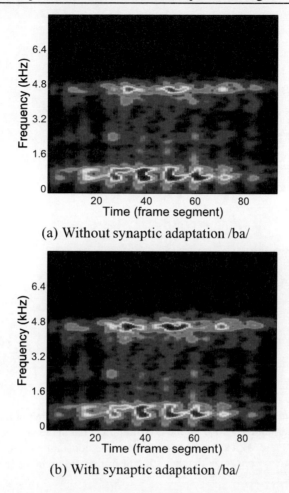

(a) Without synaptic adaptation /ba/

(b) With synaptic adaptation /ba/

Figure 9: Spectrogram of the ZCPA for the 35-th frame of the male utterance /ba/ in clean condition (a) without synaptic adaptation, and (b) with synaptic adaptation with a time constant $\tau$=250 ms. It is seen that the high frequency segments are enhanced by the application of the adaptation filtering.

cess obtained from the simulated firing pattern for the voiced plosive /ba/ in clean conditions. The plot was obtained using 120 FIR filters from the upward zero-crossing events of the waveform and was collected over a fixed derivative window of 80 ms for each frame. It has been implemented for greater detailed modelling of the the peripheral auditory system and is not suitable for speech recognition applications because of computational costs and complexities. The effect of fixed derivative windows, in contrast to channel dependent derivative windows in other implementations in this project, is a histogram bias at high frequencies which is equivalent to a pre-emphasis operation. The utterance 'ba' was chosen to emphasize the CV transitions for the plosive /b/ followed by the formants associated with the vowel /a/. The formant structures are visible as a narrowband spectrogram. In Fig. 10, the upper panel shows the base ZCPA without synaptic adaptation and the lower panel shows the same plot with temporal synaptic adaptation. It is seen in the upper panel that the burst after the closure is emphasized with temporal synaptic adaptation in the high

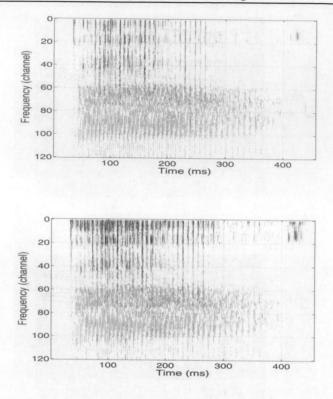

Figure 10: Spectrogram-like time-frequency plot (narrowband) of the point process obtained from the simulated firing pattern of the ZCPA for the CV utterance /ba/ in clean condition without synaptic adaptation (upper panel) and with synaptic adaptation (time constant $\tau$=250 ms)(lower panel). The lower panel shows enhanced onsets with adaptation at higher frequencies (corresponding to lower channels).

frequency regions (lower numbered channels), indicating increased discharge rate at higher frequencies.

## 3.5   CV Discriminatory Characteristics of Temporal Synaptic Adaptation

Measuring the discrimination effectiveness of feature vectors is an important method of determining robustness which aids in the selection of optimal features for a given dimensionality. Compared to conventional speech features such as MFCC and the PLP, temporal auditory models usually employ larger window lengths which is particularly sensitive to non-stationary segments of speech. These non-stationary segments such as the consonant-vowel (CV) transitions are poorly represented in such models. To test the effectiveness of the adaptation model in CV discrimination, we implemented three experiments - frequency discrimination, vowel clustering by grouped scatter plots and LDA separability measures using within class and between class scatter matrices, which are explained in the following three subsections.

The speech corpus used for the CV discrimination tasks was the UCLA-SPAPL CV corpus which is an extensive database of 1728 isolated CV utterances by four speakers

(2 males and 2 females). Each CV was spoken in 8 different annotations by each of the four speakers in 18 consonants, each consonant in three vowel contexts, thus constituting a total of 1728 utterances. For example, corresponding to the plosive /b/, the utterances are /ba/,/bee/ and /boo/ in three vowel contexts /a/,/ee/ and /oo/. The CV combinations were digitally recorded at a sampling rate of 16 kHz, and are shown labeled in ASCII in Table 1.

### 3.5.1   Frequency Discrimination by Synaptic Adaptation

The IIR adaptation filtering primarily enhances the high frequency components associated with frication and voice onsets. Since most speech energies are concentrated in the lower frequency regions, the contributions to the high frequency histograms were mainly due to the increased zero-crossing counts instead of the contributions of the interval peak values. Hence, a quantitative measure of the effects of the high pass synaptic adaptation filtering on speech perception could be obtained by analyzing the histogram counts at the output of the higher frequency channels compared to the lower frequency channels. For this discrimination, we chose a threshold frequency of 1340 Hz. The choice of this frequency is rather heuristic, and is partly based on consideration that it should be higher than the first formant, which is the dominant formant of the common vowels. Again a too high threshold may eliminate the high frequency artefacts of speech such as consonants (voiced and unvoiced plosives and the fricatives), which may compromise the experimental results.

Table 1: The UCLA-SPAPL CV corpus with the consonant types and the corresponding vowel tokens.

| Articulation | Consonants | Vowel contexts |
|---|---|---|
| Voiced plosives | /b/,/d/,/g/ | |
| Aspirated plosives | /p/,/t/,/k | /a/ as in "bought" |
| Nasals | /m/,/n/ | /ee/ as in "beat" |
| Fricatives | /s/,/Z/,/sh/,/SH/ /f/,/V/,/th/,/TH/ | /oo/ as in "boot" |
| Affricates | /j/,/ch/ | |

The vowel discrimination with synaptic adaptation was measured as the percentage increase in the histogram counts with synaptic adaptation ($ZC_{adp}$) over the histogram counts without synaptic adaptation (ZC), as obtained using the formula

$$\frac{\sum_f ZC_{adp}(f) - \sum_f ZC(f)}{\sum_f ZC(f)} \times 100\%, \qquad f \geq 1340 \quad \text{Hz.} \qquad (18)$$

The consonant types /b/,/d/,/g/,/p/,/t/,/k/,/m/,/n/,/s/,/SH/,/j/,/ch/ in the three vowel contexts /a/,/ee/and /oo/ were used in the experiment. The results are summarized in Fig. 11. It is observed that the largest increase in the histogram counts is achieved for the fricatives, which contain substantial high frequency components. As for the vowels, the largest percentage increase are recorded for the vowel /ee/ in all consonant types (14.16 % for /SHee/), followed by the vowel /oo/ in fricatives (11.49 %) and affricates (9.19 %). This may be due to the higher second formant for the vowel /ee/ (1730 Hz) compared to vowel /a/ (1090 Hz) and vowel /oo/ (870 Hz).

### 3.5.2    Vowel Clustering with Synaptic Adaptation

ASR relies to a larger extent on the correct classification of vowels than consonants [25]. The mixture likelihood approach to clustering, which is a class of unsupervised learning, is based on maximization of the likelihood estimation of finite mixture models utilizing the EM algorithm. A more simple measure of unsupervised clustering may be obtained by the linear discriminant analysis. In our experiment, a qualitative measure of clustering of the three vowel classes with synaptic adaptation was obtained by grouped scatter plots of the CV utterances in the UCLA-SPAPL database, which was represented by an utterance matrix, each row corresponding to an utterance represented by a $m$-cepstrum vector in the $m$-dimensional space. In two dimensional linear discrimination, any two fixed dimensions of the utterance matrix may be plotted as the $x$ and $y$ coordinates, with the means associated with each class as the centroid. The discrimination among the classes is essentially reflected in the extent of the correlation between these two components of the feature vector set, as exemplified by scattering from the individual class centroids. For our experiments, we selected the voiced plosives /b/,/d/,/g/ and the aspirated plosives /p/,/t/,/k/ in three vowel contexts /a/,/ee/ and /oo/, for a total of 18 utterances. The 18 CVs were spoken by 2 male and 2 female speakers, each speaker uttering the same CV in five different annotations, thus constituting a total of 360 CVs. Features were extracted from each utterance from an interval histogram at the rate of 13 cepstra per frame. These were collapsed into a single vector by taking the mean of all the frames, thus converting the 360 CVs into a single 360x13 utterance matrix.

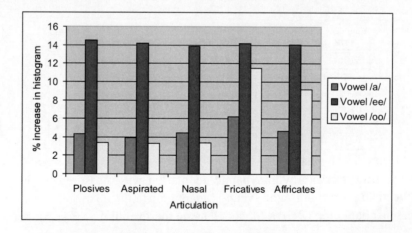

Figure 11: Graph showing effects of temporal synaptic adaptation on speech articulation as percentage increase in the high frequency histogram counts in the ZCPA with temporal synaptic adaptation ($ZC_{adp}$) over the base ZCPA.

The two dimensional grouped scatter plots of the utterance matrix are shown in Fig. 12 without synaptic adaptation in (a) and with synaptic adaptation in (b). The increased clustering of the vowel /ee/ having a higher second formant (1730 Hz) is observed in (b). However, the other vowels /aa/ and /oo/ having lower second formants (1090 Hz for /a/ and 870 Hz for /oo/) appears to be just as scattered. This further emphasizes the role of synaptic adaptation on high frequency articulation and dynamic behaviours of speech. Improved speech recognition performance may result from this effect.

## 3.6 Linear Discriminant Analysis by Class Separability Measure

Class separability measures may be used to determine the discrimination effectiveness of a particular feature vector. In Sec. 3.5.2, a qualitative representation of vowel clustering with synaptic adaptation was presented as grouped scatter plots. In this section, we present a quantitative measure of separability among the vowel classes. A quantitative measure of the separability, or divergence among the three vowel classes may be determined by one of several methods such as Kulback-Liebler distance measure between density functions, and the Brattacharayya distance. However, determination of these separability measures are feasible only when a Gaussian assumption of the distribution of the class members is valid.

A simpler and more general quantitative criterion may be obtained from the scatter characteristics of the feature vector samples in the $m$-dimensional space using the linear discriminant analysis approach based on the within-class and between-class scatter matrices [49]. It utilizes a linear transformation which maps the feature space into a lower dimensional space such that a class separability criterion is optimized.

For our experiment, we obtained the two quantitative measures of separability, $J_1$ and $J_2$, among the three vowel classes utilizing the three voiced plosives /b/,/d,/g/, each in three vowel contexts, /a/,/ee/,/oo/. The 9 CVs were uttered by 4 speakers in 5 different styles, for a total of 180 CV utterances (with 60 utterances in each of the three vowel classes). The two quantitative measures (unnormalized) of separability, $J_1$ and $J_2$ are obtained as

$$J_1 = \text{tr}(S_w^{-1} S_b) \tag{19}$$

$$J_2 = \frac{\det(S_b + S_w)}{\det(S_w)}. \tag{20}$$

where

$$S_w = \frac{1}{(N-1)} \sum_{l=1}^{L} \sum_{\mathbf{x} \in w_l} (\mathbf{x} - \mu_l)(\mathbf{x} - \mu_l)^T \tag{21}$$

$$S_b = \frac{1}{N} \sum_{l=1}^{L} N_l(\mu_l - \mu)(\mu_l - \mu)^T. \tag{22}$$

In the above equations, $\{\mathbf{x}_n\}_{n=1}^{K}$ is a set of feature vectors each of dimension $K = 13$, $N$=180 is the total number of observations in the three vowel classes, $N_l$ is the observations in each class $l$, $l \in L$, where $L$=3 is the number of classes, $\mu_l$ is the class mean vector and $\mu$ is the total mean. It is seen that $S_w$ is the covariance matrix of individual classes summed over all classes and its traces are sum of variances. $J_1$ takes large values when samples in the $l$-dimensional space are well clustered around their mean, within each class, and the clusters of the different classes are well separated. It has the advantage of being invariant under linear transformations [49]. $J_2$ gives an alternate criterion with determinants used in place of traces. This is justified for scatter matrices that are symmetric positive definite and thus

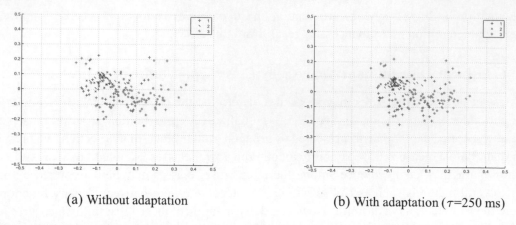

(a) Without adaptation                    (b) With adaptation ($\tau$=250 ms)

Figure 12: Scatter plots of voiced and unvoiced plosives /b/,/d/,/g/ and /p/,/t/,/k/, respectively, in three vowel contexts /a/,/ee/,/oo/ for (a) Base ZCPA and (b) ZCPA with synaptic adaptation ( $\tau$=250 ms) in clean condition. Increased clustering is observed for vowel /ee/ in (b).

their eigenvalues are positive and the trace is equivalent to the sum of the eigenvalues [49]. Hence, these measures are useful benchmarks of separability of feature vectors for speech recognition. The computed measures of separability, $J_1$ and $J_2$ (unnormalized), are shown in Table 2. It is observed that with synaptic adaptation (ZCPA _ADP) demonstrates higher between class separability than the base ZCPA for the three vowel classes /a/,/ee/,/oo/.

# 4   Speech Recognition using Two-tone Suppression

Neural two-tone suppression is a phenomenon of the human auditory system in which there is a reduction to one tone due to the presence of another tone at a nearby frequency. Two-tone suppression is a non-linear property of the cochlea and originates in the mechanical phenomena at the basilar membrane (BM) arising from an interaction between the outer hair cells and the BM [50]. Lyon [3] has proposed that although the main source of two-tone suppression is cochlear non-linearity, the nature of that non-linearity is not "saturation". It is more like an automatic gain control in which the mechanical gain gradually reduces as a function of the response level over a very wide dynamic range of input power levels. The gain control or multichannel compression by itself improves audibility. For a probe tone located at a particular CF, and a suppressor tone with frequencies both higher and lower than the CF, the magnitude of suppression increases monotonically with suppressor intensity [50]. Moreover, the rate of growth of suppression magnitude with suppressor intensity is higher for suppressors in the region below CF than for those in the region above CF. Suppression has also been observed for a probe embedded in a band of noise [51].

The gain control or multichannel compression in the auditory system may improve audibility. However, the asymmetric amplification due to compression may result in the degradation of the spectral contrast. This degradation may be prevented by introducing two-tone suppression as observed in the peripheral auditory system. The method may be applied to the speech processors of hearing aid and cochlear implant patients to improve audibility and speech intelligently through low-power analog VLSI implementations [18]. This property of spectral enhancement associated with two-tone suppression indicates that it may also be usefully utilized for performance enhancement in automatic speech recognition.

## 4.1   The Companding Architecture

A procedure to reproduce two-tone suppression in a cochlear model as observed in the biological cochlea was proposed by Kates [52] utilizing a traveling wave amplification with a cascade of adaptive-$Q$ filter sections. However, the disadvantage of such a system is that it is not only complex, but may cause interactions between the feedback and the feedforward parameters in a traveling wave architecture. As a result, Turicchia $et$ $al.$ [18] proposed an alternate methodology, the companding strategy, which performed multichannel syllabic compression and spectral contrast enhancement via two-tone suppression simultaneously. Hence, the companding strategy may be effectively used in an ASR front-end for the enhancement of recognition performance.

The principle of companding is based on the non-linear interactions between a compression block and an expansion block. It utilizes non-coupled filterbanks with the compression-expansion blocks to reproduce the compressibility effects of the two-tone suppression in the biological cochlea parametrically by a set of independent and programmable parameters. The concept of companding is not new and has been applied in other fields of speech processing, particularly for improving the signal-to-noise ratio in cases where the dominant noise occurs after the compression block. It has also been applied in novel analog filtering circuits [53],[54].

Table 2: Quantitative measures of separability (unnormalized), $J_1$ and $J_2$, among the three vowel classes /a/,/ee/ and /oo/ based on LDA of the within- and between-class scatter matrices of base ZCPA and ZCPA with adaptation.

|              | J1    | J2     |
|--------------|-------|--------|
| Base ZCPA    | 21.98 | 112.50 |
| ZCPA_ADP     | 24.49 | 120.49 |

The companding architecture is shown in Fig. 13, the detailed implementation of which is given in [18]. Every channel has a pre-filter, a compression block, a post-filter, and an expansion block. The two-tone suppression effect is produced due to the presence of the second filterbank between the compression and the expansion blocks, and the non-linear interaction between signals in the first filterbank, the compressor, and the second filterbank. The pre-filterbank and the post-filterbank have the same perceptual frequency scale, but the bandwidth are different for the two cases - the first filterbank is broadly tuned, while the second filterbank is sharply tuned. Both the compression block and the expansion block consist of a feed-forward path made up of an envelope detector (ED), a non-linear block and a multiplier. The envelope detector consists of a half-wave rectifier followed by a low-pass filter. The dynamics of the compression and the expansion is controlled by the time constant of the ED ($\tau_{ED}$), which is scaled with the resonant frequency, $f_i$, for the channel $i$ such that $\tau_{ED}=w\tau_i$, where $w=10$ and $\tau_i = 1/(2\pi f_i)$.

The compression and expansion characteristics are non-linear and are determined by the parameters $n_1$ and $n_2$, respectively as shown in Fig. 13. Particularly, the exponent $n_1$ in the compression block determines the compression for values $n_1 < 1$. However, the parameter $n_2$ determines the overall compression characteristics of the system. For values of $0 < n_2 < 1$, the effect of the channel is to implement syllabic compression with an overall compression index of $n_2$. Expansion takes place in the expansion block and depends on the ratio $n_2/n_1$ when $n_2 > n_1$.

If we represent the input by $x_0$ given by

$$x_0 = a_1 \sin(\omega_1 t) + a_2 \sin(\omega_2 t + \varphi_0) \tag{23}$$

where $\omega_1$ and $\omega_2$ are the frequencies of two tones in $x_0$, then the output, $y_0$, is given in [18] as

$$
\begin{aligned}
y_0 &= \left[ a_1^{n_2/n_1} (a_1 + f_2 a_2)^{n_2(n_1-1)/n_1} \right] \sin(\omega_1 t + \varphi_1 + \vartheta_1) \\
&= \left[ a_1 \left( \frac{a_1 + f_2 a_2}{a_1} \right)^{(n_1-1)/n_1} \right]^{n_2} \sin(\omega_1 t + \varphi_1 + \vartheta_1).
\end{aligned}
\tag{24}
$$

It is seen from Eqn. (24) that the presence of a second tone (suppressor) with amplitude $a_2$ at a frequency $\omega_2$ suppresses the tone with amplitude $a_1$ at frequency $\omega_1$. If only a single tone is present such that $a_2=0$, then for $n_2=1$, the output has the amplitude of $a_1$ only.

## 4.2   Temporal Companding in the ZCPA Auditory Model

In this section, the biologically inspired companding strategy which performs simultaneous multichannel syllabic compression and spectral contrast enhancement via two-tone suppression is implemented in a ZCPA auditory model used as an ASR front-end. There are several significant differences between this implementation and the implementation by [18]. Firstly, in [18], it is implemented in the spectral domain, whereas we implemented the companding in the time domain using a zero-crossing algorithm, which we term as temporal companding. The advantages of temporal processing of speech have been stated in Sec. 1. Secondly, we propose several enhancements to the original companding model in our temporal implementation. These are (1) The suppression model proposed in [18] utilized cascaded second order biquad filter sections with 50 channels. This is not only complex, but also computationally expensive. The temporal companding was implemented using simple linear phase FIR bandpass filters with only 16 channels for computational efficiency and hardware implementation. The FIR filterbank has been explained in detail in Sec. 3.4 for the case of synaptic adaptation. (2) In the companding scheme in [18], a final summation across all the channels were taken to obtain a summary output. This might cause interference due to phase differences across channels due to adjacent channel interferences in the filterbank outputs. The companding scheme alleviated this by applying the first order lowpass filter twice for obtaining zero phase, once in the forward time direction and once in the reverse time direction. In the ZCPA, instead of taking a final summation at the output across all channels, the usual ensemble interval histogram is constructed from the zero-crossing intervals. Since the phase information is not considered in a frequency histogram construction [13], this eliminated the additional filtering required to minimize the phase effects. (3)

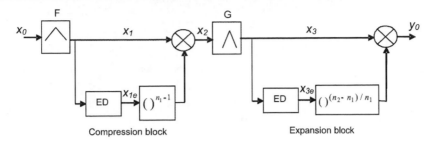

Figure 13: The companding architecture for a single channel for implementing the two-tone suppression effect. The parameters $n_1$ and $n_2$ determine the compression/expansion, that is, compression takes place for $n_1 < 1$, and expansion for $n_2 > n_1$ (from Turicchia *et al.* [18])

The method also extends the capabilities of the ZCPA auditory model with the perceptual feature of two-tone suppression.

Fig. 14 shows the ZCPA auditory model with the two-tone suppression using the temporal companding method. It consists of a companding stage followed by a ZCPA feature extraction stage. In the companding stage, two filterbanks are used - a compression filterbank, $F$, and a expansion filterbank, $G$, each consisting of 16 FIR filters spaced between 10-3500 Hz at the ERB frequency scale. However, the compression filterbank has bandwidths which are 20% higher than the second filterbank. In each channel, the compression block and the expansion block consisted of an envelope detector (ED) (a half-wave rectifier followed by a first order low-pass filter) and a non-linear unit depending on values of $n_1$ and $n_2$, as shown in Fig. 13. The filter time constant was made inversely proportional to the centre frequency of the respective channel filter ($\tau_i = 1/(2\pi f_i)$), where $i$ is the channel index. The half-wave rectifier, Eqn. (25), is given in [1] which combines the rectification process with the compressive non-linear saturation effects as observed in the biological cochlea. This being a tangent function has the characteristics of being exponential for negative inputs, linear for small input values and compressive for larger signals,

$$\begin{aligned} y &= 1 + A\tan^{-1}Bx, & x > 0 \\ &= e^{ABx}, & x \le 0 \end{aligned} \tag{25}$$

where $x$ and $y$ are the input and output, respectively, and $A$=10 and $B$=65 are constants equivalent to gain.

The half-wave rectifier removes the negative values from an input speech signal and normally can not be used for feature extraction using the zero crossing algorithm since all zero-crossings are removed. However, when used with companding, feature extraction is still possible primarily due to the presence of the forward path after the FIR filtering, and due to the presence of the multiplier in Fig. 13. The values for the compression and the expansion parameter were $n_1$=0.5 and $n_2$=1.1, respectively. For these set of parameters, the compression applied is ($n_1$-1)= -0.5, as seen from the compression block in Fig. 13. An interval histogram, $y_t$, was constructed (Eqn. (26)) from the zero-crossing intervals which were collected in 26 frequency bins spaced at the ERB frequency scale between 10-4000 Hz,

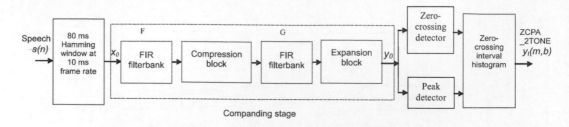

Figure 14: The ZCPA with companding for the implementation of two-tone suppression. The features are extracted into an interval histogram by a zero-crossing detector and a peak detector (from [17])

$$y_t(m,b) = Z\{y_0\} = \sum_{i=1}^{C} \sum_{k=1}^{D_i-1} \log(P_{ik}+1)\delta_{bj_k}, \qquad 1 \le b < R \qquad (26)$$

where $Z\{.\}$ is an operator for transformation by the zero-crossing algorithm, $C$ is the number of bandpass cochlear filters, $D_i$ is the number of zero-crossings in the $i$-th filter in the $m$-th frame, $\delta_{bj}$ is the Kronecker delta defined in Eqn. (12) and $R$ is the number of histogram bins indexed by $b$ and weighted by peak values $P_{ik}$ within a zero-crossing interval. Thirteen cepstra were collected from each frame at a frame rate of 10 ms.

A relationship between the variance, $\sigma_l^2$, of the time interval perturbation of the zero-crossings, and the compression and expansion parameters, $n_1$ and $n_2$ may be obtained using Eqns. (14) and (24). For any input with two tones with amplitudes $a_1$ and $a_2$ with the suppressor tone, $a_2$, fixed at a constant frequency component $l$, and the probe tone, $a_1$, at a frequency component close to $l$, the variance of the zero-crossing perturbation may be expressed using Eqn. (14) as

$$\sigma_l^2 = \frac{2A_\varphi^2 B_l/W(N-1)^2}{\left[a_1\left(\frac{a_1+f_2a_2}{a_1}\right)^{(n_1-1)/n_1}\right]^{2n_2} \pi^2 E\{D_l\}^2} \qquad (27)$$

where $A_\varphi$ is the noise amplitude, $W$ is the bandwidth of the noise power spectrum, $E\{D_l\}$ is the expected value of the zero-crossing count $D_l$, and $N$ is the total number of samples from which $D_l$ is computed. Since the companding scheme uses two filterbanks of different bandwidths, the filter bandwidth $B_l$ in the above equation may be approximated by the average bandwidth of the compression block filter and the expansion block filter.

Fig. 15 shows the synthesized short vowel /a/ for the base ZCPA and ZCPA with temporal companding for $A$=10 and $B$=65 with the two values of compression, -0.5 and -4.0 corresponding to $n_1$=1 and 4.5, respectively as shown in Fig. 13, with the expansion maintained at the same level for both the cases. It is observed that when we used a compression of -0.5 as used in [18], the dominant first formant at 730 Hz was slightly suppressed than the base ZCPA (without compression), the second formant at 1090 Hz was enhanced, and the third formant at 2240 Hz was also enhanced, but to a much larger extent. This degraded the formant contrast with respect to the first and the second formants. The greater enhancement of the third formant is due to the fact that the higher gain provided by the $A$ and $B$ parameters in the half-wave rectification (Eqn. (25)) increased the peak values contributing to the histogram weights. The higher frequencies are affected more than the lower frequencies due to the compression and expansion effects of the companding algorithm. We, therefore, increased the compression from -0.5 to -4.0 by changing the exponent for the compression block in Fig. 13 from $(n_1\text{-}1)$ to $(n_1\text{-}4.5)$, keeping $n_1$ and $n_2$ parameters the same as before. This would have the effect of increasing compression without affecting the expansion. By this strategy, it is observed that the second formant is slightly reduced while the third formant is significantly reduced, with an overall effect of improving the spectral contrasts. Therefore, a compression of -4.0 was used in all of our experiments.

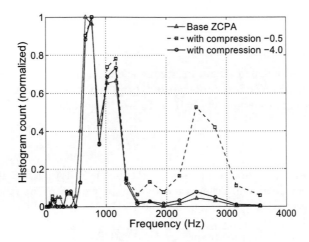

Figure 15: Comparison of the vowel /a/ with the first three formants obtained from the base ZCPA, ZCPA with temporal companding with two values of compression -0.5 and -4.0. It is seen that the third formant is emphasized significantly due to the zero-crossing effects in the temporal companding.

The two-tone suppression effect at the output of the temporal companding stage is demonstrated in Fig. 16 when excited with a pair of tones (suppressor and a probe tone). The suppressor tone was fixed at 1 kHz keeping the amplitude constant at 0 dB, while the frequency of the probe tone was varied from 100 Hz to 3 kHz, maintaining the amplitude constant at -20 dB. A compression of -4.0 was used in the companding scheme. At the output of the companding stage, the probe tone (measured in dB) demonstrated suppression effects in the vicinity of the suppressor tone for frequencies both lower and higher than the probe tone frequency. The output probe tone in the figure has a higher magnitude than the input because of the gain effects of parameters $A$ and $B$ in the half-wave rectification ( Eqn. (25)).

Since the output of the ZCPA is in the form of a histogram, we next studied the effect of two-tone suppression on the ZCPA interval histogram. In the auditory system, there is an aggregate reduction of firing rate (and an equivalent reduction in intensity) of a fibre due to the presence of a suppressor tone of a nearby frequency in another fibre. In the ZCPA, it is expected that this effect should be reflected in the reduction in the histogram count of a frequency bin in the vicinity of the frequency of a suppressor. Table 3 shows the data with

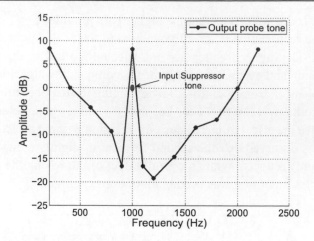

Figure 16: Two-tone suppressed output of a companding stage implemented in a ZCPA when excited with an input consisting of a pair of sinusoids (suppressor and a probe tone). A compression of -4.0 was used in the companding with $A$=10 and $B$=65 (Eqn. (25)).

Table 3: Table showing the two-tone suppression effect on the ZCPA interval histogram count. It is observed that there is a reduction of histogram counts in the vicinity of the suppressor as the probe tone approaches the stronger suppressor tone fixed at 1 kHz.

| Probe frequency $f_2$, Hz | ZCPA histogram count |
|---|---|
| 500 | 17941 |
| 800 | 17511 |
| 1000 | 17618 |
| 1200 | 17545 |
| 1500 | 17770 |
| 1800 | 18745 |

the same setup as in Fig. 16 but the output taken, instead of at the output of the companding stage, at the output of the ZCPA by summing all the bin counts of the histogram as the frequency of the probe tone is varied. It is observed from Table 3 that the histogram shows a similar suppression effect, that is, there is a reduction in the histogram counts as the probe tone approaches the stronger suppressor tone fixed at 1 kHz.

Fig. 17 shows the time-frequency plots of the ZCPA interval histogram with and without the two-tone suppression effects in Figs. (a) and (b), respectively, for the utterance of the digit 'one' in clean condition. The magnitude inhibition due to the suppression effect, which depends on the stimulus intensity within the utterance, is seen along the vertical $z$-axis. The suppression is more prominent at lower frequencies (higher histogram bins) due to the fact that the lower frequencies have higher intensities.

## 4.3   Comparison of CV Discrimination with Synaptic Adaptation and Two-Tone Suppression

We further compared the CV discrimination characteristics of the synaptic adaptation and the two-tone suppression using the UCLA-SPAPL CV corpus (Sec. 3.5). For the comparison, we define a frequency discrimination (FD) parameter as

$$FD = \frac{\sum_{f>1340Hz} ZC(f)}{\sum_{f\leq1340Hz} ZC(f)} \tag{28}$$

where ZC is the zero-crossing count as obtained from the interval histogram. A higher value of FD would indicate a high frequency enhancement or a low frequency suppression of a CV utterance, and vice versa. The high and low frequency discrimination was based on a frequency of 1340 Hz. The choice of this frequency was rather heuristic and was partly based on consideration that it should be higher than the first formant, which is the dominant formant of the common vowels. The comparison of CV discrimination by the two algorithms of synaptic adaptation and the two-tone suppression in clean conditions is given in Table 4.

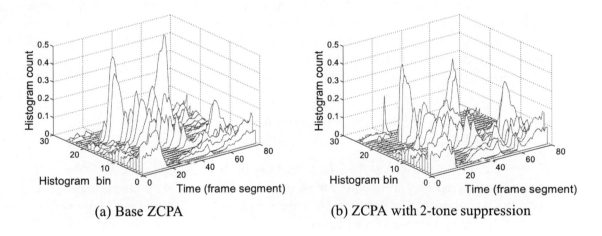

(a) Base ZCPA                    (b) ZCPA with 2-tone suppression

Figure 17: The 3-D time-frequency plots of the ZCPA histogram for (a) ZCPA and (b) ZCPA with two-tone suppressed output for the digit utterance 'one' in clean condition. The magnitude inhibition may be observed along the $z$-axis (vertical) at lower frequencies (higher histogram bins).

It is observed from Table 4 that both synaptic adaptation and two-tone suppression have a higher FD than the base ZCPA for all articulation types. Moreover, in all cases, the vowel /ee/ has a higher FD than the vowels /a/ and /oo/. This result is expected since /ee/ has higher frequency formants than /a/ and /oo/. However, a significant observation made in Table 4 is that for the vowel /ee/, the increase in FD was higher with synaptic adaptation than with two-tone suppression (3.33 vs. 2.96 for /bee/), while for vowels /a/ and /oo/, the increase in FD is higher with two-tone suppression than with synaptic adaptation (0.23 vs. 0.40 for /ba/ and 0.51 vs. 0.78 for /boo/). This result emphasizes the frequency dependence of the perceptual features in speech, with the synaptic adaptation having a greater effect on high frequency articulation, and the two-tone suppression having greater effect on low-frequency articulation. One exception to this rule is observed for /jee/ where two-tone suppression performed better than synaptic adaptation. This may be due to the fact that this CV contains substantial frication in addition to having higher formants, and the increase in FD value is mainly due to the reduction in the low frequency counts.

## 4.4   HMM Recognition Results

In this section, we make a comparison of the recognition performances of synaptic adaptation and two-tone suppression as word error rates using continuous density HMM and isolated digits TIdigits/NOISEX 92 speech corpus. The isolated digits were chosen over continuous digits to make a better comparison of the two algorithms of adaptation and two-tone suppression for speech recognition. There were 55 male speakers in the training set, each speaker with two utterances of the digits 1-9, 'oh' and 'zero' (total 1210 utterances in the training set) and a separate set of 31 male speakers in the test set, each speaker with 2 utterances of the digits 1-9, 'oh' and 'zero' (total 682 utterances in the test set). Continuous Gaussian density HMM with 15 states per digit, 5 mixture components per state with diagonal covariances were used to define each model. A 3-state silence model was inserted at the beginning of each utterance. The Baum-Welch re-estimation using a flat-start scheme and 12 estimation iterations was used for training under clean conditions. Test speech was corrupted with 4 different types of additive noise from the NOISEX 92 database - Gaussian white noise, factory noise, babble noise and Volvo noise. In the testing phase, a left-to-right Viterbi decoder using word-level lattice network, a dictionary and a token passing algorithm with dynamic programming was used for decoding.

### 4.4.1   Comparison of Recognition Performances of the Base Models - ZCPA, MFCC and PLP

We first make a comparison of the effectiveness of the base ZCPA (without the perceptual features added) auditory front-end in a speech recognition task with the standard MFCC (with the zeroth coefficient) and the more perceptual PLP. Table 5 shows the word error rates as percentage recognition of these three features in clean condition and two noise types - stationary Gaussian white noise, and non-stationary real-world factory noise. For each type of parameter, 13 cepstra were generated per frame at a frame rate of 10 ms and a sampling frequency of 20 kHz. The dynamic (delta-delta) features were not used for the following reason. It was reported that the ZCPA algorithm do not perform well with delta-delta coefficients and the contribution of dynamic features of the EIH's to performance improvements is much smaller than that of MFCC [19]. This may be due to the fact that the length of the time-window is channel dependent in the EIH's i.e., it varies inversely with the characteristic frequency of the channel. For example, the length of the time-window at the channel with the lowest characteristic frequency spans upto 80 ms, which is much longer length when compared with the frame rate of about 10 ms. Thus appropriate dynamic features cannot be obtained in the ZCPA with the derivative window of 80 ms duration [13]. Therefore, for a fair comparison with all parameters, these are compared without the dynamic coefficients.

Table 5 shows that the MFCC and PLP performs better than ZCPA in clean conditions, but ZCPA performs better than the MFCC or the PLP in white noise conditions as the noise

Table 4: Comparison of high and low frequency discrimination (FD) of CV utterances with synaptic adaptation and two-tone suppression in the ZCPA auditory model.

| | FD | | | | | FD | | |
|---|---|---|---|---|---|---|---|---|
| | Base ZCPA | ZCPA _ADP | ZCPA _2TONE | | | Base ZCPA | ZCPA _ADP | ZCPA _2TONE |
| /ba/ | 0.22 | 0.23 | 0.40 | | /SHa/ | 0.58 | 0.65 | 0.95 |
| /bee/ | 2.82 | 3.33 | 2.96 | | /SHee/ | 2.89 | 3.43 | 3.41 |
| /boo/ | 0.46 | 0.51 | 0.78 | | /SHoo/ | 1.97 | 2.28 | 2.56 |
| /pa/ | 0.28 | 0.30 | 0.46 | | /ja/ | 0.56 | 0.62 | 0.86 |
| /pee/ | 2.31 | 2.79 | 2.53 | | /jee/ | 2.51 | 2.98 | 3.19 |
| /poo/ | 0.45 | 0.50 | 0.74 | | /joo/ | 1.45 | 1.64 | 1.96 |
| /ma/ | 0.33 | 0.36 | 0.63 | | | | | |
| /mee/ | 1.92 | 2.32 | 2.10 | | | | | |
| /moo/ | 0.43 | 0.47 | 0.73 | | | | | |

increases, which is in agreement with the results of [13]. However, in factory noise, the ZCPA performs better than the MFCC only at very low SNR (0 dB).

### 4.4.2 Comparison of Recognition Performances of ZCPA with Synaptic Adaptation and with Two-Tone Suppression

Table 6 shows the word recognition results of the base ZCPA, ZCPA with adaptation (ZCPA_ADP) and ZCPA with two-tone suppression (ZCPA_2TONE). The feature extraction with adaptation were described in detail in Sec. 3.4 and in Sec. 4.2 for two-tone suppression with companding.

Table 5: Comparisons of HMM recognition rates (%) of the base ZCPA, MFCC and PLP for isolated digits (TIdigits corpus) with male speakers.

| SNR (dB) | White | | | Factory | | |
|---|---|---|---|---|---|---|
| | ZCPA | MFCC_0 | PLP | ZCPA | MFC_0 | PLP |
| Clean | 95.4 | 100.0 | 100.0 | | | |
| 30 | 81.8 | 81.8 | 81.8 | 86.3 | 100.0 | 100.0 |
| 15 | 77.3 | 21.0 | 27.3 | 81.8 | 95.4 | 95.4 |
| 10 | 68.2 | 18.2 | 21.2 | 68.2 | 86.3 | 86.3 |
| 5 | 50.0 | 11.1 | 13.6 | 50.0 | 54.5 | 81.5 |
| 0 | 40.9 | 9.1 | 9.1 | 45.4 | 27.3 | 59.1 |

It is observed from Table 6 that the performance in clean conditions is improved with synaptic adaptation and with two-tone suppression over the base ZCPA. In noise conditions, it follows the same trend as given by [13]. That is, the best performance is achieved in Volvo noise, followed by factory noise, white noise and babble noise. Thus the response depends on the type of noise, with better performance in real-world noise environments. Real-world non-Gaussian noise contain significant low frequency components and are characterized by the absence of high frequency noise perturbations which usually corrupt the lower intensity articulatory cues. Moreover due to the dominant frequency principle, the formants are

Table 6: Percentage word recognition rates with continuous density HMM with isolated digits (TIdigits) of the base ZCPA, ZCPA with synaptic adaptation and ZCPA with two-tone suppression.

| SNR (dB) | White | | | Factory | | |
|---|---|---|---|---|---|---|
| | ZCPA | ZCPA _ADP | ZCPA _2TONE | ZCPA | ZCPA _ADP | ZCPA _2TONE |
| Clean | 95.4 | 95.4 | 95.4 | | | |
| 40 | 90.9 | 95.4 | 95.4 | 95.4 | 90.9 | 95.4 |
| 30 | 81.8 | 90.9 | 54.5 | 86.3 | 81.8 | 95.4 |
| 15 | 77.3 | 72.7 | 50.0 | 81.8 | 77.3 | 90.9 |
| 10 | 68.2 | 59.1 | 45.4 | 68.8 | 72.7 | 86.3 |
| 5 | 50.0 | 31.8 | 40.9 | 50.0 | 68.8 | 72.7 |

preserved in presence of low frequency noise perturbations.

A similar trend is observed with synaptic adaptation and two-tone suppression, with the best performance observed with Volvo noise and the worst performance with babble noise. However, with synaptic adaptation, improvements are observed over the base ZCPA only in white Gaussian noise at high SNRs, with degradations observed at low SNRs. With Factory noise, a reciprocal effect, that is, a degradation at high SNRs with improvement at low SNRs, is observed. In both babble and Volvo noise, there is a degradation particularly at low SNRs. In general, synaptic adaptation performed better over the base ZCPA in stationary Gaussian white noise (except at very low SNRs), but performed poorly in non-Gaussian noise.

With two-tone suppression, the recognition results are improved over both the base ZCPA and with synaptic adaptation under all noise types and at all SNRs, except for white Gaussian noise at low SNRs. A significant observation made from the Table 6 is that synaptic adaptation performs better than two-tone suppression in stationary white Gaussian noise and worse in non-stationary non-Gaussian noise (factory and babble), whereas an opposite effect is observed with two-tone suppression. That is, two-tone suppression performs better in non-Gaussian real-world noise (factory, babble, Volvo) and worse in Gaussian white noise.

However, at very low SNR Gaussian noise, there is a degradation in recognition rates with both synaptic adaptation and the two-tone suppression. This is due to three reasons. Firstly, if the unit sample response, $h(n)$, of the FIR filter is finite in length and zero outside the interval $[0, N-1]$, then the variance (power) of the output uncorrelated white noise, $\varphi = [\varphi(0), \varphi(1), \ldots, \varphi(N-1)]$, with zero mean at the output of the $i$-th filter can be expressed as

$$\sigma_{\varphi_i}^2 = E\left\{|\varphi_i(n)|^2\right\} = \mathbf{h}^H \mathbf{R}_\varphi \mathbf{h} = \mathbf{h}^H \mathbf{C}_\varphi \mathbf{h} = \mathbf{C}_\varphi \mathbf{h}^2 \qquad (29)$$

where $\mathbf{h}$ is the vector of filter coefficients, $\mathbf{R}_\varphi$ is noise autocorrelation matrix and $\mathbf{C}_\varphi$ is autocovariance matrix whose diagonals are simply the variances of the input noise process. Thus, it is observed that the variance of the noise $\varphi(n)$ at the output of the FIR filter is obtained by multiplying the input noise variance by the square of the FIR filter coefficient vector, $\mathbf{h}$. Thus, for a large order FIR filter, output noise variances may be significantly large. Secondly, high-pass filtering of white noise is equivalent to differentiating it, by which higher frequencies get more power. Hence, the high pass adaptation filtering further increases the zero-crossing perturbation and decreases low frequency formant contrasts. Thirdly, it is observed from Eqn. (14), that the zero-crossing variance is directly proportional to the square of the noise amplitudes,

$$\sigma_l^2 \frac{A_\varphi^2}{A_l^2}. \tag{30}$$

With synaptic adaptation in non-stationary factory noise, the improvements were observed to be opposite to that with white noise with a degradation at high SNRs, which is consistent with the results in [13]. This may be due to the fact that larger window lengths would give poor estimates in time domain processing in the presence of non-stationary noise. For babble noise, the results were similar to the non-stationary factory noise, while for the pseudo-stationary Volvo (car) noise, the results were similar to white noise, but with improved response at lower SNRs due to the presence of significant low frequency components.

The fact that the performance with two-tone suppression in white noise was worse than with synaptic adaptation was due to the increased variance of the noise $\varphi(n)$ at the output of the FIR filter obtained by multiplying the noise variance by the square of the FIR filter coefficient vector, **h**, as explained above. Since the companding utilizes two FIR filterbanks, a pre-filter and a post-filter, the noise variance is substantially increased over the base ZCPA and ZCPA_ADP.

It is usually important in speech recognition tests to perform a statistical significance test to establish that the differences in error-rates between two algorithms tested on the same data set are statistically significant or not. The McNemar's test [55] can be used for this purpose, which requires the errors made by an algorithm to be independent events. This is particularly applicable for isolated word recognition, that is, when the uttered words are not context dependent or dependent on some language model. The recognition results in Table 5 and Table 6 were further tested using the McNemar's two-tail test relating to the 682 test utterances and it was found that the differences in recognition results due to the three algorithms (base ZCPA, ZCPA with synaptic adaptation and ZCPA with two-tone suppression) were statistically significant 90% in white noise, 60% in factory noise, 80% in babble noise and 70% in Volvo noise for a significance level of $\alpha=0.03$.

# 5 Conclusion

It has been reported in [13], that although the base ZCPA performs better than the MFCC in noisy conditions, the relative performance improvement for the ZCPA over the MFCC is greater in white Gaussian noise than in real-world noise, such as the factory noise. It is stated therein that the reason for this is not clear. It is shown in this paper that one reason for this may be that in the ZCPA, the zero-crossing variance is reduced more for the high frequency white noise than the lower frequency real-world (factory, car, babble) noise. Therefore, although overall the ZCPA performs better in real-world noise than in white noise, the relative improvement in performance compared to the MFCC is higher in white noise than in non-Gaussian real-world noise.

In Sec. 4.3, it is observed that synaptic adaptation has a greater effect on high frequency articulation, whereas two-tone suppression has a greater effect on low-frequency articulation. Moreover, in Table 6, it is observed that synaptic adaptation performs better in white Gaussian noise while two-tone suppression performs better in non-Gaussian real-world noise. This effect may be observed from Eqn. (13) and Eqn. (14), in which it is seen that the zero-crossing variance is reduced for the high frequency noise components and the corresponding higher zero-crossing rates, respectively. The high pass synaptic adaptation filter further enhances the high frequency components which further reduces the variance. For the case of two-tone suppression, the performance improvement is mainly due to improvement of spectral contrasts due to companding utilizing low-pass filters. Hence, two-tone suppression is a low frequency enhancement technique, whereas adaptation scheme is a high frequency enhancement technique. Consequently, with a zero-crossing algorithm, the performance with two-tone suppression is expected to be reciprocal to that obtained for the synaptic adaptation, with improved response in low-frequency real-world noise due to reduced zero-crossing variance. Another reason of improved performance is that the higher energy low frequency peak values are emphasized in the two-tone suppression. These observations are consistent with the results in Table 6. In summary, these results demonstrate the frequency dependence of the perceptual features in speech recognition utilizing temporal methods and using a zero-crossing algorithm. The synaptic adaptation has a greater effect on high frequency articulation and the two-tone suppression has a greater effect on low-frequency articulation. In noise conditions, it is observed that synaptic adaptation is more immune to white Gaussian noise than two-tone suppression while two-tone suppression is more immune to the non-Gaussian, real-world noise than synaptic adaptation. Additionally, these results may be applied to speech processing, particularly in cochlear implants and hearing aids for improved intelligibility.

In this research, a classical frame based method embedded in a hidden Markov model (HMM) technique was used to evaluate the effects of perceptual features on speech recognition performance. The classical frame-based framework (typically 25 ms) is based on the assumption that the features are stationary (or quasi stationary) within the frame window duration. However, time constants associated with perceptual features are several order higher than this duration. There may be some model-feature mismatch between the frame-based approach and auditory events like rapid adaptation, and also due to the application of wider window lengths (30 ms to 120 ms) in perceptual processing with some loss of assumption of stationarity. As a result, a frame-based approach for auditory processing using HMMs has always been a compromise. Nevertheless, frame-based HMM technique for ASR in auditory models have been shown to provide improved performances as demonstrated by several researchers [8],[12],[13],[14], and additionally in this research.

The following issues may be addressed in any future research. It was observed that in the ZCPA the application of perceptual features, such as synaptic adaptation and two-tone suppression, degraded the performance over the baseline performance in white noise at very low SNRs. The reason for this degradation was explained in Sec 4.4.2. One way the performance in white noise may be improved is by adjusting the FIR filter order for a desired filter response. For example, in the minimum variance method of spectrum estimation of a stochastic process, the noise power spectrum estimate at the filter output decreases as the filter order increases [43]. Further research may be undertaken in this direction. Proper integration of dynamic features (delta-delta) features with channel dependent variable derivative window lengths may also be explored. Effects of frame synchronous processing on forward and backward masking related to the adaptation and other perceptual features of the human auditory system may be further investigated.

# References

[1] Seneff, S. (1988). A joint synchrony/mean-rate model of auditory processing. *J. Phonetics*, 85(1), 55-76.

[2] Ghitza, O. (1988). Auditory models and human performance in tasks related to speech coding and speech recognition. *IEEE Trans. Speech Audio Process.*, 2(1), 115-132.

[3] Lyon, R.F. & Mead, C. (1988). An analog electronic cochlea. *IEEE Trans. Acoust. Speech Signal Process.*, 36(7), 1119-1134.

[4] Zhang, X., Heinz, M. G. & Carney, L. H. (1988). Nonlinear compression in an auditory-nerve model. *Proc. of The First Joint BMES/EMBS Conf. Serving Humanity, Advancing Technology*, Atlanta, Oct. 1999, 13-16.

[5] Baer, T., Moore, B. C. J. & Gatehouse, S. (1993). Spectral contrast enhancement of speech in noise for listeners with sensorineural hearing impairment: Effects on intelligibility, quality, and response times. *J. Rehabil. Res. Dev.*, 3(1), 49-72.

[6] Grayden, D. B., Burkitt, A. N., Kenny, O. P., Clarey, Paolini, J. N. A. G. & Clark, G. M. (2004). A cochlear implant speech processing strategy based on an auditory model. *Int. Conf. on Intelligent Sensors, Sensor Networks and Information Processing (ISSNIP 2004)*, Melbourne, 491-496.

[7] Hunt, M. J. & Lefebvre, C. (1986). Speech recognition using a cochlear model. *IEEE Int. Conf. Acoust. Speech, Signal Processing (ICASSP 1986)*, Tokyo.

[8] Cohen, J. R. (1989). Application of an auditory model to speech recognition. *J. Acoust. Soc. Am.*, 85(6), 2623-2629.

[9] Zwicker, E., Terhardt, E. & Poulus, E. (1979). Automatic speech recognition using psychoacoustic models. *J. Acoust. Soc. Am.*, 65(2).

[10] Searle, C. L., Jacobson, J. & Rayment, S. G. (1979). Stop consonant discrimination based on human audition. *J. Acoust. Soc. Am.*, 65, 799-809.

[11] Bloomberg, M., Carlson, R., Elenius, K. & Granstrom, B. (1984). Auditory models and isolated word recognition. *Q Prog. Stat. Rep.*, Speech Transmiss. Lab. (Royal Institute of Technology, Stockholm), 1-15.

[12] Strope, B. & Alwan, A. (1997). A model of dynamic auditory perception and its application to robust word recognition. *IEEE Trans. Speech Audio Process.*, 95(5), 451-464.

[13] Kim, D. S., Lee, S. Y. & Kil, R. M. (1999). Auditory processing of speech signals for robust speech recognition in real world noisy environments. *IEEE Trans. Speech and Audio Process.*, 7(1), 55-69.

[14] Holmberg, M., Gelbart, D. & Hemmert, W. (2006). Automatic Speech Recognition with an adaptation model motivated by auditory processing. *IEEE Trans. Audio, Speech, Lang. Process.*, 14(1), 44-49.

[15] Haque, S., Togneri, R. & Zaknich, A. (2007). A temporal auditory model with adaptation for automatic speech recognition. *Proc. IEEE Int. Conf. on Acoust. Speech, and Signal Processing (ICASSP 2007)*.

[16] Haque, S. Togneri, R. & Zaknich, A. (2006). Zero-Crossings with adaptation for automatic speech recognition. *Proc. The Eleventh Australasian International Conference on Speech Science and Technology (SST 2006)*, 199-204, Dec. 6-8, 2006, Auckland.

[17] Haque, S., Togneri, R. & Zaknich, A. (2009). Perceptual features for automatic speech recognition in noisy environments. *Speech Communication.*, 51(1), 58-75.

[18] Turicchia, L. & Sarpeshkar R. (2005). A bio-inspired companding strategy for spectral enhancement. *IEEE Trans. Speech Audio Process.*, 13(2), 243-253.

[19] Sandhu, S. & Ghitza, O. (1995). A comparative study of mel cepstra and EIH for phone classification under adverse conditions. *Proc. IEEE Int. Conf. on Acoust. Speech, and Signal Processing (ICASSP 1995)*.

[20] Abdelatty, A. M., Spiegel, J. V., Mueller, P., Haentjens, G. & Berman, J. (1999). An acoustic-phonetic feature-based system for automatic phoneme recognition in continuous speech. *Proc. IEEE Int. Conf. on Acoust. Speech, and Signal Processing (ICASSP 1999)*.

[21] Gajić, B. & Paliwal, K. K. (2003). Robust speech recognition using features based on zero-crossings with peak amplitudes. *Proc. IEEE Int. Conf. on Acoust. Speech, and Signal Processing (ICASSP 2003)*.

[22] Markel, J. D. Gray, A. H. Linear Prediction of Speech. Berlin: Springer-Verlag; 1976.

[23] Bogert, B. P., Healy, M. J. & Tukey, J. W. Title: The quefrency analysis of time series for echoes: cepstrum, pseudo-autocovariance, cross-cepstrum, and shape tracking. In: Rosenblatt, M. editor. Title: Time Series Analysis. New York: John Wiley; 1963; 209-243.

[24] Loizou, P. C. (2006). Coclear and Brainstem Implants: Speech processing in vocoder-centric cochlear implants. In: A. Moeller editor. Adv. Otorhinolaryngol. vol 64; 2006; 109-143.

[25] Pitton, J. W., Wang K. & Juang, B. (1996). Time-Frequency analysis and auditory modeling for automatic recognition of speech. *Proc. IEEE*, 84(9), 1199-1215.

[26] Ghulam, M., Fukuda, T., Horikawa, J. & Nitta, T. (2005). Pitch-synchronous ZCPA (PS-ZCPA)-based feature extraction with auditory masking. *Proc. IEEE Int. Conf. on Acoust. Speech, and Signal Processing (ICASSP 2005).*

[27] Zwicker, E., Flottorp, G. & Stevens, S. S. (1957). Critical bandwidth in loudness summation. *J. Acoust. Soc. Am.*, 29, 548-557.

[28] Hermansky, H. (1990). Perceptual linear Prediction (PLP) analysis of speech. *J. Acoust. Soc. Am.*, vol. 87, 1738-1752.

[29] Hermansky H. & Morgan, N. (1994). RASTA processing of speech. *IEEE Trans. Speech Audio Process.*, 2, 587-589.

[30] Deng, L. & O'Shaughnessy, D. Speech Processing - A Dynamic and Optimization-Oriented Approach. New York: Marcel Dekker; 2003.

[31] Sachs, M. B., Voigt, H. F. & Young, E. D. (1983). Auditory nerve representation of vowels in background noise. *J. Neurophysiology. 50(1)*.

[32] Loughlin, P., Groutage, D. & Rohrbaugh, R. (1997). Time-frequency analysis of acoustic transients. *Proc. IEEE Int. Conf. on Acoust. Speech, and Signal Processing (ICASSP 1997).*

[33] Kedem, B. (1986). Spectral analysis and discrimination by zero-crossings. *Proc. IEEE*, 74(11), 1477-1493.

[34] Hermansky, H. (1994). Speech Beyond 10 ms (Temporal Filtering in Feature Domain). *Proc. Int. Workshop on Human Interface Technology, Aizu, Japan.*

[35] Patterson, R. D. (1999). Time-interval information in the auditory representation of speech sounds. *J. Acoust. Soc. Am.*, 105(2), 1305.

[36] Pickles, J. O. An Introduction to the Physiology of Hearing, London: Academic; 1988.

[37] Smith, R. & Zwislocki, J. J. (1975). Short-term adaptation and incremental responses of single auditory-nerve fibres. *Biological Cybernetics*, 17, 169-182.

[38] Westerman, L. & Smith, R. L. (1984). Rapid and short-term adaptation in auditory nerve responses. *Hearing Research*, 15, 249-260.

[39] Meddis, R. (1988). Simulation of mechanical to neural transduction in the auditory receptor. *J. Acoust. Soc. Am.*, 79(3), 702-711.

[40] Jankowski Jr., C. R., Vo, H. H. & Lippman, R. P. (1995). A comparison of signal processing front ends for automatic word recognition. *IEEE Trans. Speech Audio Process.*, 3, 286-293.

[41] Koopmans, L. H. The Spectral Analysis of Time Series. New York: Academic Press; 1995.

[42] Oxenham, A. J. (2001). Forward masking: adaptation or integration? *J. Acoust. Soc. Am.*, 109, 732-741.

[43] Hayes, M. H. Statistical Digital Signal Processing and Modeling. New Jersey: John Wiley and Sons, Inc.; 1996.

[44] Gunawan, T. S. & Ambikairajah, E. (2006). On the use of simultaneous and temporal masking in noise suppression applications. *Proc. of 11th Int. Conf. Speech Science and Technology (SST 2006),* Auckland.

[45] Spoor, A., Eggermont, J. J. & Odenthal, D. W. Title: Comparison of human and animal data concerning adaptation and masking of eighth nerve compound action potential. In: Ruber, J. Elberling, C. & Solomon, G., editors, Title: Electrocochleography. Baltimore, University Park, MD; 1976; 183-198.

[46] Zwicker, E. & Fastl, H. Psychoacoustics: Facts and Models. 2nd Edition. New York: Springer-Verlag; 1990.

[47] Tchorz, J. & Kollmeier, B. (1999). A model of auditory perception as front-end for automatic speech recognition. *J. Acoust. Soc. Am.*, 106(4).

[48] Moore, B. C. J. & Glasberg, B. R. (1983). Suggested formulae for calculating auditory-filter bandwidths and excitation patterns. *J. Acoust. Soc. Am.*, 74(3), 750-753.

[49] Theodoridis, S. & Koutroumbas, K. Pattern recognition. San Diego: Elsevier; 1999.

[50] Ruggero, M. A., Narayan, S. S., Temchin, A. N. & Recio, A. (2000). Mechanical bases of frequency tuning and neural excitation at the base of the cochlea. *Proc. Natl. Acad. Sci., USA, vol.*, 97, 11744-11750.

[51] Rhode, W. S. (1978). Some observations on cochlear mechanics. *J. Acoust. Soc. Am.*, 64, no. 1, 158-176.

[52] Kates, J. M. (1995). Two-tone suppression in a cochlear model. *IEEE Trans. Speech Audio Process.*, 3(5), 396-406.

[53] Dolby, R. (1967). An audio noise reduction system. *J. Audio Eng. Soc.*, 15(4).

[54] Frey D., Tsividis, Y., Efthivoulidis, G. & Krishnapura, N. (2001). Syllabic- Companding log domain filters. *IEEE Trans. Circuits Syst. II.*, 48(4), 329-339.

[55] Gillick, L. & Cox, S.J. (1989). Some statistical issues in the comparison of speech recognition algorithms. *Proc. IEEE Int. Conf. on Acoust. Speech, and Signal Processing (ICASSP 1989).*

In: Deafness, Hearing Loss and the Auditory System    ISBN: 978-1-60741-259-5
Editors: D. Fiedler and R. Krause, pp.373    ©2010 Nova Science Publishers, Inc.

# COMMENTARY: ACUPUNCTURE IN THE TREATMENT OF EAR DISORDERS

## *Wong-Kein Low*

Department of Otolaryngology, Singapore General Hospital, Singapore

As part of Traditional Chinese Medicine (TCM), acupuncture is one of the oldest healing practices in the world that can be traced back at least 2,500 years. The general theory of acupuncture is based on the premise that there are patterns of energy flow (qi) through the body that are essential for health. Health is achieved through balancing the forces of yin and yang, and disease is caused by an imbalance leading to a blockage in the flow of qi along specific pathways known as meridians. Acupuncture applied at specific acupoints along the meridians, has the potential to correct imbalances of the flow of qi. There have been many studies which had attempted to find out if acupuncture is effective in treating a wide range of conditions. The 1997 NIH Consensus Statement on Acupuncture concluded that overall, the results were difficult to interpret because of problems with the size and design of the studies.

By targeting the relevant acupoints on the meridians associated with the ear, acupuncture has been used to treat ear-related symptoms such as hearing loss, vertigo and tinnitus. A meridian which is of particular interest, is that of the kidney. According to TCM, the kidney opens into the ear, and kidney disorders can manifest in the ear. It can be argued that this is not logical, given that the ear and the kidney are located at almost opposite ends of the torso! Let us pause and ponder. The kidney and ear lobe share a similar shape, but probably by chance. It is, however, no coincidence that the ear and kidney have certain associations in Western Medicine. Medications such as gentamicin have toxic side effects, which specifically target the inner ear and kidney. Some congenital malformations of the ear, for example, the branchio-oto-renal syndrome, also affect the kidney. These observations may suggest an embryological relationship between the two organ systems. The TCM concept of using acupuncture on the kidney meridian as a means to treat certain ear conditions, may not be that far-fetched after all.

It remains to be seen if the use of acupuncture in the treatment of ear disorders can be supported by solid well-designed research. Although it is unrealistic to expect it to work in established hearing defects due to cochlear hair-cell loss, it will be interesting to find out if it is of value in treating potentially reversible conditions such as early sudden hearing loss and Meniere's disease.

# INDEX

## D

## F

## G

# H

## I

## K

## L

## M

# P

## Ω

## R

## S

## T